COVID-19 and the Dermatologist

Editors

ESTHER E. FREEMAN
DEVON E. MCMAHON

DERMATOLOGIC CLINICS

www.derm.theclinics.com

Consulting Editor
BRUCE H. THIERS

October 2021 • Volume 39 • Number 4

ELSEVIER

1600 John F. Kennedy Boulevard • Suite 1800 • Philadelphia, Pennsylvania, 19103-2899

http://www.theclinics.com

DERMATOLOGIC CLINICS Volume 39, Number 4
October 2021 ISSN 0733-8635, ISBN-13: 978-0-323-83600-5

Editor: Lauren Boyle
Developmental Editor: Karen Justine Solomon

Dermatologic Clinics (ISSN 0733-8635) is published quarterly by Elsevier Inc., 360 Park Avenue South, New York, NY 10010-1710. Months of publication are January, April, July, and October. Business and editorial offices: 1600 John F. Kennedy Blvd., Suite 1800, Philadelphia, PA 19103-2899. Customer service office: 11830 Westline Drive, St. Louis, MO 63146. Periodicals postage paid at New York, NY, and additional mailing offices. Subscription prices are USD 416.00 per year for US individuals, USD 1,000.00 per year for US institutions, USD 456.00 per year for Canadian individuals, USD 1,055.00 per year for Canadian institutions, USD 510.00 per year for international individuals, USD 1,055.00 per year for international institutions, USD 100.00 per year for US students/residents, USD 100.00 per year for Canadian students/residents, and USD 240 per year for international students/residents. International air speed delivery is included in all *Clinics* subscription prices. All prices are subject to change without notice. **POSTMASTER:** Send address changes to *Dermatologic Clinics*, Elsevier Health Sciences Division, Subscription Customer Service, 3251 Riverport Lane, Maryland Heights, MO 63043. **Customer Service: 1-800-654-2452 (U.S. and Canada); 314-447-8871 (outside U.S. and Canada). Fax: 314-447-8029. E-mail: journalscustomerservice-usa@elsevier.com (for print support); journalsonlinesupport-usa@elsevier.com (for online support).**

Reprints. For copies of 100 or more, of articles in this publication, please contact the Commercial Reprints Department, Elsevier Inc., 360 Park Avenue South, New York, New York 10010-1710. Tel.: 212-633-3874; Fax: 212-633-3820; Email: reprints@elsevier.com.

The *Dermatologic Clinics* is covered in *MEDLINE/PubMed (Index Medicus), Current Contents/Clinical Medicine, Excerpta Medica, Chemical Abstracts,* and *ISI/BIOMED.*

Contributors

CONSULTING EDITOR

BRUCE H. THIERS, MD
Professor and Chairman Emeritus, Department of Dermatology and Dermatologic Surgery, Medical University of South Carolina, Charleston, South Carolina, USA

EDITORS

ESTHER E. FREEMAN, MD, PhD
Department of Dermatology, Medical Practice Evaluation Center, Mongan Institute, Massachusetts General Hospital, Harvard Medical School, Boston, Massachusetts, USA

DEVON E. McMAHON, MD
Department of Dermatology, Massachusetts General Hospital, Harvard Medical School, Boston, Massachusetts, USA

AUTHORS

SELLI ABDALI, MS
Philadelphia College of Osteopathic Medicine, Philadelphia, Pennsylvania, USA

RITESH AGNIHOTHRI, MD
Complex Medical Dermatology Fellow, Department of Dermatology, University of California San Francisco, San Francisco, California, USA

APRIL W. ARMSTRONG, MD, MPH
University of Southern California Keck School of Medicine, Los Angeles, California, USA

JOAO AVANCINI, MD
Department of Dermatology, Hospital das Clínicas of the University of Sao Paulo, Sao Paulo, Brazil

ESTHER A. BALOGH, MD
Center for Dermatology Research, Department of Dermatology, Wake Forest School of Medicine, Winston-Salem, North Carolina, USA

FRANCISCO BRAVO, MD
Departments of Dermatology and Pathology, Universidad Peruana Cayetano Heredia, Hospital Cayetano Heredia, Lima, Peru

LESLIE CASTELO-SOCCIO, MD, PhD
Section of Pediatric Dermatology, Children's Hospital of Philadelphia, Philadelphia, Pennsylvania, USA

GRACE C. CHAMBERLIN, BA
Medical Practice Evaluation Center, Mongan Institute, Massachusetts General Hospital, Boston, Massachusetts, USA

JULIANA CHOI, MD, PhD
Assistant Professor, University of Pennsylvania, Philadelphia, Pennsylvania, USA

ALVIN H. CHONG, MBBS, MMed, FACD
Skin Health Institute, Carlton, Victoria, Australia; Department of Medicine (Dermatology), St Vincent's Hospital Melbourne, University of Melbourne, Victoria, Australia

KELLY M. CORDORO, MD
Department of Dermatology, University of
California San Francisco, San Francisco,
California, USA

SEEMAL R. DESAI, MD
Innovative Dermatology, Plano, Texas, USA;
Department of Dermatology, The University of
Texas Southwestern Medical Center, Dallas,
Texas, USA

MYTRANG H. DO, PhD
Weill Cornell Medicine, New York, New York,
USA

RONI P. DODIUK-GAD, MD
Bruce Rappaport Faculty of Medicine,
Technion - Institute of Technology, Haifa,
Israel; Department of Dermatology, Emek
Medical Center, Afula, Israel; Division of
Dermatology, Department of Medicine,
Sunnybrook Health Sciences Centre,
University of Toronto, Toronto, Ontario,
Canada

FABRIZIO FANTINI, MD
Department of Dermatology, Dermatology
Unit, ASST Lecco, Alessandro Manzoni
Hospital, Lecco, Italy

MARLYS S. FASSETT, MD, PhD
Department of Microbiology and Immunology,
Department of Dermatology, University of
California San Francisco, San Francisco,
California, USA

RAMIE FATHY, AB
Perelman School of Medicine, University of
Pennsylvania, Philadelphia, Pennsylvania, USA

STEVEN R. FELDMAN, MD, PhD
Center for Dermatology Research, Department
of Dermatology, Wake Forest School of
Medicine, Winston-Salem, North Carolina,
USA

CARSTEN FLOHR, MD, PhD
Unit for Population-Based Dermatology
Research, St John's Institute of Dermatology,
King's College London and Guy's and St
Thomas' NHS Foundation Trust, London,
United Kingdom

AMY FORRESTEL, MD
Assistant Professor, Department of
Dermatology, Hospital of the University of
Pennsylvania, Philadelphia, Pennsylvania, USA

LINDY P. FOX, MD
Professor, Department of Dermatology,
University of California San Francisco, San
Francisco, California, USA

ESTHER E. FREEMAN, MD, PhD
Department of Dermatology, Medical Practice
Evaluation Center, Mongan Institute,
Massachusetts General Hospital, Harvard
Medical School, Boston, Massachusetts, USA

LARS E. FRENCH, MD
Department of Dermatology, University
Hospital, Munich University of Ludwig
Maximilian, Munich, Germany; Dr. Philip Frost
Department of Dermatology and Cutaneous
Surgery, University of Miami Miller School of
Medicine, Miami, Florida, USA

LUCINDA CLAIRE FULLER, MA, FRCP(UK)
Consultant Dermatologist, Chelsea and
Westminster Hospital NHS Foundation Trust,
International Foundation for Dermatology,
London, United Kingdom

ANTONIA E. GALLMAN, PhD
Department of Microbiology and Immunology,
Medical Scientist Training Program, University
of California San Francisco, San Francisco,
California, USA

CRISTINA GALVÁN, MD
Department of Dermatology, Hospital
Universitario de Móstoles, Madrid, Spain

CHRISTOPHER E.M. GRIFFITHS, MD
Dermatology Centre, Salford Royal Hospital,
NIHR Manchester Biomedical Research
Centre, University of Manchester, Manchester,
United Kingdom

YASMIN GUTIERREZ, BS
University of California Riverside School of
Medicine, Riverside, California, USA

CLAIRE HANNAH, MD
Resident of Dermatology and Internal
Medicine, Departments of Dermatology and

Internal Medicine, Hospital of the University of Pennsylvania, Philadelphia, Pennsylvania, USA

JOANNA HARP, MD
Associate Professor of Dermatology, Weill Cornell Medicine, NewYork-Presbyterian Hospital, New York, New York, USA

NAILAH HARVEY, BS
Philadelphia College of Osteopathic Medicine Philadelphia, Pennsylvania, USA

ELENA B. HAWRYLUK, MD, PhD
Department of Dermatology, Massachusetts General Hospital, Harvard Medical School, Boston Children's Hospital, Boston, Massachusetts, USA

GEORGE J. HRUZA, MD, MBA
Department of Dermatology, Saint Louis University, St Louis, Missouri, USA

ALAN D IRVINE, MD, DSc
Clinical Medicine, Trinity College Dublin, Dublin, Ireland

MADISON E. JONES, BA
University of Southern California Keck School of Medicine, Los Angeles, California, USA

RAYVA KHANNA, BA
Georgetown University School of Medicine, Washington, District of Columbia, USA

ALISON H. KOHN, BS
Florida Atlantic University Charles E Schmidt College of Science, Boca Raton, Florida, USA

ROHAN KRISHNAN
Department of Dermatology, Perelman School of Medicine, University of Pennsylvania, Philadelphia, Pennsylvania, USA

IRENE LARA-CORRALES, MD, MSc
Section of Pediatric Dermatology, Hospital for Sick Children, Toronto, Canada

JULES B. LIPOFF, MD
Assistant Professor, Department of Dermatology, Perelman School of Medicine, Leonard Davis Institute of Health Economics, University of Pennsylvania, Philadelphia, Pennsylvania, USA

MICHELLE A. LOWES, MBBS, PhD
Department of Dermatology, The Rockefeller University, New York, New York, USA

SATVEER K. MAHIL, MD, PhD
St John's Institute of Dermatology, King's College London and Guy's and St Thomas' NHS Foundation Trust, London, United Kingdom

ANGELO V. MARZANO, MD
Dermatology Unit, Fondazione IRCCS Ca' Granda Ospedale Maggiore Policlinico, Department of Pathophysiology and Transplantation, Università degli Studi di Milano, Milan, Italy

DEVON E. McMAHON, MD
Department of Dermatology, Massachusetts General Hospital, Harvard Medical School, Boston, Massachusetts, USA

AMY J. McMICHAEL, MD
Wake Forest School of Medicine, Winston-Salem, North Carolina, USA

NEKMA MEAH, MD, FACD
St Helens and Knowsley NHS Trust, St Helens, United Kingdom

DENISE MIYAMOTO, MD, PhD
Department of Dermatology, Hospital das Clínicas of the University of Sao Paulo, Sao Paulo, Brazil

HALEY B. NAIK, MD, MHSc
Department of Dermatology, University of California San Francisco, San Francisco, California, USA

HOLLY NEALE, BS
Department of Dermatology, Massachusetts General Hospital, Boston, Massachusetts, USA; University of Massachusetts Medical School, Worcester, Massachusetts, USA

CHOON CHIAT OH, MD
Department of Dermatology, Singapore General Hospital, Singapore, Singapore

DAVID M. OZOG, MD
Department of Dermatology, Henry Ford Health System, Detroit, Michigan, USA

SARAH P. POURALI, BS
Vanderbilt University School of Medicine,
Nashville, Tennessee, USA

NOUFAL RABOOBEE, MD
Department of Dermatology, Westville
Hospital, Westville, South Africa

JEFFREY R. RAJKUMAR, BS
University of Illinois College of Medicine at
Chicago, Chicago, Illinois, USA

SAREM RASHID, BS
Department of Dermatology, Wellman Center
for Photomedicine, Massachusetts General
Hospital, Boston University School of
Medicine, Boston, Massachusetts, USA

SEBASTIANO RECALCATI, MD
Department of Dermatology, Dermatology
Unit, ASST Lecco, Alessandro Manzoni
Hospital, Lecco, Italy

MISHA ROSENBACH, MD
Associate Professor, University of
Pennsylvania, Philadelphia, Pennsylvania, USA

ILANA S. ROSMAN, MD
Associate Professor, Washington University, St
Louis, Missouri, USA

SARA SAMIMI, MD
Assistant Professor, University of
Pennsylvania, Philadelphia, Pennsylvania, USA

JOSE A. SANCHES, MD, PhD
Department of Dermatology, Hospital das
Clínicas of the University of Sao Paulo, Sao
Paulo, Brazil

RODNEY SINCLAIR, MBBS, MD, FACD
Sinclair Dermatology, East Melbourne,
Victoria, Australia

CATHERINE H. SMITH, MD
St John's Institute of Dermatology, King's
College London and Guy's and St Thomas'
NHS Foundation Trust, London, United
Kingdom

PHYLLIS I. SPULS, MD, PhD
Department of Dermatology, Amsterdam
University Medical Center, Amsterdam Public
Health, Immunity and Infections, University of
Amsterdam, Amsterdam, The Netherlands

CLAIRE R. STEWART, BA
Weill Cornell Medicine, New York, New York,
USA

POONKIAT SUCHONWANIT, MD
Division of Dermatology, Faculty of Medicine,
Ramathibodi Hospital, Mahidol University,
Bangkok, Thailand

QISI SUN, MD
Department of Dermatology, Yale School of
Medicine, New Haven, Connecticut, USA

QIUNING SUN, MD
Department of Dermatology, Peking Union
Medical College Hospital, Peking Union
Medical College, Chinese Academy of Medical
Sciences, Beijing, China

KEYUN TANG, BS
Department of Dermatology, Peking Union
Medical College Hospital, Peking Union
Medical College, Chinese Academy of Medical
Sciences, Beijing, China

ANGELI ELOISE TORRES, MD
Department of Dermatology, Makati Medical
Center, Makati City, Philippines; Department of
Dermatology, Henry Ford Health System,
Detroit, Michigan, USA

HENSIN TSAO, MD, PhD
Department of Dermatology, Wellman Center
for Photomedicine, Massachusetts General
Hospital, Boston, Massachusetts, USA

PEARL O. UGWU-DIKE, BS
Department of Dermatology, Massachusetts
General Hospital, Harvard Medical School,
Boston, Massachusetts, USA

DMITRI WALL, MB BCh BAO, MRCP, MSc
Hair Restoration Blackrock, National and
International Skin Registry Solutions (NISR),
Charles Institute of Dermatology, School of
Medicine, University College Dublin, Dublin,
Ireland

ANNELIESE WILLEMS, MBBS, FRACGP
Skin Health Institute, Carlton, Victoria, Australia

VICTORIA WILLIAMS, MD
Adjunct Faculty, Department of Dermatology,
Hospital of the University of Pennsylvania,
Philadelphia, Pennsylvania, USA; Director,

Global Regulatory Affairs, Vaccines and Infectious Diseases, Merck & Co, Inc, Upper Gwynedd, Pennsylvania, USA

CASSANDRA B. YEBOAH, BS, MBS
Philadelphia College of Osteopathic Medicine, Philadelphia, Pennsylvania, USA

REBECCA M. YIM, BA
University of Southern California Keck School of Medicine, Los Angeles, California, USA

JIADE YU, MD
Assistant Professor, Department of Dermatology, Massachusetts General Hospital, Harvard Medical School, Boston, Massachusetts, USA

HANLIN ZHANG, BS
Department of Dermatology, Peking Union Medical College Hospital, Peking Union Medical College, Chinese Academy of Medical Sciences, Beijing, China

Contents

Coronavirus disease 2019 (COVID-19), an emergent disease caused by severe acute respiratory syndrome coronavirus 2 (SARS-CoV-2), has rapidly spread since its discovery in 2019. This article reviews the broad spectrum of cutaneous manifestations reported in association with SARS-CoV-2 infection. The most commonly reported cutaneous manifestations associated with COVID-19 infection include pernio (chilblain)-like acral lesions, morbilliform (exanthematous) rash, urticaria, vesicular (varicella-like) eruptions, and vaso-occlusive lesions (livedo racemosa, retiform purpura). It is important to consider SARS-CoV-2 infection in the differential diagnosis of a patient presenting with these lesions in the appropriate clinical context.

Children are a unique subset of patients in relation to the COVID-19 pandemic, often presenting asymptomatically, mildly, or atypically. Manifestations of the skin may be a primary (or the only) presenting sign. Recognizing cutaneous manifestations of COVID-19 in the pediatric population is important to guiding precautions, testing, and management for patients and close contacts. Whereas some dermatologic signs in children overlap with those in adults, other skin findings are reported with higher frequency in children and may be clues to multisystemic sequelae. This article describes presentation, pathophysiologic theories, and management strategies for cutaneous manifestations of COVID-19 in children.

Cutaneous findings have increasingly been reported in patients with coronavirus disease 2019 (COVID-19). This review discusses associated skin findings in patients with COVID-19 in the inpatient setting, ranging from vasculopathy-related lesions associated with high hospitalization rate and poor prognosis to inflammatory vesicular and urticarial eruptions that are rarely associated with prolonged hospitalization. We also discuss other reported COVID-19 cutaneous manifestations such as Sweet's syndrome, purpuric eruptions, and Multisystem Inflammatory Syndrome in Children. Although the relationship between dermatologic changes and COVID-19 disease progression is not fully elucidated, familiarity with cutaneous manifestations is valuable for physicians caring for patients hospitalized with COVID-19 and may help improve disease recognition and care.

Esther E. Freeman, Grace C. Chamberlin, Devon E. McMahon, George J. Hruza, Dmitri Wall, Nekma Meah, Rodney Sinclair, Esther A. Balogh, Steven R. Feldman, Michelle A. Lowes, Angelo V. Marzano, Haley B. Naik, Leslie Castelo-Soccio, Irene Lara-Corrales, Kelly M. Cordoro, Satveer K. Mahil, Christopher E.M. Griffiths, Catherine H. Smith, Alan D. Irvine, Phyllis I. Spuls, Carsten Flohr, and Lars E. French

During the COVID-19 pandemic, the rapid collection of real-world evidence is essential for the development of knowledge and subsequent public health response. In dermatology, provider-facing and patient-facing registries focused on COVID-19 have been important sources of research and new information aimed at guiding optimal patient care. The 7 dermatology registries in this update now include more than 8000 case reports sourced from physicians and patients from countries all over the world.

Angeli Eloise Torres, David M. Ozog, and George J. Hruza

The impact of the COVID-19 pandemic on dermatology practice cannot be overstated. At its peak, the pandemic resulted in the temporary closure of ambulatory sites as resources were reallocated towards pandemic response efforts. Many outpatient clinics have since reopened and are beginning to experience a semblance of pre-pandemic routine, albeit with restrictions in place. We provide an overview of how COVID-19 has affected dermatology practice globally beginning with the rise of teledermatology. A summary of expert recommendations that shape the "new normal" in various domains of dermatology practice, namely, dermatology consultation, procedural dermatology, and phototherapy, is also provided.

Cassandra B. Yeboah, Nailah Harvey, Rohan Krishnan, and Jules B. Lipoff

The accelerated implementation and use of teledermatology during the coronavirus disease 2019 pandemic has met with successes and challenges. This review explores how telemedicine was used in dermatology before the pandemic, the regulatory adaptions made in response to the pandemic, and the effectiveness of the rapid implementation of teledermatology during the coronavirus disease 2019 pandemic, and, finally, how teledermatology has expanded in response to the pandemic. This review examines lessons learned and how teledermatology's reliance on digital technologies might paradoxically exacerbate health care disparities, and finally, considers the future outlook.

Sara Samimi, Juliana Choi, Ilana S. Rosman, and Misha Rosenbach

COVID-19 has created challenges across medicine, including in medical education, with deeply rooted impacts in the dermatology residency experience. Its effects are both acute and chronic, including: shifts to virtual education and conferences, skewed clinical experiences, negatively impacted wellness, and uncertainty in the future. As educators and mentors, it is important to recognize and address these issues so that we may remain transparent, adaptable, and engaged as we continue to build a better tomorrow for our resident trainees.

In this article, we discuss the impact of the COVID-19 pandemic on various areas of global health dermatology, including patient care, neglected tropical diseases, education, and collaborations. Information was collected from literature review and informal interviews with more than 20 dermatologists from around the world. Many of the setbacks and hardships experienced by the global health community in the last year highlight long-standing global interdependencies and systems that perpetuate ethnic, economic, and social inequalities on local and global scales. The pandemic has brought discussions on global health colonialism and domestic health inequality to the forefront.

The COVID-19 pandemic has presented a unique set of challenges to cancer care centers around the world. Diagnostic and treatment delays associated with lockdown periods may be expected to increase the total number of avoidable skin cancer deaths. During this unprecedented time, dermatologists have been pressed to balance early surgical interventions for skin cancer with the risk of viral transmission. This article summarizes evidenced-based recommendations for the surgical management of cutaneous melanoma, keratinocyte cancer, and Merkel cell carcinoma during the COVID-19 pandemic. Additional long-term studies are required to determine the effect of COVID-19 on skin cancer outcomes.

Coronavirus disease 2019 (COVID-19) brought the world to its knees, shifting the medical and scientific landscape permanently. In particular, COVID-19 has challenged and transformed the field of dermatology and the way we practice. In this article, dermatologists from 11 countries share insights gained from local experience on redeployment, caring for COVID-19 skin manifestations, practice management, and telemedicine. These global perspectives will help provide a better framework for delivering quality dermatologic care and understanding how the field has evolved during this medical crisis.

In 2021, we entered a new phase of the COVID-19 pandemic. As mass vaccinations are underway and more vaccines are approved, it is important to recognize cutaneous adverse events. We review the dermatologic manifestations of COVID-19 vaccines as reported in clinical trial data and summarize additional observational reports of skin reactions to COVID-19 vaccines. Early-onset local injection reactions were the most common cutaneous side effects observed in clinical trials; delayed injection reactions were the most common cutaneous side effect reported outside of clinical trials. Understanding the landscape of cutaneous manifestations to COVID-19 vaccines is key to providing appropriate vaccine guidance.

DERMATOLOGIC CLINICS

SERIES OF RELATED INTEREST

Medical Clinics
https://www.medical.theclinics.com/
Immunology and Allergy Clinics
https://www.immunology.theclinics.com/
Clinics in Plastic Surgery
https://www.plasticsurgery.theclinics.com/

THE CLINICS ARE AVAILABLE ONLINE!
Access your subscription at:
www.theclinics.com

Preface
COVID-19 and Dermatology: One Year in Review

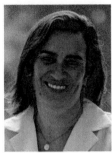
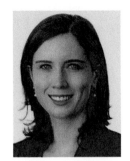

Esther E. Freeman, MD, PhD   Devon E. McMahon, MD

Editors

COVID-19 has fundamentally altered health care, from the direct impacts of severe acute respiratory syndrome coronavirus 2 (SARS-CoV-2) infection and spread, to resulting changes in medical practice.[1] Dermatologists have played an important role in all aspects of the COVID-19 pandemic, from identification of cutaneous manifestations of the virus, to restructuring clinical practice to accommodate lockdown and social distancing measures, and now to vaccine roll out and management of cutaneous vaccine side effects.[2–6]

Despite a year of loss and disruption for so many, one silver lining of the COVID-19 pandemic has been collaboration across the medical and scientific community, ultimately leading to a substantial body of literature on SARS-CoV-2 genomics, pathogenesis, epidemiology, and now vaccination. Scientific progress has been accelerated not just by novel research techniques but also through collaboration across institutions and countries, with results disseminated more rapidly with the growth of preprint publishing, virtual conferences, and use of social media.[7] Although disruptions in medical practice due to lockdowns had negative results for many patients, this change also prompted a surge in telemedicine use, which has many important applications for delivering timely and more equitable care.[8]

Undoubtedly, the COVID-19 pandemic has also heightened the medical community's attention to the important topics of health care disparities and structural racism, in addition to awareness of the rise in anti-Asian sentiment.[1,9,10] Lockdown measures and school closures have also taken an unprecedented toll on women in medicine and scientific fields, raising the important issue of gender inequity in medicine.[11]

In this issue of *Dermatologic Clinics of North America*, we have invited experts in COVID-19 dermatology to review multiple important issues in this emerging field of study. In these articles, our authors describe cutaneous morphologies of COVID-19 vaccine reactions and SARS-CoV-2 infection, as well as cutaneous manifestations specific to pediatric patients and hospitalized patients. We recognize how images of COVID-19 cutaneous manifestations have been underrepresented in patients with skin of color. We investigate dermatoses related to increased personal protective equipment use by both medical professionals and the public. We further explore some of the immunologic underpinnings of COVID-19 cutaneous manifestations, as well as recommendations for dermatology patients on biologic medications during the pandemic. We reflect on how COVID-19 has transformed dermatology practice as a whole, from changes in clinic flow, to advances in teledermatology, to delays in skin cancer management, as well as impacts on dermatology residency and the residency selection process. We examine how COVID-19 has changed the global landscape of dermatology across multiple countries and had far-reaching effects for global dermatology training programs. We then discuss updates of multiple dermatology COVID-19 registries, which have collected real-world evidence from providers and patients to inform patient care. Last, we examine cutaneous

Dermatol Clin 39 (2021) xv–xvi
https://doi.org/10.1016/j.det.2021.06.001
0733-8635/21/© 2021 Published by Elsevier Inc.

derm.theclinics.com

side effects of the novel COVID-19 vaccines and provide recommendations for patients who experienced a cutaneous reaction to their first vaccine dose.

Thank you to all the dermatologists and trainees who have made this special issue possible. This collaboration across multiple institutions and countries in many ways reflects the larger collaborative spirit we have been privileged to be a part of during the COVID-19 pandemic. Although the pandemic and its effects are far from over,[12] the amount of scientific knowledge on COVID-19 dermatology we have been able to gather in a year is remarkable.

Esther E. Freeman, MD, PhD
Massachusetts General Hospital
55 Fruit Street
Boston, MA 02114, USA

Devon E. McMahon, MD
Department of Dermatology
Massachusetts General Hospital
Harvard Medical School
Boston, MA 02114, USA

E-mail addresses:
efreeman@mgh.harvard.edu (E.E. Freeman)
devon_mcmahon@hms.harvard.edu
(D.E. McMahon)

REFERENCES

1. Woolf SH, Chapman DA, Sabo RT, et al. Excess deaths from COVID-19 and other causes, March-July 2020. JAMA 2020;324:1562–4.
2. Freeman EE, McMahon DE, Hruza GJ, et al. International collaboration and rapid harmonization across dermatologic COVID-19 registries. J Am Acad Dermatol 2020;83:e261–6.
3. Freeman EE, McMahon DE. Creating dermatology guidelines for COVID-19: the pitfalls of applying evidence-based medicine to an emerging infectious disease. J Am Acad Dermatol 2020;82:e231–2.
4. Freeman EE, McMahon DE, Fitzgerald ME, et al. The American Academy of Dermatology COVID-19 registry: Crowdsourcing dermatology in the age of COVID-19. J Am Acad Dermatol 2020;83(2):509–10.
5. Freeman EE, McMahon DE, Lipoff JB, et al. The spectrum of COVID-19-associated dermatologic manifestations: an international registry of 716 patients from 31 countries. J Am Acad Dermatol 2020;83:1118–29.
6. McMahon DE, Amerson E, Rosenbach M, et al. Cutaneous reactions reported after Moderna and Pfizer COVID-19 vaccination: A registry-based study of 414 cases. J Am Acad Dermatol 2021; 85(1):46–55.
7. Kadakia KT, Beckman AL, Ross JS, et al. Leveraging open science to accelerate research. N Engl J Med 2021;384(17):e61.
8. Mehrotra A, Bhatia RS, Snoswell CL. Paying for telemedicine after the pandemic. JAMA 2021;325:431–2.
9. Lopez L 3rd, Hart LH 3rd, Katz MH. Racial and ethnic health disparities related to COVID-19. JAMA 2021;325:719–20.
10. Lee JH. Combating anti-Asian sentiment—a practical guide for clinicians. N Engl J Med 2021; 384(25):2367–9.
11. Armstrong K. Covid-19 and the investigator pipeline. N Engl J Med 2021;385(1):7–9.
12. McMahon DE, Gallman AE, Hruza GJ, et al. Long COVID in the skin: a registry analysis of COVID-19 dermatological duration. Lancet Infect Dis 2021; 21(3):313–4.

Clinical Patterns and Morphology of COVID-19 Dermatology

Ritesh Agnihothri, MD, Lindy P. Fox, MD*

KEYWORDS

- COVID-19 • SARS-CoV-2 • Dermatology • Morphology

KEY POINTS

- Numerous skin manifestations associated with COVID-19 have been reported. Dermatologists should be aware of these cutaneous manifestations, which may help with diagnosis, management, and prognosis.
- The most commonly reported cutaneous manifestations associated with COVID-19 infection include pernio (chilblain)-like acral lesions, morbilliform (exanthematous) rash, urticaria, vesicular (varicella-like) eruptions, and vaso-occlusive lesions (livedo racemosa, retiform purpura).
- It is important to consider COVID-19 on the differential diagnosis for these disease entities in the proper clinical context, as dermatologic findings of COVID-19 can be a presenting sign in an otherwise minimally or asymptomatic individual.

INTRODUCTION

In December 2019, unexplained pneumonia cases were reported in Wuhan, China. The new pathogen, named SARS-CoV-2 (severe acute respiratory syndrome coronavirus 2), was isolated from samples of the respiratory tract of infected patients, and the resulting disease was called COVID-19 (coronavirus disease 2019). The virus traveled rapidly throughout the globe and was characterized as a pandemic by the World Health Organization on March 11, 2020.

It was soon recognized that COVID-19 patients were experiencing myriad clinical manifestations involving multiple organ systems (including the central nervous, gastrointestinal, and cardiovascular systems), as well as viral illness-induced coagulopathy.[1–4] Initial case series rarely documented skin changes, possibly due to the lack of dermatologists caring for patients with COVID-19 infection as well as the inability to perform complete skin examinations in critically ill patients. Dermatologists also experienced significant challenges collecting samples and taking clinical images while maintaining strict infection prevention techniques, particularly with a widespread limited supply of personal protective equipment.[5] In an early cohort study of 1099 patients with laboratory-confirmed COVID-19, only 2 patients were noted to have "skin rash."[6]

Shortly thereafter, small cohorts of patients were being reported to have cutaneous findings possibly associated with COVID-19 infection.[7,8] The reported findings ranged from those more commonly seen in viral infections, such as morbilliform eruptions and urticaria, to more unique, such as pernio and varicelliform eruptions. A large case series describing patterns of skin manifestations among 375 patients highlighted 5 predominant morphologic patterns: maculopapular, urticarial, pernio-like, vesicular, and livedoid.[9] This series also provided for the first time, a temporal relationship between cutaneous lesions, systemic symptoms, as well as severity of disease. As COVID-19 testing was initially only available to

Department of Dermatology, University of California San Francisco, 1701 Divisadero Street, 3rd Floor, San Francisco, CA 94115, USA
* Corresponding author.
E-mail address: lindy.fox@ucsf.edu

Dermatol Clin 39 (2021) 487–503
https://doi.org/10.1016/j.det.2021.05.006
0733-8635/21/© 2021 Elsevier Inc. All rights reserved.

those with severe disease, the true incidence of cutaneous manifestations with COVID-19 infection is not yet known. The pandemic has encouraged broad collaboration among physicians and scientists around the world,[10] facilitated by multiple registries, which are helping us increase our understanding of dermatologic manifestations in patients with COVID-19.[11,12]

Virology/Immunology

SARS-CoV-2 is a single-stranded RNA virus composed of 16 nonstructural proteins, each of which plays a specific role in replication.[13] SARS-CoV-2 binds to angiotensin-converting enzyme 2 (ACE2) receptors, which is known to be found in the lungs (surfactant producing alveolar type 2 cells) as well as the cardiovascular, gastrointestinal, pulmonary, and renal systems.[14] Expression of ACE2 in the skin is highest in keratinocytes, followed by sweat glands. The widespread expression of ACE2 in the skin is just one of the potential reasons for cutaneous manifestations seen with COVID-19 infection.[15,16]

Pernio (chilblain)-Like Acral Lesions

Since the outbreak of SARS-CoV-2, reports of pernio-like acral lesions have rapidly accumulated. Pernio (chilblains) is an idiopathic cold-sensitive inflammatory disorder that manifests as pink to violaceous macules, papules, plaques, or nodules at sites of cold exposure, commonly on the fingers or toes.[17] Chilblains may be idiopathic or may be associated with autoimmune conditions (ie, chilblains lupus), hematologic malignancies, genetic mutations, and less commonly infections, such as Epstein-Barr virus (EBV).[18] When EBV-associated, cold agglutinins are thought to play a role in pathogenesis.[18] Skin findings may be accompanied by pruritus, pain, burning, and sometimes blistering or ulceration. When making a diagnosis of chilblains, it is important to rule out Parvovirus B19 infection, which can present with acral purpuric lesions.

The first report of pernio-like lesions thought to be associated with COVID-19 was of an Italian adolescent (with family members suspected of having COVID-19 infection) who developed purpuric lesions on the feet before developing systemic symptoms such as fever and myalgias.[19] Reports of young adults with skin lesions on hands and feet identical to chilblains began appearing, seemingly later in the course of their infection.[9] Analysis of Google Trends data, which illustrates popularity of search trends over a period in a particular location, demonstrated that there were sharp increases in search terms including chilblains, fingers, and toes in early 2020.[20,21] As this phenomenon became better known and circulated on social media, it was colloquialized as "COVID-toes," although the precise relationship with SARS-CoV-2 continues to be elucidated. The association was first suspected for multiple reasons: there was a spike in cases during the pandemic, at an atypical time of year for symptoms to occur (spring), in temperate areas, and in patients typically at low risk (ie, no known comorbid conditions associated with chilblains such as autoimmunity,[22] connective tissue disease such as lupus erythematosus, Raynaud phenomenon/syndrome, or a history of chilblains).

Before the pandemic, pernio was uncommon; one case series reported an average of 9 to 10 diagnoses per year across an entire tertiary academic center.[18] Since the onset of the pandemic, studies from around the world have reported numerous individuals with pernio-like lesions thought to be associated with COVID-19 infection. In a French retrospective study on skin manifestations during the early COVID-19 outbreak, pernio-like lesions were noted in 38.3% (106 of 277) of dermatologic outpatients.[23] More recently, an international registry of COVID-19 dermatologic manifestations has recorded 619 cases of pernio in patients with suspected or confirmed COVID-19 infection.[24] Patients with pernio-like lesions are noted to present with pruritus and pain of their toes (less often fingers or heels), which progresses to pink-red papules or plaques and then to violaceous purpuric lesions.[25] Rarely, pernio-like lesions have been reported in other acral sites, such as on the ear.[26] In addition to pernio-like lesions, variations in morphologies have been reported, including erythema multiforme (EM)-like (round, maculopapular, or targetoid lesions), punctiform purpuric lesions, diffuse vascular erythema, and edema of the dorsum/sole of foot or palms.[27] Patients with COVID-19 who develop pernio have relatively mild courses; with 2% to 16% of patients with pernio-like lesions being hospitalized.[9,28–32] This can be compared to other dermatologic manifestations associated with more severe disease such as retiform purpura, where 100% of patients were hospitalized, with 82% of patients developing acute respiratory distress syndrome.[28] Pernio-like acral lesions should be recognized as distinct from acroischemic lesions. The two terms were initially used synonymously, but acroischemic lesions are now known to represent a separate manifestation seen among critically ill patients with hypercoagulopathy and/or disseminated intravascular coagulation.[8]

Histopathology of pernio-like lesions is similar to that of idiopathic or systemic disease-associated chilblains. Pathology frequently contains vascular changes, dermal edema, and a superficial and deep perivascular lymphocytic infiltrate. In select reports, immunohistochemistry has confirmed vasculitis of dermal vessels, deposition of immunoglobulins or complement on dermal vessels, and platelet aggregation.[22,31] When histologic findings of pernio-like lesions in multiple reports were reviewed, it appears that these lesions are primarily inflammatory, nonischemic, and not reflective of systemic coagulopathy, unlike retiform purpura or acral ischemia.[28] Furthermore, the microthrombi seen in a small subset of patients with chilblains are likely secondary to the inflammation and clinically correlate with a bullous or necrotic phenotype.[33]

In a study of dermoscopy features of COVID-19–related chilblains in children and adolescents, dermoscopic findings were found to correlate with clinical and histopathologic findings of COVID-19–related chilblains. For example, the background color noted on dermoscopy is an indicator of vascular macules, hemosiderin, and inflammatory cells in the dermis; gray areas may be indicative of an ischemic phenomenon, and globules likely representing damaged vessels with extravasated red cells. The specificity of these findings, however, is unclear as there is no dermoscopic study of primary chilblains or chilblains secondary to other causes.[34,35]

Overall, pernio-like lesions are typically seen in patients with relatively mild COVID-19 disease courses and resolve within 2 to 8 weeks (median 12 days in laboratory-confirmed cases).[32,36,37] However, persistent and recurrent lesions have been reported. Recent data illustrate a subset of patients with "long COVID" in the skin who had dermatologic signs of COVID-19 that persisted longer than 60 days, including 7 of 103 cases of pernio.[37] Recurrent pernio-like lesions in the absence of reinfection have also been noted, with patients who complained of pernio in the fall experiencing an absence of symptoms in the summer, despite surges of COVID-19 infections in the warmer months.[24] Of note, pernio lesions in type I interferonopathies are also known to flare with cold exposure.[38]

There are increasing number of reports suggesting a direct association between pernio-like lesions and SARS-CoV-2. Positive anti–SARS-CoV-2 immunostaining and viral spike protein have been demonstrated in lesional skin biopsy specimens (endothelial cells and eccrine glands) in adult and pediatric patients with pernio-like lesions.[39–41] However, owing to lack of specificity,

some authors have suggested that these findings be interpreted with caution.[42–44]

The pathogenesis of pernio-like lesions is not well understood but is thought to be predominantly an inflammatory process similar to idiopathic and autoimmune-related chilblains. The striking similarity of pernio-like lesions to those observed in type 1 interferonopathies (ie, Aicardi-Goutieres syndrome and STING-associated vasculopathy) has raised the suspicion of the important role of interferon (IFN) despite the absence of other manifestations of interferonopathies in patients with COVID-19 infection.[45–47] One group demonstrated induction of the type I IFN pathway in lesional sections of COVID-19–associated chilblain-like lesions.[48] Type I interferon is known to have an important role in the pathogenesis of lupus erythematosus.[49,50] Furthermore, interferons are also thought to induce microangiopathic changes contributing to the development of chilblains lupus.[46,47]

As mounting evidence suggests a direct association with SARS-CoV-2, pernio-like lesions are currently believed to represent a postviral or late-onset finding after COVID-19 infection, especially in those who can mount a robust IFN response. In a report by Freeman and colleagues, 80 of 318 cases developed pernio-like lesions after the onset of other symptoms of COVID-19 infection; a similar finding has been noted in at least one other study.[9,32] Conversely, pernio-like lesions have also been reported to occur concurrently with RT-PCR test positivity.[32,51] Negative nasopharyngeal reverse-transcription polymerase chain reaction (RT-PCR) or anti–SARS-CoV-2 serologies in many patients[52–58] created uncertainty early in the pandemic regarding the precise relationship.[39,54,57–59] Indeed, some patients who were RT-PCR negative after developing pernio, were later found to have positive COVID-19 antibodies (immunoglobulin M, G, or A).[24,26,32,60,61]

What was initially surprising, however, was that serologic testing for IgM or IgG antibodies was often negative. There is increased understanding of this mechanism:

I. Early in the pandemic, interpretation of RT-PCR/antibody results in patients with skin rash and probable COVID-19 was difficult due to lack of understanding of timing and antibody kinetics. Much of the available antibody data were drawn from patients with more severe illness as widespread testing was not available. Many patients with pernio-like lesions were undergoing serologic evaluation for SARS-CoV-2 antibodies early in the disease course. In one study, patients had antibody testing between 3 and 30 days after pernio developed, with most evaluated less than 15 days after pernio onset.[57] It is now appreciated that delayed antibody development after infection with SARS-CoV-2 is common.[62] In one early report, positive antibodies were detected a median of 30 days from disease onset, beyond the typical 14- to 21-day testing window.[63]

II. Population level antibody testing from the past year has revealed that there is a relationship between disease severity and the level of SARS-CoV-2 antibodies. In one particular hospital, for both IgG and IgA isotypes, patients with moderate/severe infection had significantly higher antibody titers within the first 1.5 months after diagnosis compared to those with milder disease.[64] As previously discussed, it is now well-established that those with COVID-19 who develop chilblains have relatively mild clinical courses and may not mount a marked antibody response, similar to others with minimal symptoms of infection.[60] Despite a more muted antibody response, data suggest that patients with milder SARS-CoV-2 infection are able to elicit in vitro neutralizing antibodies (preventing the virus from entering epithelial cells).[65] Negative RT-PCR on nasopharyngeal swabs is supportive of the notion that pernio-like lesions are a late symptom of COVID-19.[28]

III. Most serologic testing for SARS-CoV-2 currently is against SARS-CoV-2 IgM and IgG. It is appreciated that the host immune response to SARS-CoV-2 infection includes synthesis of several types of virus-specific antibodies including IgM, IgG, and IgA.[66,67] There are also reports that some patients with pernio-like lesions have positive serology for anti–SARS-CoV-2 IgA.[55,60] The authors postulated that children with mild or asymptomatic infection may develop an IgA humoral response, rather than IgG. Secretory IgA plays a vital role in host protection of mucosal surfaces by preventing entry and subsequent infection by respiratory viruses including influenza; elevated levels are also associated with improved influenza vaccine efficacy.[68] With SARS-CoV-2, a pathogen that first interacts with the immune system at mucosal surfaces/lungs due to person-to-person respiratory transmission, a robust IgA response appears before IgG. IgA serum levels reach their peak earlier than IgG (10–14 days) suggesting that both IgA and IgG are part of the initial humoral immune response. Given that currently widely used commercial antibody tests do not look for IgA, a "negative antibody test" may not truly reflect the absence of prior infection and/or antibody production.

IV. The kinetics of early interferon production may determine overall COVID-19 disease severity and antibody production. Interferons are early antiviral response proteins that interfere with intracellular viral replication, recruit other cells for antiviral response, and cause "flu-like symptoms" such as fever and muscle pain. It is thought that robust production of interferon-I is associated with early viral control, suppressed antibody response, and mild COVID-19 infection. This may be an additional explanation for why some patients fail serologic detection.[69] Conversely, patients with severe COVID-19 have notably depressed/absent interferon responses or interferon deficiency that can lead to severe, life-threatening COVID-19 infection.[70–73] Several authors hypothesize that chilblains, specifically, could be the cutaneous expression of a strong type I interferon response.[74–77] This could therefore explain the absence of antibodies in patients with chilblains.

There is a correlation between the severity of COVID and the timing of appearance of COVID-antigen–specific CD4 T-cells in circulation. Patients with the early expansion of antigen-specific CD4 T-cells (2 days after symptom onset) seem to have mild COVID and those who have a late response (CD4 appearance >20 days after symptoms) have severe disease, suggesting that an early CD4 T-cell response is important in fighting SARS-CoV-2 infection.[78] Sekine and colleagues have demonstrated T-cell immunity to SARS-CoV-2 in those with mild COVID-19 infection who were also subsequently seronegative.[79]

Morbilliform Eruptions

Morbilliform (maculopapular) eruptions frequently arise as a result of viral infections or adverse drug reactions, and are the most commonly reported cutaneous manifestation of COVID-19 with a prevalence as high as 47%.[7,9,23,28,80] Predominantly involving the trunk, the rash has been noted either at disease onset, or more frequently, after hospital discharge, with a reported median duration of 7 days.[7,37,81] Morbilliform eruptions are associated with intermediate severity of disease.[82] It is difficult to definitively associate morbilliform eruptions with SARS-CoV-2 infection as many reported patients may have received concomitant drug therapy for their infection. Although medications given as a part of COVID-19 treatment (ie, ribavarin, IVIG, and antiretroviral drugs) may cause morbilliform eruptions, this manifestation has been noted in patients with no new medications.[83,84] Taking a detailed history is critical, and it is important to consider COVID-19 testing in patients when the eruption is not better explained by medications or other infections.

Urticarial Eruptions

Urticaria (hives) is a common feature among COVID-19 patients who experienced rashes. Acute urticaria, defined as a self-limited lesion lasting less than 6 weeks, has been reported as a presenting sign of COVID-19 infection, although it can also occur later in the disease course.[7,9,23,28,45] COVID-associated urticaria has also been reported to present with fever as an early prodromal sign in otherwise asymptomatic individuals.[85–87] Acute urticaria can be triggered by infections, medications, insect bites/stings, and type I immune reactions. It has been hypothesized that viral IgM/IgG can cross-react with mast cell IgE and cause mast cell degranulation, which could explain urticaria in the setting of COVID-19 infection.[88] It is important to note that urticaria is also a possible side-effect for numerous medications used to treat COVID-19.[84] COVID-19–associated urticarial eruptions are reported to last a median of 4 days with a maximum duration of 28 days.[37] Although the specificity of urticaria to COVID-19 infection is low, in patients with new onset urticaria developing during the pandemic, one should consider evaluation for COVID-19 infection with RT-PCR and serologic studies.

Vesicular Eruptions

Vesicles are fluid-filled collections in the epidermis less than $1/2$ cm in diameter. Vesicles can be caused by a variety of viral infections including varicella-zoster, herpes simplex, echovirus, and coxsackievirus infections.[89] Most patients with COVID-19 presenting with varicella-like exanthem also have general respiratory and general symptoms of COVID-19 infection. One Italian study including 22 patients reported vesicular, varicelliform lesions, which developed on average 3 days after onset of COVID-19 symptoms.[90] Although more often being reported as developing early after onset of systemic signs of COVID-19 infection (up to 79.2%),[91] 15% of patients in one study developed this rash before other symptoms.[9] The papulovesicular exanthems noted in association with COVID-19 infection differ from true varicella infection with their truncal involvement, scattered distribution, and minimal pruritus.[90] Vesicular lesions are thought to be associated with moderate severity of COVID-19.[9,91] In the appropriate clinical context, COVID-19 testing (in addition to HSV/VZV PCR) should be performed in a patient presenting with varicelliform cutaneous eruption.

Two morphologies of COVID-associated vesicular eruption have been described: localized, monomorphic lesions typically involving the trunk or back, and a more diffuse polymorphic eruption notable for small papules, vesicles, and pustules of varying sizes.[91] The distribution of lesions involving the trunk and back mimics Grover disease (transient acantholytic dermatosis), a benign condition seen in older Caucasian men with crusted papules and papulovesicles on the trunk and back. COVID-19–associated varicella-like exanthem can share some histologic similarity to Grover disease. In one report of 3 cases, a prominent nonballooning acantholysis with intraepidermal vesicle and eosinophilic dyskeratosis without nuclear atypia was noted, leading to the suggestion that this entity would be better termed "COVID-19–associated acantholytic rash."[92] Conversely, in other histologic reports of COVID-19–associated vesicular eruptions, histology was consistent with viral infection, with vacuolar degeneration of the basal layer with multinucleate, hyperchromatic keratinocytes and dyskeratotic cells.[90,93]

Erythema Multiforme-like Lesions

EM is an acute, typically self-limited hypersensitivity reaction involving the skin and mucous membranes presenting with concentric three-ring targetoid plaques on acral surfaces. It is clinically characterized as presenting with acute onset of concentric (targetoid) plaques. In adults, more than 90% of EM is thought to be triggered by infection, particularly the herpes simplex virus. EM-like eruptions of targetoid lesions with either truncal or acral predominance have been observed in association with SARS-CoV-2 infection in adults and children.[9,94–97] Children with COVID-19 who develop EM generally have mild respiratory/gastrointestinal symptoms or are otherwise asymptomatic.[98] In one series, 2 of 4 children with suspected COVID-related EM underwent skin biopsies with positive immunohistochemistry staining of endothelium to SARS-CoV-2 spike protein.[99] Another study reported 4 hospitalized women with COVID-19 infection who developed pink truncal papules evolving to targetoid lesions, which resolved in all 4 patients within 2 to 3 weeks.[94] A 60-year-old woman with fixed urticarial eruption (nonevanescent) underwent skin biopsy, which was notable for slight vacuolar-type interface dermatitis with necrotic keratinocytes and no eosinophils, most consistent with an EM-like pattern, highlighting that not all EM-like lesions present as targets.[100]

Pityriasis Rosea-like Eruption

Pityriasis rosea (PR) is a common papulosquamous eruption presenting with ovoid patches and plaques with fine collarettes of scale. In classic cases, a solitary lesion (herald patch) precedes the development of a more diffuse eruption. Lesions are classically formed along skin fold lines on the trunk. PR-like eruptions have been noted to be occurring in greater frequency and in association with SARS-CoV-2 infection.[101–107] An atypical digitate papulosquamous variant in an elderly patient with COVID-19 infection has also been reported.[108] Although the exact cause of typical PR is unclear, viral etiologies, including human herpesvirus (HHV)-6 and 7 have been favored. Reactivation of HHV-6 and EBV has been demonstrated in one patient with COVID-19 infection and PR.[109] A recent report demonstrated 2 patients with PR-like rash and urticaria-like rash with COVID-19 infection with SARS-CoV-2 spike protein present in the endothelium of dermal blood vessels of affected skin.[110] It is unclear if the increased incidence of PR is due to direct viral infection of SARS-CoV-2, reactivation of HHV-6/7, or other factors. Testing for infection is recommended in a patient who presents with this characteristic eruption in the appropriate clinical context.

Pediatric COVID-19

Despite more than 3.85 million testing positive for COVID-19 since the onset of the pandemic, children have been relatively spared from severe COVID-19–related complications, with less frequent infection, less severe respiratory sequelae, and generally a milder course.[111,112] This milder course is attributed to children having fewer predisposing factors for severe disease (ie, cardiovascular disease, diabetes mellitus), healthy vascular endothelium, strong antiviral innate immunity, and fewer ACE receptors in nasal and lung epithelium, making viral entry and infection more difficult.[113]

In children, cutaneous signs of COVID-19 may be the predominant or only clue of infection and, in fact, are not uncommon. Cutaneous lesions of COVID-19 occur in more than 8% of hospitalized children[114] and are the 7th most common extrapulmonary manifestation.[115] There are several case reports and case series of various cutaneous eruptions in COVID-positive children. Children with COVID-19 and skin manifestations carry an overall better prognosis than those without.[116]

Multisystem Inflammatory Syndrome in Children (MIS-C)

Since April 2020, there have been multiple reports worldwide of severe pediatric disease several weeks (median 25 days) after SARS-CoV-2 infection with fevers, multiorgan involvement, and characteristics of Kawasaki disease (KD).[117–119] This syndrome has been called MIS-C and is thought to be a postviral consequence of COVID-19 infection. There is confirmed laboratory evidence of COVID-19 infection in 99% of cases, antibody testing is positive, and RT-PCR tends to be negative. The US Centers for Disease Control and Prevention (CDC) has developed a case definition of MIS-C (**Table 1**).[120]

MIS-S shares some features of KD and toxic shock syndrome, including fever and skin, mucous membrane, and distal extremity changes. However, it is considered a distinct disease. In contrast to KD, MIS-C is being seen in older children and adolescents (median age 9 years) and non-Hispanic black and Hispanic children, whereas KD more commonly affects children younger than 5 years who are of East Asian descent. In addition, children with MIS-C experience more gastrointestinal symptoms and less than 50% meet formal criteria for KD.[121,122]

The pathogenesis of MIS-C is thought to be multifactorial, including the robust immune system of children, immune complex activation, and the superantigen activity of SARS-CoV-2 spike protein all leading to cytokine storm and systemic inflammation.[123–125] MIS-C cases and deaths unfortunately continue to accumulate; although most children with this condition require intensive care, patients with MIS-C carry a good prognosis, with current mortality estimated at 2%.

Although many studies have described cutaneous involvement with MIS-C, the type of rash, distribution, and clinical course needs to be studied further. Greater than 50% of cases of MIS-C are reported to have mucocutaneous changes. Reported mucocutaneous findings include morbilliform, scarlatiniform, urticarial, and reticulated patterns, as well as periorbital edema, malar rash, and reticulated exanthems similar to erythema infectiosum.[126] In addition, distal extremity changes, oral mucous membrane changes,

Table 1
Case definition for Multisystem Inflammatory Syndrome in Children (MIS-C) associated with COVID-19 infection[120]

Criteria	Additional Information	
Age <21 y		
Fever	Fever ≥38.0°C for ≥24 h, or report of subjective fever lasting ≥24 h	
Laboratory evidence of inflammation	Including, but not limited to, one or more of the following: an elevated CRP, ESR, fibrinogen, procalcitonin, D-dimer, ferritin, LDH, or IL-6, elevated neutrophils, reduced lymphocytes, and low albumin	
Multisystem (≥2) organ involvement (cardiac, renal, respiratory, hematologic, gastrointestinal, dermatologic, or neurologic)	*Organ system*	*Examples of involvement[130,131]*
	Gastrointestinal	Abdominal pain, diarrhea, nausea, vomiting, abnormal hepatobiliary markers
	Hematologic	Fever, myalgias, lymphadenopathy, fatigue, abnormal blood counts
	Neurologic	Headache, irritability, altered mental status, dizziness
	Dermatologic	Cutaneous eruption, conjunctivitis, edema, mucositis
	Respiratory	Dyspnea, upper respiratory infection-like signs, cough, wheezing, respiratory failure, pulmonary infiltrates
	Cardiovascular	Shock, chest pain, myocarditis, coronary artery dilatation/ aneurysm, elevated cardiac enzyme markers
	Renal	Acute kidney injury
No alternative plausible diagnoses; AND		
Positive for current or recent SARS-CoV-2 infection by RT-PCR, serology, or antigen test; or exposure to a suspected or confirmed COVID-19 case within the 4 wk before the onset of symptoms.		

Abbreviations: CRP, C-reactive protein; ESR, erythrocyte sedimentation rate; IL-6, interleukin 6; LDH, lactic acid dehydrogenase.

conjunctivitis, and purpura are reported.[127] The molecular mechanisms underlying the relationship between COVID-19 and MIS-C are poorly understood. There are increasing numbers of adults being reported to have COVID-19–associated MIS-C, characterized by multiorgan dysfunction (particularly cardiac) in the absence of severe respiratory illness.[128,129]

Vascular Lesions

Petechiae and purpura

Petechiae and purpura (visible hemorrhage into the skin or mucous membranes) are among the less commonly described cutaneous manifestations of COVID-19 infection. The first COVID-19–associated cutaneous manifestation with purpuric features was reported by Joob and colleagues, who described a petechial rash misdiagnosed as dengue in a COVID-19 patient.[132] Only 3% of patients in a French study of 277 patients had petechial skin lesions.[23] Petechial eruptions can have many etiologies including platelet deficiency or dysfunction, disorders of coagulation, and loss of vascular wall integrity. This morphology is associated with certain viral infections including enterovirus, parvovirus B19, and dengue virus.[133] COVID-19–associated petechial and purpuric lesions have been noted on acral surfaces, intertriginous regions, extremities, or diffusely.[9,23,134–136] When secondary to vasculitis, lesions can progress to form blisters.[137] Henoch-Schonlein Purpura and IgA vasculitis has been reported to be triggered by SARS-CoV-2 infection.[138–140]

Livedo reticularis-like lesions

Livedo reticularis (LR) is a transient finding that classically presents with a blue-purple reticulated vascular pattern. LR results from alterations in vascular flow, which results in accumulation of deoxygenated blood in the cutaneous venous plexis. LR has been observed in association with COVID-19 infection.[141–143] Although cases of LR were grouped with more severe necrosis in a major early study,[9] more recent reports estimate that this manifestation was present in 3.5% of patients.[28]

Fixed livedo racemosa, retiform purpura, and necrotic vascular lesions

Vaso-occlusive lesions (livedo racemosa, thrombotic retiform purpura, and acral ischemia) have been noted in elderly, critically ill patients with severe COVID-19 infection.[9,28,144] These clinical entities exist at the opposite end of the disease severity spectrum compared to perniosis, which occurs in those with mild or asymptomatic disease. Patients with this clinical finding have been noted to have markedly elevated D-dimer levels and disseminated intravascular coagulation.[8,144] Skin biopsy of a COVID patient with retiform purpuric patches showed multiple occlusive thrombi in most small vessels of the superficial and mid-dermis.[145] Direct immunofluorescence in this patient was notable for IgM, C3 and C9 deposition within dermal vessel walls.[145] In a subsequent study of a series of COVID patients with retiform purpura, terminal complements C5b-9 and other complement components were found in the microvasculature. This may be suggestive of systemic complement activation and pathophysiology similar to atypical hemolytic uremic syndrome or other microthrombotic syndromes.[144] Pauci-inflammatory purpuric (most often on buttocks) pressure ulcers have also been noted in several critically ill COVID patients with limited mobility, incontinence, and malnutrition.[146] Histopathology of these purpuric pressure ulcers were consistent with pressure necrosis (epidermal necrosis, eccrine gland necrosis); SARS-CoV-2 RNA in-situ hybridization of all 4 skin biopsies was negative. The reported patients did not have any laboratory evidence of coagulopathy such as disseminated intravascular coagulation.[146] It is important to recognize that this clinical finding is distinct from the thrombotic vasculopathy noted by Magro and colleagues[144]

In a recent review of the literature, vaso-occlusive lesions were found to be the least commonly reported cutaneous manifestation with COVID-19 infection but may portend a worse prognosis with the highest mortality rate of all COVID-associated cutaneous manifestations (18.2%).[82,147]

OTHER REPORTED CUTANEOUS MANIFESTATIONS/ASSOCIATIONS

Cutaneous Manifestation	Subtype, if Applicable	Morphology	Additional Clinical Findings
Alopecia	Androgenetic alopecia	Hair loss from the anterior hairline moving posteriorly or thinning at the vertex scalp	Associated with worse clinical outcomes in some studies[148,149]
	Telogen effluvium	Diffuse hair shedding 2–3 mo after a stressor[150,151]	

(continued on next page)

(continued)

Cutaneous Manifestation	Subtype, if Applicable	Morphology	Additional Clinical Findings
Gianotti-Crosti-like rash		Pruritic erythematous papules and vesicles on elbows, anterior thighs, and bilateral popliteal fossa coalescing into plaques.[152]	Rash started 18 d after onset of symptoms, 13 d after +COVID test, and 3 d after resolution of all respiratory and systemic symptoms.
SDRIFE-like		Erythematous rash on bilateral axillae and antecubital fossae, which subsequently extended to trunk and inner thighs[153,154]	
Grover-disease-like		Red papules and papulovesicles distributed on the trunk[155] Note: some evidence suggests clinical overlap with vesicular, or "varicella-like" eruptions	
Erythema elevatum diutinum-like		Firm symmetric smooth nodules on extensor surfaces, particularly joints[156]	
Reactive infectious mucocutaneous eruption (formerly known as *Mycoplasma*-induced rash and mucositis)		Shallow erosions of the vermilion lips, hard palate, periurethral glans penis.[157]	Reported patient with +COVID PCR 1 wk before rash onset, and again positive at rash onset. Mycoplasma PCR negative, IgM negative, IgG positive (consistent with past exposure).
Enanthems (eruptions of the mucous membranes)		83% (5 patients) with petechial enanthem ± macular enanthem[158]	Recorded from a group of 21 patients with COVID-19 and skin rash ranging from papulovesicular, purpuric periflexural, and erythema multiforme-like.
Oral lesions		Aphthous-like, ulcerations, and macules, tongue depapillation, angular cheilitis, ulcers, blisters, white plaques, dark pigmentations.[159]	Etiology postulated to be multifactorial. Hypotheses include direct action of SARS-CoV-2 on oral mucosal cells, coinfection, immunity impairment, or adverse drug reactions[160]
Acute genital ulcers (Lipschütz ulcers)		Necrotic ulcers with raised, sharply demarcated borders of the labia minora with no evidence of "kissing lesions."[161]	Single oral aphtha was also observed, with no cutaneous involvement
Transient rash in newborns		Transient "rash" (morphology not described) in babies born to mothers with COVID-19.[162] Mottling noted in a neonate with sepsis and +COVID-19.[163]	

Abbreviation: SDRIFE, symmetric drug-related intertriginous and flexural exanthema.

DISCUSSION

As the novel SARS-CoV-2 virus rapidly spread throughout the world, the scientific and medical community has worked with remarkable pace to understand its full clinical effects. Early in the pandemic, scarcity of diagnostic assays limited our ability to confirm infection in patients presenting with an array of cutaneous manifestations. Most young patients presenting with pernio-like lesions had mild clinical courses, which precluded them from having access to COVID-19 testing early in the pandemic when diagnostic resources were limited.

Viral infections are known to produce a variety of clinical findings due not only to their direct action on human cells but also to the host immune response and resulting inflammatory cascade. Further complicating the clinical picture, patients with COVID-19 infections were often treated with a multitude of medications, many of which can be associated with the reported cutaneous manifestations. Now with relative widespread availability of RT-PCR assays and serologic testing, we are beginning to understand the utility and limitations of testing (including timing in relation to a patient's infection course and imperfect sensitivities and specificities of available tests).[62,164] It is now understood that a negative swab or antibody test at one point in time does not necessarily rule out SARS-CoV-2 as a causative agent.[164] Data derived from a UK COVID Symptoms Study app suggest that those with cutaneous rash are more likely to test positive for SARS-CoV-2 (odds ratio 1.67).[165] Although less prevalent than fever, the authors also found rash to be more specific for COVID-19 infection, which lends support to the diagnostic value of cutaneous manifestations of SARS-CoV-2 infection.[165]

The most commonly reported cutaneous manifestations associated with COVID-19 infection include pernio-like, urticarial, morbilliform, and retiform purpura. As previously discussed, identifying cutaneous eruptions and their possible association with SARS-CoV-2 infection can allow for early identification of infection, sometimes even before onset of more classic symptoms such as respiratory distress.[82] As seen in **Fig. 1**, Jamshidi and colleagues in their systematic review found that vesicular and urticarial eruptions are seen

early relative to other COVID-19 symptoms. Maculopapular, papulosquamous, vascular lesions tend to occur around the time that a patient is symptomatic. Pernio-like lesions occur later in the disease course.[82] Certain cutaneous morphologies are noted to correlate to severity of illness and overall prognosis. According to a study by Galvan and colleagues, pernio-like, vesicular, urticarial, maculopapular, and livedoid/necrotic lesions were associated with progressively increasing disease severity.[9] This has been corroborated by another study by Freeman and colleagues, which demonstrated cutaneous manifestations associated with a spectrum of severity, with pernio-like lesions noted in mild disease, vesicular/urticarial/macular erythema/morbilliform eruption in intermediate severity, and retiform purpura in critically ill patients.[28] Similarly, pernio-like lesions and morbilliform eruptions are associated with the highest survival rates (98.7% and 98.2%, respectively), whereas vaso-occlusive lesions are associated with the lowest survival rate of 78.9%.[147] It is important to consider SARS-CoV-2 infection in the differential diagnosis of a patient presenting with these lesions (ie, new onset pernio-like lesions, vesicular or morbilliform eruption) in the appropriate clinical context, as cutaneous manifestations may be present in otherwise asymptomatic individuals, or present before developing other symptoms of infection.

The coronavirus pandemic has been found to disproportionally affect people of color in both the United States and the United Kingdom, yet registry data on cutaneous manifestations in this population is lacking.[28] A systematic review of literature describing cases of cutaneous manifestations associated with COVID-19 found a significant paucity of reports and photographs of manifestations in skin of color, and no published photos of cutaneous manifestations in Fitzpatrick type V or VI skin.[166] A recent study suggests there are geographic differences in the morphology and prevalence of COVID-19–associated skin manifestations.[147] More work must be done to better understand the true prevalence of skin findings in COVID-19 across all populations and ethnicities.

SUMMARY

The clinical phenotype of COVID-19 includes a broad spectrum of cutaneous manifestations of varying degrees of severity and specificity. Although initially thought to be an infection with primarily internal/systemic manifestations, COVID-19 has taught us that dermatologists play an important role in the treatment of COVID-19 patients, as well as in the broad scientific

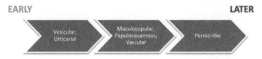

EARLY   LATER

Vesicular, Urticarial   Maculopapular, Papulosquamous, Vascular   Pernio-like

Fig. 1. Timing of skin lesions relative to other COVID-19 symptoms.[82]

collaboration to learn more about the pathophysiology of infection. Widespread availability of COVID-19 tests, as well as improved diagnostic assays, will further assist our understanding of how skin manifestations are related to this viral infection, and parse out potential confounding factors such as concurrent pharmacotherapy or lifestyle changes.

CLINICS CARE POINTS

- Cutaneous manifestations of COVID-19 are generally benign and self-limited. These manifestations have prognostic significance depending on type of skin lesion. Pernio (chilblain)-like acral lesions are generally associated with mild disease; retiform purpura is typically seen in patients on the severe end of the disease severity spectrum.

- Cutaneous manifestations may be present in otherwise asymptomatic individuals, or present before developing other symptoms of infection.

- With increased access to diagnostic testing, we are beginning to understand the utility and limitations of currently available assays.

DISCLOSURE

The authors have nothing to disclose.

REFERENCES

1. Hajifathalian K, Mahadev S, Schwartz RE, et al. SARS-COV-2 infection (coronavirus disease 2019) for the gastrointestinal consultant. World J Gastroenterol 2020;26(14):1546–53.

2. Helms J, Kremer S, Merdji H, et al. Neurologic Features in Severe SARS-CoV-2 Infection. N Engl J Med 2020;382(23):2268–70.

3. Bikdeli B, Madhavan MV, Jimenez D, et al. COVID-19 and Thrombotic or Thromboembolic Disease: Implications for Prevention, Antithrombotic Therapy, and Follow-Up: JACC State-of-the-Art Review. J Am Coll Cardiol 2020;75(23):2950–73.

4. Batlle D, Soler MJ, Sparks MA, et al. Acute kidney injury in COVID-19: Emerging evidence of a distinct pathophysiology. J Am Soc Nephrol 2020; 31(7):1380–3.

5. Fernandez-Nieto D, Ortega-Quijano D, Segurado-Miravalles G, et al. Comment on: Cutaneous manifestations in COVID-19: a first perspective. Safety concerns of clinical images and skin biopsies. J Eur Acad Dermatol Venereol 2020;34(6):e252–4.

6. Guan W, Ni Z, Hu Y, et al. Clinical Characteristics of Coronavirus Disease 2019 in China. N Engl J Med 2020;382(18):1708–20.

7. Recalcati S. Cutaneous manifestations in COVID-19: a first perspective. J Eur Acad Dermatol Venereol 2020;34(5):e212–3.

8. Zhang Y, Cao W, Xiao M, et al. Clinical and coagulation characteristics in 7 patients with critical COVID-2019 pneumonia and acro-ischemia. Zhonghua Xue Ye Xue Za Zhi 2020;41(4):302–7.

9. Galván Casas C, Català A, Carretero Hernández G, et al. Classification of the cutaneous manifestations of COVID-19: a rapid prospective nationwide consensus study in Spain with 375 cases. Br J Dermatol 2020;183(1):71–7.

10. Robinson PC, Yazdany J. The COVID-19 Global Rheumatology Alliance: collecting data in a pandemic. Nat Rev Rheumatol 2020;16(6):293–4.

11. Freeman EE, McMahon DE, Fitzgerald ME, et al. The American Academy of Dermatology COVID-19 registry: Crowdsourcing dermatology in the age of COVID-19. J Am Acad Dermatol 2020;83(2):509–10.

12. Freeman EE, McMahon DE, Hruza GJ, et al. International collaboration and rapid harmonization across dermatologic COVID-19 registries. J Am Acad Dermatol 2020;83(3):e261–6.

13. Chen Y, Liu Q, Guo D. Emerging coronaviruses: Genome structure, replication, and pathogenesis. J Med Virol 2020;92(4):418–23.

14. Prompetchara E, Ketloy C, Palaga T. Immune responses in COVID-19 and potential vaccines: Lessons learned from SARS and MERS epidemic. Asian Pac J Allergy Immunol 2020;38(1):1–9.

15. Li MY, Li L, Zhang Y, et al. Expression of the SARS-CoV-2 cell receptor gene ACE2 in a wide variety of human tissues. Infect Dis Poverty 2020;9(1). https://doi.org/10.1186/s40249-020-00662-x.

16. Xue X, Mi Z, Wang Z, et al. High Expression of ACE2 on Keratinocytes Reveals Skin as a Potential Target for SARS-CoV-2. J Invest Dermatol 2021; 141(1):206–9.e1.

17. Hedrich CM, Fiebig B, Hauck FH, et al. Chilblain lupus erythematosus - A review of literature. Clin Rheumatol 2008;27(8):949–54.

18. Cappel JA, Wetter DA. Clinical characteristics, etiologic associations, laboratory findings, treatment, and proposal of diagnostic criteria of pernio (chilblains) in a series of 104 patients at Mayo Clinic, 2000 to 2011. Mayo Clin Proc 2014;89(2): 207–15.

19. Mazzotta F, Troccoli T. Acute Acro-ischemia in the Child at the time of COVID-19. Eur J Pediat Dermatol 2020;30(2):71–4.

20. Kluger N, Scrivener JN. The use of Google Trends for acral symptoms during COVID-19 outbreak in

France. J Eur Acad Dermatol Venereol 2020;34(8): e358–60.

21. Hughes M, Rogers S, Lepri G, et al. Further evidence that chilblains are a cutaneous manifestation of COVID-19 infection. Br J Dermatol 2020; 183(3):596–8.

22. Kanitakis J, Lesort C, Danset M, et al. Chilblain-like acral lesions during the COVID-19 pandemic ("COVID toes"): Histologic, immunofluorescence, and immunohistochemical study of 17 cases. J Am Acad Dermatol 2020;83(3):870–5.

23. de Masson A, Bouaziz JD, Sulimovic L, et al. Chilblains is a common cutaneous finding during the COVID-19 pandemic: A retrospective nationwide study from France. J Am Acad Dermatol 2020; 83(2):667–70.

24. Freeman EE, McMahon DE, Lipoff JB, et al. Cold and COVID: recurrent pernio during the COVID-19 pandemic. Br J Dermatol 2021. https://doi.org/10.1111/bjd.19894.

25. Hubiche T, Cardot-Leccia N, Le Duff F, et al. Clinical, Laboratory, and Interferon-Alpha Response Characteristics of Patients with Chilblain-like Lesions during the COVID-19 Pandemic. JAMA Dermatol 2020. https://doi.org/10.1001/jamadermatol. 2020.4324.

26. Proietti I, Tolino E, Bernardini N, et al. Auricle perniosis as a manifestation of Covid-19 infection. Dermatol Ther 2020;33(6). https://doi.org/10.1111/dth. 14089.

27. Le Cleach L, Dousset L, Assier H, et al. Most chilblains observed during the COVID-19 outbreak occur in patients who are negative for COVID-19 on PCR and serology testing. Br J Dermatol 2020. https://doi.org/10.1111/bjd.19377.

28. Freeman EE, McMahon DE, Lipoff JB, et al. The spectrum of COVID-19–associated dermatologic manifestations: An international registry of 716 patients from 31 countries. J Am Acad Dermatol 2020;83(4):1118–29.

29. Fernandez-Nieto D, Jimenez-Cauhe J, Suarez-Valle A, et al. Characterization of acute acral skin lesions in nonhospitalized patients: A case series of 132 patients during the COVID-19 outbreak. J Am Acad Dermatol 2020;83(1):e61–3.

30. Andina D, Noguera-Morel L, Bascuas-Arribas M, et al. Chilblains in children in the setting of COVID-19 pandemic. Pediatr Dermatol 2020; 37(3):406–11.

31. Kolivras A, Dehavay F, Delplace D, et al. Coronavirus (COVID-19) infection–induced chilblains: A case report with histopathologic findings. JAAD Case Rep 2020;6(6):489–92.

32. Freeman EE, McMahon DE, Lipoff JB, et al. Pernio-like skin lesions associated with COVID-19: A case series of 318 patients from 8 countries. J Am Acad Dermatol 2020;83(2):486–92.

33. Baeck M, Herman A, Peeters C, et al. Are chilblains a skin expression of COVID-19 microangiopathy? J Thromb Haemost 2020;18(9):2414–5.

34. Navarro L, Andina D, Noguera-Morel L, et al. Dermoscopy features of COVID-19-related chilblains in children and adolescents. J Eur Acad Dermatol Venereol 2020;34(12):e762–4.

35. Piccolo V, Bassi A, Argenziano G, et al. Dermoscopy of chilblain-like lesions during the COVID-19 outbreak: A multicenter study on 10 patients. J Am Acad Dermatol 2020;83(6):1749–51.

36. Marzano AV, Genovese G, Moltrasio C, et al. The clinical spectrum of COVID-19-associated cutaneous manifestations: an Italian multicentre study of 200 adult patients. J Am Acad Dermatol 2021. https://doi.org/10.1016/j.jaad.2021.01.023.

37. McMahon DE, Gallman AE, Hruza GJ, et al. Long COVID in the skin: a registry analysis of COVID-19 dermatological duration. Lancet Infect Dis 2021. https://doi.org/10.1016/s1473-3099(20) 30986-5.

38. Orcesi S, La Piana R, Fazzi E. Aicardi-Goutieres syndrome. Br Med Bull 2009;89(1):183–201.

39. Colmenero I, Santonja C, Alonso-Riaño M, et al. SARS-CoV-2 endothelial infection causes COVID-19 chilblains: histopathological, immunohistochemical and ultrastructural study of seven paediatric cases. Br J Dermatol 2020;183(4):729–37.

40. Santonja C, Heras F, Núñez L, et al. COVID-19 chilblain-like lesion: immunohistochemical demonstration of SARS-CoV-2 spike protein in blood vessel endothelium and sweat gland epithelium in a polymerase chain reaction-negative patient. Br J Dermatol 2020;183(4):778–80.

41. Gambichler T, Reuther J, Stücker M, et al. SARS-CoV-2 spike protein is present in both endothelial and eccrine cells of a chilblain-like skin lesion. J Eur Acad Dermatol Venereol 2021;35(3): e187–9.

42. Ko CJ, Harigopal M, Damsky W, et al. Perniosis during the COVID-19 pandemic: Negative anti-SARS-CoV-2 immunohistochemistry in six patients and comparison to perniosis before the emergence of SARS-CoV-2. J Cutan Pathol 2020;47(11): 997–1002.

43. Baeck M, Hoton D, Marot L, et al. Chilblains and COVID-19: why SARS-CoV-2 endothelial infection is questioned. Br J Dermatol 2020;183(6): 1152–3.

44. Brealey JK, Miller SE. SARS-CoV-2 has not been detected directly by electron microscopy in the endothelium of chilblain lesions. Br J Dermatol 2021;184(1):186.

45. Bouaziz JD, Duong TA, Jachiet M, et al. Vascular skin symptoms in COVID-19: a French observational study. J Eur Acad Dermatol Venereol 2020; 34(9):e451–2.

46. Rodero MP, Crow YJ. Type I interferonâ-mediated monogenic autoinflammation: The type i interferonopathies, a conceptual overview. J Exp Med 2016;213(12):2527–38.

47. Papa R, Volpi S, Gattorno M. Monogenetic causes of chilblains, panniculitis and vasculopathy: The Type I interferonopathies. G Ital di Dermatologia e Venereol 2020;155(5):590–8.

48. Aschoff R, Zimmermann N, Beissert S, et al. Type I Interferon Signature in Chilblain-Like Lesions Associated with the COVID-19 Pandemic. Dermatopathology 2020;7(3):57–63.

49. Saeed M. Lupus pathobiology based on genomics. Immunogenetics 2017;69(1):1–12.

50. Ivashkiv LB, Donlin LT. Regulation of type i interferon responses. Nat Rev Immunol 2014;14(1):36–49.

51. Guarneri C, Venanzi Rullo E, Gallizzi R, et al. Diversity of clinical appearance of cutaneous manifestations in the course of COVID-19. J Eur Acad Dermatol Venereol 2020;34(9):e449–50.

52. Baeck M, Peeters C, Herman A. Chilblains and COVID-19: further evidence against a causal association. J Eur Acad Dermatol Venereol 2021;35(1):e2–3.

53. Colonna C, Genovese G, Monzani NA, et al. Outbreak of chilblain-like acral lesions in children in the metropolitan area of Milan, Italy, during the COVID-19 pandemic. J Am Acad Dermatol 2020; 83(3):965–9.

54. Denina M, Pellegrino F, Morotti F, et al. All that glisters is not COVID: Low prevalence of seroconversion against SARS-CoV-2 in a pediatric cohort of patients with chilblain-like lesions. J Am Acad Dermatol 2020;83(6):1751–3.

55. El Hachem M, Diociaiuti A, Concato C, et al. A clinical, histopathological and laboratory study of 19 consecutive Italian paediatric patients with chilblain-like lesions: lights and shadows on the relationship with COVID-19 infection. J Eur Acad Dermatol Venereol 2020;34(11). https://doi.org/10.1111/jdv.16682.

56. Garcia-Lara G, Linares-González L, Ródenas-Herranz T, et al. Chilblain-like lesions in pediatrics dermatological outpatients during the COVID-19 outbreak. Dermatol Ther 2020;33(5). https://doi.org/10.1111/dth.13516.

57. Herman A, Peeters C, Verroken A, et al. Evaluation of Chilblains as a Manifestation of the COVID-19 Pandemic. JAMA Dermatol 2020;156(9):998–1003.

58. Stavert R, Meydani-Korb A, de Leon D, et al. Evaluation of SARS-CoV-2 antibodies in 24 patients presenting with chilblains-like lesions during the COVID-19 pandemic. J Am Acad Dermatol 2020; 83(6):1753–5.

59. Roca-Ginés J, Torres-Navarro I, Sánchez-Arráez J, et al. Assessment of Acute Acral Lesions in a Case Series of Children and Adolescents during the COVID-19 Pandemic. JAMA Dermatol 2020; 156(9):992–7.

60. Hubiche T, Le Duff F, Chiaverini C, et al. Negative SARS-CoV-2 PCR in patients with chilblain-like lesions. Lancet Infect Dis 2020. https://doi.org/10.1016/s1473-3099(20)30518-1.

61. Papa A, Salzano AM, Di Dato MT, et al. Images in Practice: Painful Cutaneous Vasculitis in a SARS-Cov-2 IgG-Positive Child. Pain Ther 2020;9(2):805–7.

62. Sethuraman N, Jeremiah SS, Ryo A. Interpreting Diagnostic Tests for SARS-CoV-2. JAMA - J Am Med Assoc 2020;323(22):2249–51.

63. Freeman EE, McMahon DE, Hruza GJ, et al. Timing of PCR and antibody testing in patients with COVID-19–associated dermatologic manifestations. J Am Acad Dermatol 2021;84(2):505–7.

64. Ma H, Zeng W, He H, et al. Serum IgA, IgM, and IgG responses in COVID-19. Cell Mol Immunol 2020;17(7):773–5.

65. Robbiani DF, Gaebler C, Muecksch F, et al. Convergent antibody responses to SARS-CoV-2 in convalescent individuals. Nature 2020;584(7821):437–42.

66. Long QX, Liu BZ, Deng HJ, et al. Antibody responses to SARS-CoV-2 in patients with COVID-19. Nat Med 2020;26(6):845–8.

67. Sterlin D, Mathian A, Miyara M, et al. IgA dominates the early neutralizing antibody response to SARS-CoV-2. Sci Transl Med 2021;(577):13.

68. Abreu RB, Clutter EF, Attari S, et al. IgA Responses Following Recurrent Influenza Virus Vaccination. Front Immunol 2020;11:902.

69. Baeck M, Herman A. COVID toes: Where do we stand with the current evidence? Int J Infect Dis 2021;102:53–5.

70. Hadjadj J, Yatim N, Barnabei L, et al. Impaired type I interferon activity and inflammatory responses in severe COVID-19 patients. Science 2020; 369(6504):718–24.

71. Meffre E, Iwasaki A. Interferon deficiency can lead to severe COVID. Nature 2020;587(7834):374–6.

72. Magro CM, Mulvey JJ, Laurence J, et al. The differing pathophysiologies that underlie COVID-19-associated perniosis and thrombotic retiform purpura: a case series. Br J Dermatol 2021; 184(1):141–50.

73. Park A, Iwasaki A. Type I and Type III Interferons – Induction, Signaling, Evasion, and Application to Combat COVID-19. Cell Host Microbe 2020;27(6):870–8.

74. Lipsker D. A chilblain epidemic during the COVID-19 pandemic. A sign of natural resistance to SARS-CoV-2? Med Hypotheses 2020;144:109959.

75. Battesti G, El Khalifa J, Abdelhedi N, et al. New insights in COVID-19–associated chilblains: A

comparative study with chilblain lupus erythematosus. J Am Acad Dermatol 2020;83(4):1219–22.

76. Damsky W, Peterson D, King B. When interferon tiptoes through COVID-19: Pernio-like lesions and their prognostic implications during SARS-CoV-2 infection. J Am Acad Dermatol 2020;83(3): e269–70.

77. Rodríguez-Villa Lario A, Vega-Díez D, González-Cañete M, et al. Histological findings in chilblain lupus-like COVID lesions: in search of an answer to understand their aetiology. J Eur Acad Dermatol Venereol 2020;34(10):e572–4.

78. Sette A, Crotty S. Adaptive immunity to SARS-CoV-2 and COVID-19. Cell 2021;184(4):861–80.

79. Sekine T, Perez-Potti A, Rivera-Ballesteros O, et al. Robust T Cell Immunity in Convalescent Individuals with Asymptomatic or Mild COVID-19. Cell 2020; 183(1):158–68.e14.

80. Najarian DJ. Morbilliform exanthem associated with COVID-19. JAAD Case Rep 2020;6(6):493–4.

81. Rubio-Muniz CA, Puerta-Peña M, Falkenhain-López D, et al. The broad spectrum of dermatological manifestations in COVID-19: clinical and histopathological features learned from a series of 34 cases. J Eur Acad Dermatol Venereol 2020;34(10):e574–6.

82. Jamshidi P, Hajikhani B, Mirsaeidi M, et al. Skin Manifestations in COVID-19 Patients: Are They Indicators for Disease Severity? A Systematic Review. Front Med 2021;8:634208.

83. Reymundo A, Fernáldez-Bernáldez A, Reolid A, et al. Clinical and histological characterization of late appearance maculopapular eruptions in association with the coronavirus disease 2019. A case series of seven patients. J Eur Acad Dermatol Venereol 2020;34(12):e755–7.

84. Türsen Ü, Türsen B, Lotti T. Cutaneous side-effects of the potential COVID-19 drugs. Dermatol Ther 2020;33(4). https://doi.org/10.1111/dth.13476.

85. Hassan K. Urticaria and angioedema as a prodromal cutaneous manifestation of SARS-CoV-2 (COVID-19) infection. BMJ Case Rep 2020;13(7). https://doi.org/10.1136/bcr-2020-236981.

86. van Damme C, Berlingin E, Saussez S, et al. Acute urticaria with pyrexia as the first manifestations of a COVID-19 infection. J Eur Acad Dermatol Venereol 2020;34(7):e300–1.

87. Quintana-Castanedo L, Feito-Rodríguez M, Valero-López I, et al. Urticarial exanthem as early diagnostic clue for COVID-19 infection. JAAD Case Rep 2020;6(6):498–9.

88. Imbalzano E, Casciaro M, Quartuccio S, et al. Association between urticaria and virus infections: A systematic review. Allergy Asthma Proc 2016; 37(1):18–22.

89. Drago F, Ciccarese G, Gasparini G, et al. Contemporary infectious exanthems: An update. Future Microbiol 2017;12(2):171–93.

90. Marzano AV, Genovese G, Fabbrocini G, et al. Varicella-like exanthem as a specific COVID-19–associated skin manifestation: Multicenter case series of 22 patients. J Am Acad Dermatol 2020;83(1): 280–5.

91. Fernandez-Nieto D, Ortega-Quijano D, Jimenez-Cauhe J, et al. Clinical and histological characterization of vesicular COVID-19 rashes: a prospective study in a tertiary care hospital. Clin Exp Dermatol 2020;45(7):872–5.

92. Mahé A, Birckel E, Merklen C, et al. Histology of skin lesions establishes that the vesicular rash associated with COVID-19 is not 'varicella-like. J Eur Acad Dermatol Venereol 2020;34(10):e559–61.

93. Trellu LT, Kaya G, Alberto C, et al. Clinicopathologic Aspects of a Papulovesicular Eruption in a Patient with COVID-19. JAMA Dermatol 2020;156(8): 922–4.

94. Jimenez-Cauhe J, Ortega-Quijano D, Carretero-Barrio I, et al. Erythema multiforme-like eruption in patients with COVID-19 infection: clinical and histological findings. Clin Exp Dermatol 2020;45(7): 892–5.

95. Gargiulo L, Pavia G, Facheris P, et al. A fatal case of COVID-19 infection presenting with an erythema multiforme-like eruption and fever. Dermatol Ther 2020;33(4). https://doi.org/10.1111/dth.13779.

96. Bapst T, Romano F, Romano F, et al. Special dermatological presentation of paediatric multisystem inflammatory syndrome related to COVID-19: Erythema multiforme. BMJ Case Rep 2020; 13(6):e236986.

97. Janah H, Zinebi A, Elbenaye J. Atypical erythema multiforme palmar plaques lesions due to Sars-Cov-2. J Eur Acad Dermatol Venereol 2020;34(8): e373–5.

98. De Giorgi V, Recalcati S, Jia Z, et al. Cutaneous manifestations related to coronavirus disease 2019 (COVID-19): A prospective study from China and Italy. J Am Acad Dermatol 2020;83(2):674–5.

99. Torrelo A, Andina D, Santonja C, et al. Erythema multiforme-like lesions in children and COVID-19. Pediatr Dermatol 2020;37(3):442–6.

100. Rodríguez-Jiménez P, Chicharro P, De Argila D, et al. Urticaria-like lesions in COVID-19 patients are not really urticaria – a case with clinicopathological correlation. J Eur Acad Dermatol Venereol 2020;34(9):e459–60.

101. Kutlu Ö, Metin A. Relative changes in the pattern of diseases presenting in dermatology outpatient clinic in the era of the COVID-19 pandemic. Dermatol Ther 2020;33(6). https://doi.org/10.1111/dth.14096.

102. Merhy R, Sarkis A, Stephan F. Pityriasis rosea as a leading manifestation of COVID-19 infection. J Eur Acad Dermatol Venereol 2020. https://doi.org/10.1111/jdv.17052.

103. Ehsani AH, Nasimi M, Bigdelo Z. Pityriasis rosea as a cutaneous manifestation of COVID-19 infection. J Eur Acad Dermatol Venereol 2020;34(9): e436–7.

104. Dursun R, Temiz SA. The clinics of HHV-6 infection in COVID-19 pandemic: Pityriasis rosea and Kawasaki disease. Dermatol Ther 2020;33(4). https://doi.org/10.1111/dth.13730.

105. Veraldi S, Spigariolo CB. Pityriasis rosea and COVID-19. J Med Virol 2020. https://doi.org/10.1002/jmv.26679.

106. Veraldi S, Romagnuolo M, Benzecry V. Pityriasis rosea-like eruption revealing COVID-19. Australas J Dermatol 2020. https://doi.org/10.1111/ajd.13504.

107. Martín Enguix D, Salazar Nievas M del C, Martín Romero DT. Pityriasis rosea Gibert type rash in an asymptomatic patient that tested positive for COVID-19. Med Clínica (English Ed 2020;155(6): 273.

108. Sanchez A, Sohier P, Benghanem S, et al. Digitate Papulosquamous Eruption Associated with Severe Acute Respiratory Syndrome Coronavirus 2 Infection. JAMA Dermatol 2020;156(7): 819–20.

109. Drago F, Ciccarese G, Rebora A, et al. Human herpesvirus-6, -7, and Epstein-Barr virus reactivation in pityriasis rosea during COVID-19. J Med Virol 2020. https://doi.org/10.1002/jmv.26549.

110. Welsh E, Cardenas-de la Garza JA, Cuellar-Barboza A, et al. SARS-CoV-2 Spike Protein Positivity in Pityriasis Rosea-like and Urticaria-like Rashes of COVID-19. Br J Dermatol 2021. https://doi.org/10.1111/bjd.19833.

111. Children and COVID-19: State-Level Data Report. Available at: https://services.aap.org/en/pages/2019-novel-coronavirus-covid-19-infections/children-and-covid-19-state-level-data-report/. Accessed May 13, 2021.

112. Assaker R, Colas AE, Julien-Marsollier F, et al. Presenting symptoms of COVID-19 in children: a meta-analysis of published studies. Br J Anaesth 2020;125(3):e330–2.

113. Zimmermann P, Curtis N. Why is COVID-19 less severe in children? A review of the proposed mechanisms underlying the age-related difference in severity of SARS-CoV-2 infections. Arch Dis Child 2020. https://doi.org/10.1136/archdischild-2020-320338.

114. Kilani MM, Odeh MM, Shalabi M, et al. Clinical and laboratory characteristics of SARS-CoV2-infected paediatric patients in Jordan: serial RT-PCR testing until discharge. Paediatr Int Child Health 2021; 41(1):83–92.

115. Pousa PA, Mendonça TSC, Oliveira EA, et al. Extrapulmonary manifestations of COVID-19 in children: a comprehensive review and pathophysiological considerations. J Pediatr (Rio J 2021;97(2):116–39.

116. Rekhtman S, Tannenbaum R, Strunk A, et al. Mucocutaneous disease and related clinical characteristics in hospitalized children and adolescents with COVID-19 and multisystem inflammatory syndrome in children. J Am Acad Dermatol 2021;84(2): 408–14.

117. Galeotti C, Bayry J. Autoimmune and inflammatory diseases following COVID-19. Nat Rev Rheumatol 2020;16(8):413–4.

118. Verdoni L, Mazza A, Gervasoni A, et al. An outbreak of severe Kawasaki-like disease at the Italian epicentre of the SARS-CoV-2 epidemic: an observational cohort study. Lancet 2020;395: 1771–8.

119. Feldstein LR, Tenforde MW, Friedman KG, et al. Characteristics and Outcomes of US Children and Adolescents with Multisystem Inflammatory Syndrome in Children (MIS-C) Compared with Severe Acute COVID-19. JAMA - J Am Med Assoc 2021;325(11):1074–87.

120. Information for Healthcare Providers about Multisystem Inflammatory Syndrome in Children (MIS-C) | CDC. Available at: https://www.cdc.gov/mis-c/hcp/. Accessed May 13, 2021.

121. Multisystem Inflammatory Syndrome in Children (MIS-C) | CDC. Available at: https://www.cdc.gov/mis-c/. Accessed May 13, 2021.

122. Yasuhara J, Watanabe K, Takagi H, et al. COVID-19 and multisystem inflammatory syndrome in children: A systematic review and meta-analysis. Pediatr Pulmonol 2021;56(5):837–48.

123. Yonker LM, Neilan AM, Bartsch Y, et al. Pediatric Severe Acute Respiratory Syndrome Coronavirus 2 (SARS-CoV-2): Clinical Presentation, Infectivity, and Immune Responses. J Pediatr 2020;227: 45–52.e5.

124. Roe K. A viral infection explanation for Kawasaki disease in general and for COVID-19 virus-related Kawasaki disease symptoms. Inflammopharmacology 2020;28(5):1219–22.

125. Multisystem Inflammatory Syndrome in Children in the United States. N Engl J Med 2020;383(18): 1793–6.

126. Young TK, Shaw KS, Shah JK, et al. Mucocutaneous Manifestations of Multisystem Inflammatory Syndrome in Children during the COVID-19 Pandemic. JAMA Dermatol 2020. https://doi.org/10.1001/jamadermatol.2020.4779.

127. Whittaker E, Bamford A, Kenny J, et al. Clinical Characteristics of 58 Children with a Pediatric Inflammatory Multisystem Syndrome Temporally Associated with SARS-CoV-2. J Am Med Assoc 2020;324(3):259–69.

128. Shaigany S, Gnirke M, Guttmann A, et al. An adult with Kawasaki-like multisystem inflammatory

syndrome associated with COVID-19. Lancet 2020; 396(10246):e8–10.

129. Morris SB, Schwartz NG, Patel P, et al. Morbidity and Mortality Weekly Report Case Series of Multisystem Inflammatory Syndrome in Adults Associated with SARS-CoV-2 Infection-United Kingdom and United States. 2020. Available at: https://www.cdc.gov/mis-c/pdfs/hcp/mis-c-form-fillable.pdf. Accessed May 13, 2021.

130. Feldstein LR, Rose EB, Horwitz SM, et al. Multisystem Inflammatory Syndrome in U.S. Children and Adolescents. N Engl J Med 2020;383(4): 334–46.

131. Ahmed M, Advani S, Moreira A, et al. Multisystem inflammatory syndrome in children: A systematic review. EClinicalMedicine 2020;26. https://doi.org/10.1016/j.eclinm.2020.100527.

132. Joob B, Wiwanitkit V. COVID-19 can present with a rash and be mistaken for dengue. J Am Acad Dermatol 2020;82(5):e177.

133. McGrath A, Barrett MJ. Petechiae. In: StatPearls [Internet]. Treasure Island (FL): StatPearls Publishing; 2021.

134. Askin O, Altunkalem RN, Altinisik DD, et al. Cutaneous manifestations in hospitalized patients diagnosed as COVID-19. Dermatol Ther 2020;33(6). https://doi.org/10.1111/dth.13896.

135. Karaca Z, Yayli S, Çalışkan O. A unilateral purpuric rash in a patient with COVID-19 infection. Dermatol Ther 2020;33(4). https://doi.org/10.1111/dth.13798.

136. Silva DHM, Oppenheimer AR, Cunha T do AC. Purpuric rash on the legs of a patient with coronavirus disease. Rev Soc Bras Med Trop 2020;53: e20200464.

137. Negrini S, Guadagno A, Greco M, et al. An unusual case of bullous haemorrhagic vasculitis in a COVID-19 patient. J Eur Acad Dermatol Venereol 2020;34(11):e675–6.

138. Suso AS, Mon C, Oñate Alonso I, et al. IgA Vasculitis With Nephritis (Henoch–Schönlein Purpura) in a COVID-19 Patient. Kidney Int Rep 2020;5(11): 2074–8.

139. AlGhoozi DA, AlKhayyat HM. A child with Henoch-Schonlein purpura secondary to a COVID-19 infection. BMJ Case Rep 2021;14(1). https://doi.org/10.1136/bcr-2020-239910.

140. Jacobi M, Lancrei HM, Brosh-Nissimov T, et al. Purpurona: A Novel Report of COVID-19-Related Henoch-Schonlein Purpura in a Child. Pediatr Infect Dis J 2021;40(2):e93–4.

141. García-Gil MF, Monte Serrano J, Lapeña-Casado A, et al. Livedo reticularis and acrocyanosis as late manifestations of COVID-19 in two cases with familial aggregation. Potential pathogenic role of complement (C4c). Int J Dermatol 2020;59(12): 1549–51.

142. Khalil S, Hinds BR, Manalo IF, et al. Livedo reticularis as a presenting sign of severe acute respiratory syndrome coronavirus 2 infection. JAAD Case Rep 2020;6(9):871–4.

143. Manalo IF, Smith MK, Cheeley J, et al. A dermatologic manifestation of COVID-19: Transient livedo reticularis. J Am Acad Dermatol 2020; 83(2):700.

144. Magro C, Mulvey JJ, Berlin D, et al. Complement associated microvascular injury and thrombosis in the pathogenesis of severe COVID-19 infection: A report of five cases. Transl Res 2020; 220:1–13.

145. Bosch-Amate X, Giavedoni P, Podlipnik S, et al. Retiform purpura as a dermatological sign of coronavirus disease 2019 (COVID-19) coagulopathy. J Eur Acad Dermatol Venereol 2020;34(10): e548–9.

146. Chand S, Rrapi R, Lo JA, et al. Purpuric ulcers associated with COVID-19: A case series. JAAD Case Rep 2021;11:13–9.

147. Tan SW, Tam YC, Oh CC. Skin manifestations of COVID-19: A worldwide review. JAAD Int 2021;2: 119–33.

148. Wambier CG, Vaño-Galván S, McCoy J, et al. Androgenetic alopecia in COVID-19: Compared to age-matched epidemiologic studies and hospital outcomes with or without the Gabrin sign. J Am Acad Dermatol 2020;83(6):e453–4.

149. Wambier CG, McCoy J, Goren A. Male balding as a major risk factor for severe COVID-19: A possible role for targeting androgens and transmembrane protease serine 2 to protect vulnerable individuals. J Am Acad Dermatol 2020;83(6):e401–2.

150. Olds H, Liu J, Luk K, et al. Telogen effluvium associated with <scp>COVID</scp> -19 infection. Dermatol Ther 2021;e14761. https://doi.org/10.1111/dth.14761.

151. Domínguez-Santás M, Haya-Martínez L, Fernández-Nieto D, et al. Acute telogen effluvium associated with SARS-CoV-2 infection. Aust J Gen Pract 2020;49. https://doi.org/10.31128/ajgp-covid-32.

152. Brin C, Sohier P, L'honneur AS, et al. An isolated peculiar gianotti-crosti rash in the course of a covid-19 episode. Acta Derm Venereol 2020; 100(16):1–2.

153. Chicharro P, Rodríguez-Jiménez P, Muñoz-Aceituno E, et al. SDRIFE-like rash associated with COVID-19, clinicopathological correlation. Australas J Dermatol 2020. https://doi.org/10.1111/ajd.13444.

154. Mahé A, Birckel E, Krieger S, et al. A distinctive skin rash associated with coronavirus disease 2019? J Eur Acad Dermatol Venereol 2020;34(6): e246–7.

155. Boix-Vilanova J, Gracia-Darder I, Saus C, et al. Grover-like skin eruption: another cutaneous

manifestation in a COVID-19 patient. Int J Dermatol 2020;59(10):1290–2.

156. Català A, Galván-Casas C, Carretero-Hernández G, et al. Maculopapular eruptions associated to COVID-19: A subanalysis of the COVID-Piel study. Dermatol Ther 2020;33(6). https://doi.org/10.1111/dth.14170.

157. Holcomb ZE, Hussain S, Huang JT, et al. Reactive Infectious Mucocutaneous Eruption Associated With SARS-CoV-2 Infection. JAMA Dermatol 2021; 157(5). https://doi.org/10.1001/jamadermatol.2021.0385.

158. Jimenez-Cauhe J, Ortega-Quijano D, De Perosanz-Lobo D, et al. Enanthem in Patients with COVID-19 and Skin Rash. JAMA Dermatol 2020;156(10):1134–6.

159. Brandini DA, Takamiya AS, Thakkar P, et al. Covid-19 and oral diseases: Crosstalk, synergy or association? *Rev Med Virol* Published Online 2021. https://doi.org/10.1002/rmv.2226.

160. La Rosa GRM, Libra M, De Pasquale R, et al. Association of Viral Infections With Oral Cavity Lesions: Role of SARS-CoV-2 Infection. Front Med 2021;7. https://doi.org/10.3389/fmed.2020.571214.

161. Falkenhain-López D, Agud-Dios M, Ortiz-Romero PL, et al. COVID-19-related acute genital ulcers. J Eur Acad Dermatol Venereol 2020; 34(11):e655–6.

162. Zimmermann P, Curtis N. COVID-19 in Children, Pregnancy and Neonates: A Review of Epidemiologic and Clinical Features. Pediatr Infect Dis J 2020;39(6):469–77.

163. Kamali Aghdam M, Jafari N, Eftekhari K. Novel coronavirus in a 15-day-old neonate with clinical signs of sepsis, a case report. Infect Dis (Auckl) 2020;52(6):427–9.

164. Freeman EE, McMahon DE, Fox LP. Emerging Evidence of the Direct Association Between COVID-19 and Chilblains. JAMA Dermatol 2020. https://doi.org/10.1001/jamadermatol.2020.4937.

165. Visconti A, Bataille V, Rossi N, et al. Diagnostic value of cutaneous manifestation of SARS-CoV-2 infection. Br J Dermatol 2021;(5):184. https://doi.org/10.1111/bjd.19807.

166. Lester JC, Jia JL, Zhang L, et al. Absence of images of skin of colour in publications of COVID-19 skin manifestations. Br J Dermatol 2020; 183(3):593–5.

COVID-19 Pediatric Dermatology

Holly Neale, BS[a,b], Elena B. Hawryluk, MD, PhD[a,c,d],*

KEYWORDS

- MIS-C • Pediatric dermatology • COVID-19 children • Perniosis • Pernio-like lesions

KEY POINTS

- The robust immune system in younger individuals may be protective from traditional respiratory symptoms of COVID-19 but also may underlie cutaneous responses like those seen in multisystem inflammatory syndrome and pernio-like lesions.
- Cutaneous manifestations reported in children are diverse and include (but are not limited to) macular, papular, morbilliform, vesicular, urticarial, and vascular morphologies.
- The prognosis of pediatric patients who manifest COVID-19 cutaneously is excellent and usually self-limiting.

INTRODUCTION

During the coronavirus disease 2019 (COVID-19) pandemic, people of all ages are susceptive to infection with severe acute respiratory syndrome coronavirus 2 (SARS-CoV-2). Diagnoses in more than 3 million children beginning in the neonatal period have been made as of April 2021.[1,2] When compared with adults, however, pediatric patients manifest with less severe respiratory sequelae and higher frequencies of no, mild, or atypical symptoms.[3–6]

Reasons behind the contrasting presentation of COVID-19 in youth compared with aged individuals are multifactorial.[7] Children are less likely to have predisposing factors for severe disease, such as underlying medical comorbidities[8] or damaged endothelium.[9] Moreover, young people demonstrate differing antibody responses to SARS-CoV-2 infection[10] and possess stronger antiviral innate and adaptive immunity compared with older adults (including more cytokines, increased production of interferons,[11] increased CD4+/CD8+ T cells, and a more vigorous CD8+ T-cell response to new antigens).[12] Although these inherent protections likely aid in preventing the serious respiratory sequelae of COVID-19 in most children,[13] robust immune mechanisms also might contribute to alternate manifestations observed, such as cutaneous eruptions.

Lack of traditional or severe signs can heighten attention to nontraditional presentations, making dermatologic manifestations particularly relevant in children. Cutaneous signs sometimes are the predominant or only clue toward pediatric COVID-19 infection.[14,15] One of the earliest exemplifications of pediatric dermatoses related to the pandemic is the acral skin eruption, known as COVID toes.[16] Many children and adolescents since have presented with various acral and nonacral skin findings in connection to SARS-CoV-2 infection; cutaneous manifestations are recognized as the seventh most common extrapulmonary COVID-19 association in children.[17] Greater than 8% of hospitalized COVID-19 positive pediatric patients have a cutaneous eruption,[18] and dermatologic manifestations may be a component of a serious, systemic pediatric presentation, such as multisystem inflammatory syndrome in children (MIS-C). Thus, although cutaneous signs of

The authors have no conflicts of interest of funding sources to disclose.
a Department of Dermatology, Massachusetts General Hospital, Boston, MA, USA; b University of Massachusetts Medical School, Worcester, MA, USA; c Harvard Medical School, Boston, MA, USA; d Boston Children's Hospital, Boston, MA, USA
* Corresponding author. Department of Dermatology, Massachusetts General Hospital, Boston, MA.
E-mail address: ehawryluk@partners.org

Dermatol Clin 39 (2021) 505–519
https://doi.org/10.1016/j.det.2021.05.012
0733-8635/21/© 2021 Elsevier Inc. All rights reserved.

COVID-19 infection often are a form of mild disease in children, it also is necessary to consider the possibility of more serious complications.

Herein, the clinical presentation, demographic trends, pathophysiologic theories, implications, and management strategies for dermatologic presentations of COVID-19 are addressed with respect to MIS-C, acral eruptions, and various vascular, inflammatory, and nonspecific skin findings. Through descriptions of COVID-19 pediatric cutaneous manifestations, this article demonstrates the role of the dermatologist and importance of prompt recognition.

MULTISYSTEM INFLAMMATORY SYNDROME

- MIS-C is a serious and sometimes life-threatening response to COVID-19 infection in children, leading to organ dysfunction, shock, and often the need for intensive care and circulatory support.
- Skin and/or mucous membrane changes may be present in more than half of children affected by MIS-C and appear with various morphologies and distributions.
- Although most require intensive care, patients with MIS-C carry a good prognosis, with mortality estimated at 2%.

Definition

To date, one of the most severe pediatric consequences of COVID-19 infection is MIS-C. Initially recognized approximately 1 month after the first COVID-19 pandemic surge,[19] MIS-C is a hyperinflammatory response to SARS-CoV-2 infection in pediatric patients that leads to dysfunction in several organs. The Centers for Disease Control and Prevention (CDC) has defined MIS-C as an individual under 21 years old with current or recent SARS-CoV-2 infection (or exposure), a fever lasting greater than 24 hours, laboratory inflammatory marker evidence, and the presence of severe illness involving greater than 2 organs (cardiac, respiratory, gastrointestinal, dermatologic, renal, hematologic, or neurologic), requiring hospital admission that cannot be explained by other illness (**Fig. 1**).[20,21]

Demographics

Since the earliest reported cases in England,[22] more than 3000 children have been affected by MIS-C, as of April 2021.[23] A majority of children who develop MIS-C previously were healthy.[24] Cases have been reported as young as 1 month old[25] to 20 years old,[26] with median age estimated between 5 years and 11.5 years old.[20] There is a slight male predominance, and minority races/ethnicities are affected by MIS-C more commonly than non-Hispanic white children.[19,24]

Pathogenesis

Due to temporal emergence of MIS-C with the pandemic in addition to confirmed laboratory evidence of SARS-Co-V-2 infection in 99% of cases,[23] it is highly suggestive that MIS-C indeed is a consequence of COVID-19 infection. Specifically, it is thought that MIS-C is a late or postviral complication due to trends revealing a higher likelihood of SARS-CoV-2 antibody positivity compared with viral RNA detection.[27–30] Children who report milder viral symptoms before MIS-C onset support the notion of MIS-C being a later sequelae; the median time to onset has been reported at 25 days.[24]

Although the exact mechanisms are not yet understood, MIS-C is described as the result of a cytokine storm in response to COVID-19 infection.[31] Pathogenesis theories include the role of an overly robust pediatric innate and/or cellular immune response,[27] superantigen region on the SARS-CoV-2 spike protein,[32,33] and immune-complex development from viral antigens (type III hypersensitivity)[34] inciting strong cytokine cascade. A pediatric biorepository has been established with one main goal to better understand the complex immunologic mechanisms underpinning MIS-C.[35]

Cutaneous Presentation

MIS-C demonstrates a wide spectrum of cutaneous associations (**Fig. 2**). Mucocutaneous findings are a component of MIS-C in 50% to 83% of children,[19,24,29,36,37] which are variable and polymorphic (**Table 1**). Purpuric, targetoid, erythematous, retiform, reticular, livedoid, urticarial, scarlatiniform, papular, macular, maculopapular, desquamative, erythema multiforme (EM)-like, and morbilliform exanthems have been described.[37–41] Eruptions may be generalized or localized, such as to the trunk, face, periorbital area, extremities, or diaper area.[29,38,40,41] In 1 series of 7 MIS-C patients with cutaneous findings, 57% had lesions described as urticarial-like plaques, all had involvement of the lower extremities, and 29% experienced mild pruritis.[37]

The hands and feet frequently are a site of cutaneous symptoms; findings include erythema, swelling (edema), and desquamation.[28,38–40] Mucositis in the forms of papillitis of the tongue (strawberry tongue),[29,41] cheilitis (lips appearing erythematous, swollen, dry, or cracked/

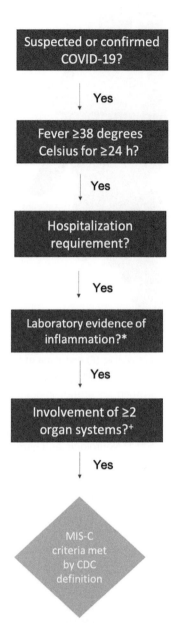

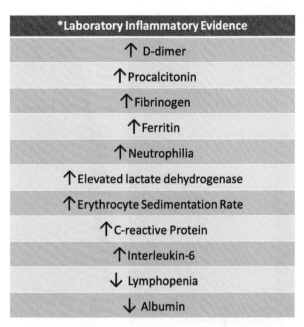

*Laboratory Inflammatory Evidence
↑ D-dimer
↑ Procalcitonin
↑ Fibrinogen
↑ Ferritin
↑ Neutrophilia
↑ Elevated lactate dehydrogenase
↑ Erythrocyte Sedimentation Rate
↑ C-reactive Protein
↑ Interleukin-6
↓ Lymphopenia
↓ Albumin

+Organ System	Examples of involvement
Gastrointestinal	Abdominal pain, diarrhea, nausea, vomiting, abnormal hepatobiliary markers
Hematologic	Fever, myalgias, lymphadenopathy, fatigue, abnormal blood counts
Neurologic	Headache, irritability, altered mental status, dizziness
Dermatologic	Cutaneous eruption, conjunctivitis, edema, mucositis
Respiratory	Dyspnea, upper respiratory infection-like signs, cough, wheezing, respiratory failure, pulmonary infiltrates
Cardiovascular	Shock, chest pain, myocarditis, coronary artery dilatation/aneurysm, elevated cardiac enzyme markers
Renal	Acute kidney injury

Fig. 1. CDC diagnostic criteria for MIS-C. An individual aged less than 21 with SARS-CoV-2 (confirmed or suspected within prior 4 weeks), a fever for greater than or equal to 24 hours, involvement of at least 2 organ systems (+gastrointestinal, hematologic, neurologic, dermatologic, respiratory, cardiovascular, or renal), laboratory evidence of inflammation, severity requiring hospitalization, and no other explanation must be present.[21] (*Laboratory markers of inflammation include but are not limited to elevations in fibrinogen, ferritin, D-dimer, erythrocyte sedimentation rate, C-reactive protein, procalcitonin, interleukin-6, neutrophils, lactic acid dehydrogenase, and/or low albumin or lymphocytes[21]; examples of hepatobiliary markers: AST/ALT[119]; examples of hematologic markers: neutrophil, lymphocytes, platelets, hemoglobin[119]; examples of cardiac markers: troponin, brain natriuretic proenzyme[21]; and examples of renal markers: creatinine,[119] blood urea nitrogen, electrolytes.)

fissured),[28,39,40,42] and/or conjunctivitis[29,41] frequently are observed.

Although some investigations have found no correlation between mucocutaneous findings and worsened disease severity,[29,41] 1 study reported that mucocutaneous signs were a risk factor for intensive care unit admission, more severe inflammatory marker derangement (C-reactive protein

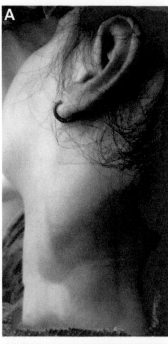 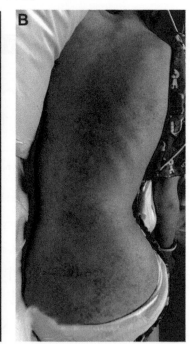 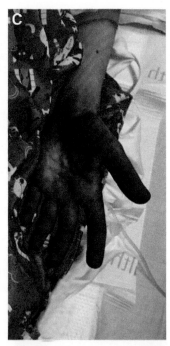

Fig. 2. Cutaneous eruptions in patients with MIS-C. (*A*) An erythematous plaque of the neck on a 7-year-old girl. (*B*) A 12-year-old boy with a maculopapular eruption of the trunk and extremities as well as (*C*) erythema of the palms. (*From* Fludiona Naka, Laura Melnick, Mark Gorelik, Kimberly D. Morel, A dermatologic perspective on multisystem inflammatory syndrome in children, Clinics in Dermatology, 2020.)

[CRP], D-dimer, and lymphopenia), and poor presentation with severe tachycardia.[43] Mucocutaneous manifestations typically resolve with treatment of underlying MIS-C.[37] Importantly, mucocutaneous findings associated with fever in a child are nonspecific, and in the setting of negative COVID-19 testing can pose a diagnostic challenge.

Extracutaneous Presentation

In addition to dermatologic presentation, awareness of the most common extra-mucocutaneous findings of MIS-C is necessary when evaluating a child for skin eruption in the COVID-19 pandemic. Fever, a critical component of the MIS-C diagnosis,[21] usually precedes mucocutaneous findings but can occur after or during acute presentation.[29] Other vital sign changes in the form of tachycardia, tachypnea, and hypotension are presenting signs in more than three-quarters of affected children.[26,36]

The gastrointestinal system is the most common organ system involved in MIS-C, and signs in the form of abdominal pain, vomiting, and/or diarrhea are noted in 80% to 92% of cases.[24,26] Respiratory symptoms, such as dyspnea, upper respiratory infection-like signs, and respiratory insufficiency, are observed in 21% to 70% of cases.[24,26,29] Cardiovascular involvement may present clinically as hypotension, shock, or, less commonly, chest pain.[44,45] Neurologic and hematologic abnormalities manifest with various signs and symptoms, such as headache, dizziness, mental status change, fatigue, lymphadenopathy, lethargy, and myalgias.[26,44]

With accumulating cases, an analysis of 570 children reported to the CDC allowed the identification of 3 distinct subgroups based on patient underlying features. Rash and mucocutaneous findings were prominent in a group of "MIS-C overlapping with Kawasaki disease (KD)," that was characterized by younger patients (median age 6 years) and lower frequency of myocardial dysfunction or shock. In contrast, the other groups represented "MIS-C without overlap with acute COVID-19 or KD" (median age 9 years) with prominent cardiovascular and gastrointestinal symptoms, and "MIS-C overlapping with severe acute COVID-19" (median age 10 years) with prominent respiratory symptoms.[30,46]

Work-up

The CDC recommended laboratory work-up for suspected MIS-C includes a SARS-CoV-2 reverse-transcriptase polymerase chain reaction (RT-PCR) test and serologic testing (prior to treatment initiation) when available.[21] Inflammatory marker elevation is a critical component of

Table 1 Mucocutaneous findings in multisystem inflammatory syndrome in children	
Location	Descriptors
Generalized[40,109] Perineal[40] Trunk[100] Face[29] Ears[109] Periorbital area[29,109] Extremities[41]	Urticarial[41] Papular[38] Maculopapular[38] Macular[39] Morbilliform[39] Desquamative[40] Edematous[39] Erythematous[41] Purpuric[38] Targetoid[41] Retiform[41] Reticular[38] Scarlatiniform[40] Petechiae[28] Livedoid[37] EM-like[37]
Hands Feet	Edematous[40] Erythematous[40] Desquamative[40] Purpuric[38] Petechiae[28]
Tongue	Papillitis[41] Strawberry tongue[40] De-epithelialized[28]
Lips	Cracked/fissured[39,41] Erythematous[29]
Eyes	Injected[29,109] Swollen[39] Nonpurulent discharge[39]

diagnosis, and markers to test include erythrocyte sedimentation rate, CRP, fibrinogen, procalcitonin, ferritin, lactic acid dehydrogenase, D-dimer, interleukin-6, and albumin.[21] Additionally, a complete blood cell count to look for lymphocytopenia, neutrophilia, and/or thrombocytopenia is warranted, because hematologic abnormalities are present in the majority cases.[24] A comprehensive metabolic panel may reveal end organ impacts, such as acute kidney injury or abnormal hepatobiliary markers.[38,44]

Usually, children receive cardiac work-up, including cardiac enzyme biomarkers, brain natriuretic peptide, echocardiogram, and/or electrocardiogram[21] due to a known relationship between MIS-C and myocarditis, cardiac dysfunction, and/or coronary artery dilatation/aneurysm.[30,47] When clinically warranted, radiologic assessment of the chest or abdomen is performed and may reveal further systemic effects, such as pulmonary infiltrates, lymphadenopathy, pleural effusion, hepatosplenomegaly, ascites, or ileitis.[38,47,48]

Differential Diagnosis

Many features of MIS-C presentation resemble KD in children, making KD a top differential diagnosis. Findings, such as high fever, conjunctivitis, lymphadenopathy, cheilitis, skin rash, myocarditis, and coronary artery aneurysms,[24,36] occur in both KD and MIS-C. Although the features of MIS-C overlap with KD and incomplete KD, many children do not meet the full diagnostic criteria,[24,25,36,41] and distinguishing demographic trends in age and geography are apparent between the 2 diseases (**Table 2**).

A severe COVID-19 infection (without meeting criterion for MIS-C) also is possible. A retrospective comparison of MIS-C versus severe COVID-19 in 1116 hospitalized patients ages 21 and under revealed MIS-C patients presented more frequently with mucocutaneous signs than those with severe COVID-19. MIS-C cases showed greater laboratory inflammation, and complications were more likely to involve the cardiac system.[48]

In addition to KD, the differential for MIS-C includes systemic illnesses, such as macrophage-activation syndrome, toxic-shock syndrome, bacterial sepsis, and scarlet fever.[40,49] Depending on the clinical picture, drug hypersensitivity, vasculitis, or other viral infections may be considered.[38]

Prognosis and Management

MIS-C is a serious complication of COVID-19 in children, requiring intensive care unit admission in up to 80% of cases[24,26] and often supportive care, including vasopressors, fluids, and/or mechanical ventilation.[48,49] Treatment includes intravenous immunoglobulin and corticosteroids; many patients also receive anticoagulants and/or antiplatelet agents.[48] Medications, such as antivirals, cytokine blockers, and various immunomodulatory agents, have been used.[19,48,50] Few children may improve without any immunomodulatory therapy.[25] The median hospital stay is approximately 1 week,[24] and a large majority of MIS-C patients enter remission. There have been reports of death, however, due to MIS-C following COVID-19 infection[24,42]; mortality is estimated at 2%.[24,26]

The post-hospitalization sequelae of MIS-C are just beginning to be appreciated. Coronary artery abnormalities were identified in a notable percentage of patients in all 3 clinical presentations/subgroups of MIS-C, described previously, ranging from 16% to 21%,[46] which has an impact on patient return to baseline activities. It has been observed that a majority of MIS-C patients with severe cardiac complications recover within 1 months to 3 months.[48] Although impacts on hair are not robustly documented in pediatric patients

Table 2
Kawasaki disease compared with multisystemic inflammatory syndrome in children

	Kawasaki Disease	Multisystem Inflammatory Syndrome in Children[44]
Demographics		
Age	Younger children (90% of cases under age 5)[110]	Mean age 9 years old
Geography	More common in Asia (Japan, South Korea, and Taiwan)[111]	Majority of reports from the US and Europe
Race/ethnicity	Most common in Asian and Pacific Islanders[112]	>65% of cases in Hispanic/Latino or non-Hispanic black children
Gender	Male predominance[110]	Slight male predominance
Clinical signs		
Fever	Unexplained fever lasting ≥5 d must be present[112]	Fever lasting >24 h must be present
Conjunctivitis Oral mucosal change Distal extremity changes Skin rash Cervical lymphadenopathy	4 of 5 are part of diagnostic criteria (or 3 of 5 for incomplete KD)[112]	<50% meet criteria for KD
Gastrointestinal involvement	Present in 61%[113]	Present in 87%
Respiratory involvement	Slightly less common Present in 35%[113]	Slightly more common Present in 41%
Cardiovascular shock	Less common Present in <10%[114]	More common Present in 66%

with MIS-C, there are reports of alopecia areata and telogen effluvium, which may be related to the infection, a postinfectious sequelae of disease, or associated stress.[51]

Although skin findings are nonspecific and nondiagnostic, dermatologists must be aware of MIS-C and potential downstream sequalae. Children who present with a new skin eruption, swollen extremities, or mucous membrane changes during the COVID-19 era benefit from a full review of systems, vital signs, and in-person examination. If a presentation is suspicious for MIS-C but the patient otherwise is stable, it is appropriate to obtain laboratory testing to assess for COVID-19 infection and markers of inflammation for signs of multiorgan dysfunction, and/or consult subspecialists.[52] Stable patients with cutaneous eruption of unknown etiology during the pandemic may be counseled to monitor for development of accompanying signs of MIS-C. Severely ill children must be evaluated by emergency/critical care for immediate further work-up and management.

PERNIO (CHILBLAINS)-LIKE LESIONS

- Pernio-like lesions are an inflammatory response to COVID-19 resulting in purpuric and erythematous acral cutaneous surfaces.

- Children and young adults are more likely to manifest with pernio-like lesions than older adults.
- Pernio-like lesions typically are self-limiting with excellent prognosis, although recurrent skin sequelae are being appreciated.

Evolution of COVID-19 Toes

Traditional pernio, also called chilblains, is an inflammatory reaction of the superficial vasculature on acral cutaneous surfaces (fingers, toes, nose, and ears) that often is idiopathic and triggered by cool and/or damp temperatures (primary pernio) or, less commonly, is due to an underlying autoimmune or systemic inflammatory disease (secondary pernio).[53] Outside of the COVID-19 era, pernio is considered a relatively uncommon disease[54]; 1 study reported only 8 pediatric cases in 10 years,[55] although many consider this reaction to be clinically identified and readily managed with supportive care.

Following the start of the COVID-19 pandemic, thousands of children and young adults with no prior history of acral skin changes began to develop asymptomatic, painful, and/or pruritic lesions with striking resemblance to pernio: erythematous, purpuric papules, and macules affecting the toes, feet, fingers, and hands (**Fig. 3** morphologies are discussed in further detail in Ritesh Agnihothri and Lindy P. Fox's article, "Clinical Patterns and Morphology of COVID-19 Dermatology," in this issue). The temporal relationship of increased pernio-like cases coinciding with the pandemic alluded to a possible relationship. Thus, the terms, COVID toes and COVID fingers, were coined, and pernio-like lesions since have become the cutaneous manifestation in confirmed or suspected COVID-19 infected individuals across the globe reported most frequently.[56]

Why Youth?

Younger, healthy people tend to present with pernio-like lesions at higher frequencies than older adults.[57] The median age of pernio-like lesions is the mid-20s to-late 20s,[56,58] and 29% of those with pernio-like lesions are children or adolescents.[59] Leading theories aid in explaining the demographical trend toward healthy youth. The immune system of younger individuals has higher amounts of interferon compared with older adults,[11] which provides innate immunity against viruses.[60] It is known that constitutive type 1 interferon responses lead to autoinflammatory manifestations, including chilblains.[61] Thus, it is possible that when infected with COVID-19, healthy children and young adults mount a strong interferon response, clearing the virus,[62] and subsequently develop pernio-like lesions as a delayed consequence of inflammation.[63,64]

Supporting this theory, it has been found that individuals with pernio-like lesions respond with significantly higher blood levels of interferon alpha when stimulated with immune ligands compared with patients with acute COVID-19 infection.[65] Higher rates of antibody test positivity compared with rates of RNA detection in individuals with pernio-like lesions,[65] in addition to the tendency for delayed presentation of lesions in relation extracutaneous symptoms (**Table 3**),[56,59] provide additional support of pernio-like lesions as a postviral manifestation of COVID-19 infection. Biopsies of pernio-like lesions offer evidence of a primarily inflammatory process.[66]

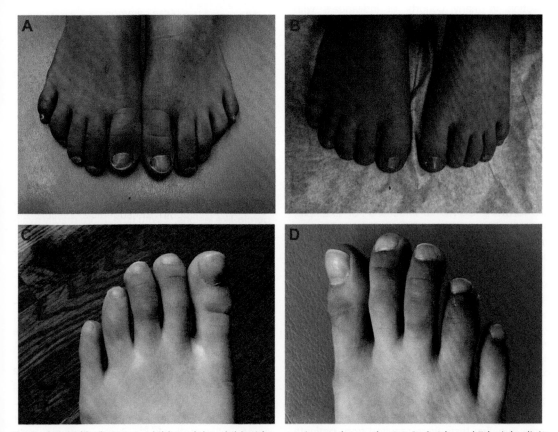

Fig. 3. Pernio-like lesions in children. (A) A child with purpuric papules on the 1st, 2nd, 4th, and 5th right digits and 2nd proximal left digit and (B) Digits on the same child appearing with increased erythema. (C) Right toes of a child appearing with pink and dusky papules and plaques, also involving (D) the child's left digits.

Table 3
Clinical presentation of pernio-like lesions in children[66,67,80,115–117]

Lesion Location	Lesion Color	Primary Lesion Morphology	Secondary Lesion Features	Associated Symptoms	Extracutaneous Symptoms[b]
Toes[a]	Red	Papules	Edema	None	Fever
Feet	Purple	Macules	Erosion	Pruritis	Cough
Ankles	Brown	Vesicles	Crust	Pain	Sore throat
Fingers	Red-bluish	Bullae			Nasal congestion
Hands	Gray	Patches			Rhinorrhea
		Plaques			Chills
					Diarrhea
					Abdominal pain
					Dyspnea
					Myalgia
					Weakness

[a] Including nail involvement.
[b] If extracutaneous signs are present, they precede cutaneous findings more than half the time[59,80,117].

Relationship to COVID-19

SARS-CoV-2 nasopharyngeal RNA and/or serologic results often fail to demonstrate COVID-19 infection in many cohorts of individuals with pernio-like lesions,[58,67–69] leading to theories that the increase in cases may be coincidental, due to patient/provider/media awareness (confirmation bias),[70] or a result of pandemic lifestyle changes (such as walking barefoot at home more often).[71] Lack of laboratory positivity, however, may speak more to testing nuances rather than lack of true infection.[72] Cleared infections[59]; failure to look for IgG, IgM, and/or IgA antibodies in serologic testing[73]; and improper timing of testing in relation to disease (ie, the window between cleared infection and detectable antibodies)[74] are potential reasons why viral testing may read negative following COVID-19 infection. For example, given the theory that pernio-like lesions are a post-viral manifestation, for a child presenting with pernio-like lesions 10 days after a mild cough, RNA testing would be negative if the infection was cleared (the median time to undetectable RNA is 14 days, meaning 50% of individuals test negative before then),[75] and antibodies may not yet be detectable (average length to mount response is 1–3 weeks),[76] thus, possible that neither test would be positive. In separate analysis of 906 reported cases of confirmed or suspected COVID-19-associated skin manifestations, COVID-19 tests were more likely to be positive if performed earlier in the disease course, and some negative tests were resulted from patients whose skin biopsies demonstrated SARS-CoV-2 RNA.[72] Mounting evidence supports that a negative test does not necessarily rule out an association of pernio skin lesions with COVID-19,[77] and optimal testing times remain an area of ongoing research.

Although it is possible that select patients manifest idiopathic pernio, the dramatic surge in cases (including in temperate climates),[65] and clustering in families and close contacts,[66] in addition to emerging evidence from larger cohorts,[59] support a connection between pernio-like lesions cases and COVID-19. Of patients with pernio-like lesions during the pandemic, 72% have a suspected COVID-19 infection,[59] and up to 30% of those with serologic testing have antibodies to SARS-CoV-2[59,65] (compared with <10% in the general US population.)[78] In a series of 7 pediatric cases, COVID-19 viral particles were observed in endothelial cells using electron microscopy of biopsied pernio-like lesions.[79] With time, more readily available COVID-19 tests, and emerging data, it is anticipated that the relationship between the pandemic and pernio-like lesions will become more clear.

Pediatric Outcomes and Management

It is overall reassuring that regardless of etiology, pernio-like lesions usually are self-limited.[65] The lesions and associated symptoms often last 1 week to 3 weeks,[59,80,81] although, in some patients, persistence or recurrence may occur.[82] First-line management is observation[83]; topical corticosteroids, topical antibiotics, and nonsteroidal anti-inflammatory agents may be useful for acute inflammation.[67,84] Some patients with increased pain and symptoms require additional pain management, and topical anesthetics and analgesics, such as topical gabapentin, diclofenac, ketamine, JAK inhibitors, lidocaine patches, and ointment are reasonable choices. The long-term outcomes and recurrence rate of lesions will become apparent with time. With the temporal second wave of COVID-19 cases, there has been another increase in reported cases of pernio-like lesions.[85]

Clinical judgment should be used in the decision to test children for SARS-CoV-2 with consideration to timing from symptoms and pretest probability. Previously healthy children with no history of acral cutaneous disease and lack of overt risk factors for traditional pernio may benefit from RT-PCR testing if they are presenting during the COVID-19 era, particularly if they are evaluated promptly upon lesion onset.

NONSPECIFIC COVID-19 DERMATOSES

- Cutaneous eruptions can be a sole presenting sign of COVID-19, be accompanied by mild extracutaneous disease, or be seen in hospitalized COVID-19 children.
- Various inflammatory, vascular, and nonspecific cutaneous morphologies have been described.

In addition to the well-reported cases of MIS-C and pernio-like lesions in children, various other cutaneous eruptions have been reported. **Table 4** summarizes the different skin findings by etiology that may be related to COVID-19 infection in pediatric patients.

Nonperniotic Acral Cutaneous Eruptions

Some acral manifestations overlap or coexist with pernio-like lesions and are a matter of subtle and/or subjective classification. For example, EM-like lesions have been found on the acral surfaces of children with pernio-like lesions[86] and may present with purpuric morphology.[87] The EM-like pattern of acral eruptions are distinguished from pernio-like lesions as round, coalescing erythematous macules and vesicles, observed more frequently in younger children.[88] Similarly, ecchymotic eruptions of the toes and feet are reported with a distinct description from pernio-like lesions in children: petechial lesions on the sole, plantar singular toes, and/or heels.[89]

In addition to ecchymotic patterns, other vascular morphologies on the acral surfaces, like reticulated purpura of the soles of an infant[90] and acrocyanosis/livedo reticularis of the extremities in children and adolescents,[91] are thought to be late SARS-CoV-2 manifestations. Immunohistochemical positivity for SARS-CoV-2 has been found in EM-like, reticulated purpura, and perniotic-like acral lesions.[86,90] Young individuals with such acral manifestations tend to have an uncomplicated disease course and excellent outcomes.

Nonacral Cutaneous Eruptions

Nonacral surfaces also are involved in cutaneous eruptions related to COVID-19 infection in children. Some manifestations that are observed in COVID-positive adults, such as erythematous, vesicular, or urticarial exanthems,[92] also can present in infants and children with suspected or confirmed SARS-CoV-2 infection.[15,93–95] Petechiae, which are associated with several other viral illness in children,[96] have been observed in 1% to 2% of hospitalized COVID-19 positive children and may be widespread or localized.[14] Case reports of children with COVID-19 further demonstrate the various forms of potential mucocutaneous changes, such as erythematous and purpuric macules on the face,[97] swelling and papillitis of the tongue,[98] vesicular oral eruption,[99] a roseola-like rash,[100] and a pruritic maculopapular rash.[100] These case reports do not support causality between COVID-19 and cutaneous eruptions, because there are many potential causes for exanthems in children. The virus has been further implicated, however, by its demonstration in biopsy tissue from various eruptions, including patients with EM[86] and purpuric and livedoid eruptions.[90]

Although most cases of young individuals with cutaneous manifestations have a mild and uncomplicated disease course, some case reports demonstrate more serious forms of disease. MIS-C, as discussed previously, is one such

---

Table 4
Acral and non-acral potential cutaneous manifestations of pediatric COVID-19

Acral	Nonacral
Pernio-like lesions[59]	Urticaria[95]
	Erythematous patches[118]
EM-like lesions[88]	EM-like lesions[86]
	Vesicles/papulovesicles[15]
Plantar papules[14]	Herpetiform oral eruption[99]
	Roseola-like rash[100]
Retiform purpura[41]	Maculopapular rash[100]
	Macular eruption[14,98]
Ecchymotic-like lesions[89]	Lingual papillitis[97]
	Eccrine hidradenitis[93]
Livedo reticularis[91]	Erythema nodosum[93]
	Petechiae[14]
MIS-C findings (see **Table 1**)	Purpura[97]
	MIS-C findings (see **Table 1**)

example. Other examples in previously healthy COVID-positive children include that of a neonate with mottling skin rash and respiratory distress requiring neonatal intensive care[101] and a 12-year-old girl with nonspecific skin rash, fever, and headache who went on to develop respiratory failure and was found to have encephalomyelitis.[102] Despite acute systemic presentations, both of these patients improved by hospital discharge.

SUMMARY

The COVID-19 era has brought many advances to the understanding of interplay between viral disease, the pediatric immune system, and the skin. Evolving understanding of the mechanisms of MIS-C and pernio demonstrate the unique ways the young immune system operates; although likely protective from the traditional COVID-19 consequences like severe respiratory deterioration, the immune profile of younger individuals may holster a role in delayed inflammatory cutaneous presentations.

Although many cutaneous eruptions in children during the COVID-19 pandemic may not be related directly to infection, the possibility is an important consideration, particularly for patients with risk factors and/or highly impacted communities. Because children often present with no or mild symptoms, dermatologic manifestations of COVID-19 may be presenting signs,[14] serving as a subtle clue toward the highly contagious infection. Even in the absence of more classic signs of COVID-19 like respiratory symptoms, children with COVID-19 still may spread the virus and infect others who are susceptible to a more severe disease course.[103] Thus, dermatologists have an important role in containing the pandemic by appropriately counseling patients and testing for acute infection if indicated. Appropriate social distancing, mask-wearing, and hand-washing should be encouraged in children during the pandemic, especially those with risk factors, regardless of the presence or absence of extracutaneous symptoms.

Whereas some pediatric dermatologic manifestations of SARS-CoV-2, such as the polymorphous rash, mucositis, and conjunctivitis seen in MIS-C, may serve a clue toward serious sequalae, a majority of cutaneous eruptions in relation to the pandemic are benign. Despite the continually evolving understanding of COVID-19 and its potential manifestations, cutaneous eruptions fortunately most often are self-limited and not associated with poor outcomes; some studies even report children with skin rashes have a better prognosis than children with COVID-19 and no rash.[41] With ongoing cases and data reports, the interaction between COVID-19 and the skin in pediatric patients will become better understood. Beyond the dermatologic manifestations of COVID-19 in the pediatric population, children and adolescents face numerous consequences of the pandemic and some are only starting to be appreciated, ranging from physical impacts, such as obesity associated with changes in diet and activity or progression of myopia during home confinement to a wide range of psychosocial consequences of school closures and home/health stressors.[104]

As new, potentially more contagious, strains of COVID-19 arise, such as the B.1.1.7 variant, there has been concern for how this has an impact on the pediatric population. From February 2021 to April 2021, there was more than double the frequency of pediatric cases (all age groups) in Michigan,[105] with several other states following similar trends.[106] Although these rises coincide with the emergence of new variants, there is no evidence that new variants preferentially infect children.[107] It is likely that such increases in pediatric cases reflect vaccination and social trends. Currently (as of April 2021), the 2-dose mRNA Pfizer-BioNTech vaccine is approved in children 16 years and older, and clinical trials are under way for younger populations.[108] As schools open and sporting activities resume, it is important to counsel pediatric patients on appropriate social distancing measures, regardless of vaccination status.

CLINICS CARE POINTS

- A thorough skin exam in children suspected to have COVID-19 may be useful in identifying cutaneous manifestations.

- Clinical judgment must be used when deciding to test a child with new cutaneous findings for COVID-19 based on pre-test probability and test availability.

- It can be challenging to ascertain causality between cutaneous eruptions and COVID-19 infection, thus children should be encouraged to practice social distancing and good hygiene.

- The skin and mucous membranes can provide clues and/or be part of the diagnostic criteria for the serious pediatric complication of MIS-C.

- Children suspected to have MIS-C should seek emergency care.
- Most cutaneous manifestations of COVID-19, such as pernio-like lesions and non-specific eruptions limited to the skin, are self-limited.

REFERENCES

1. Children and COVID-19: State-Level Data Report. Available at: https://services.aap.org/en/pages/2019-novel-coronavirus-covid-19-infections/children-and-covid-19-state-level-data-report/. Accessed January 27, 2021.
2. Xiong Y, Zhang Q, Zhao L, et al. Clinical and imaging features of COVID-19 in a neonate. Chest 2020; 158(1):e5–7.
3. Assaker R, Colas AE, Julien-Marsollier F, et al. Presenting symptoms of COVID-19 in children: a meta-analysis of published studies. Br J Anaesth 2020;125(3):e330–2.
4. Poline J, Gaschignard J, Leblanc C, et al. Systematic severe acute respiratory syndrome coronavirus 2 screening at hospital admission in children: a French prospective multicenter study. Clin Infect Dis 2020. https://doi.org/10.1093/cid/ciaa1044.
5. Lu X, Zhang L, Du H, et al. SARS-CoV-2 infection in children. N Engl J Med 2020;382(17):1663–5.
6. Dong Y, Mo X, Hu Y. Epidemiological characteristics of 2143 pediatric patients with 2019 coronavirus disease in China. J Pediatr Cit 2020. https://doi.org/10.1542/peds.2020-0702.
7. Zimmermann P, Curtis N. Why is COVID-19 less severe in children? A review of the proposed mechanisms underlying the age-related difference in severity of SARS-CoV-2 infections. Arch Dis Child 2020. https://doi.org/10.1136/archdischild-2020-320338.
8. Zhou F, Yu T, Du R, et al. Clinical course and risk factors for mortality of adult inpatients with COVID-19 in Wuhan, China: a retrospective cohort study. Lancet 2020;395(10229):1054–62.
9. Celermajer DS, Sorensen KE, Spiegelhalter DJ, et al. Aging is associated with endothelial dysfunction in healthy men years before the age-related decline in women. J Am Coll Cardiol 1994;24(2):471–6.
10. Weisberg SP, Connors TJ, Zhu Y, et al. Distinct antibody responses to SARS-CoV-2 in children and adults across the COVID-19 clinical spectrum. Nat Immunol 2021;22(1):25–31.
11. Metcalf TU, Cubas RA, Ghneim K, et al. Global analyses revealed age-related alterations in innate immune responses after stimulation of pathogen recognition receptors. Aging Cell 2015;14(3): 421–32.
12. Carr EJ, Dooley J, Garcia-Perez JE, et al. The cellular composition of the human immune system is shaped by age and cohabitation. Nat Immunol 2016;17(4):461–8.
13. Rao VUS, Arakeri G, Subash A, et al. COVID-19: Loss of bridging between innate and adaptive immunity? Med Hypotheses 2020;144:109861.
14. Klimach A, Evans J, Stevens J, et al. Rash as a presenting complaint in a child with COVID-19. Pediatr Dermatol 2020;37(5):966–7.
15. Genovese G, Colonna C, Marzano AV. Varicella-like exanthem associated with COVID-19 in an 8-year-old girl: A diagnostic clue? Pediatr Dermatol 2020;37(3):435–6.
16. Mazzotta F, Troccoli T. Acute acro-ischemia in the child at the time of COVID-19. Eur J Pediatric Dermatol. Vol 30.; 2020. doi:10.26326/2281-9649.30.2.2102
17. Pousa PA, Mendonça TSC, Oliveira EA, et al. Extrapulmonary manifestations of COVID-19 in children: a comprehensive review and pathophysiological considerations. J Pediatr (Rio J) 2020. https://doi.org/10.1016/j.jped.2020.08.007.
18. Kilani MM, Odeh MM, Shalabi M, et al. Clinical and laboratory characteristics of SARS-CoV2-infected paediatric patients in Jordan: serial RT-PCR testing until discharge. Paediatr Int Child Health 2020. https://doi.org/10.1080/20469047.2020.1804733.
19. Felsenstein S, Willis E, Lythgoe H, et al. Presentation, treatment response and short-term outcomes in paediatric multisystem inflammatory syndrome temporally associated with SARS-CoV-2 (PIMS-TS). J Clin Med 2020;9(10):3293.
20. McMurray JC, May JW, Cunningham MW, et al. Multisystem inflammatory syndrome in children (MIS-C), a post-viral myocarditis and systemic vasculitis—A critical review of its pathogenesis and treatment. Front Pediatr 2020;8. https://doi.org/10.3389/fped.2020.626182.
21. Information for healthcare providers about multisystem inflammatory syndrome in children (MIS-C) | CDC. Available at: https://www.cdc.gov/mis-c/hcp/. Accessed January 16, 2021.
22. Riphagen S, Gomez X, Gonzalez-Martinez C, et al. Hyperinflammatory shock in children during COVID-19 pandemic. Lancet 2020;395(10237): 1607–8.
23. Health department-reported cases of multisystem inflammatory syndrome in children (MIS-C) in the United States|CDC. Available at: https://www.cdc.gov/mis-c/cases/index.html. Accessed February 26, 2021.
24. Feldstein LR, Rose EB, Horwitz SM, et al. Multisystem inflammatory syndrome in U.S. children and adolescents. N Engl J Med 2020;383(4):334–46.
25. Lee PY, Day-Lewis M, Henderson LA, et al. Distinct clinical and immunological features of SARS–CoV-2–induced multisystem inflammatory syndrome in children. J Clin Invest 2020;130(11):5942–50.

26. Dufort EM, Koumans EH, Chow EJ, et al. Multisystem inflammatory syndrome in children in New York state. N Engl J Med 2020;383(4):347–58.

27. Yonker LM, Neilan AM, Bartsch Y, et al. Pediatric severe acute respiratory syndrome coronavirus 2 (SARS-CoV-2): clinical presentation, infectivity, and immune responses. J Pediatr 2020;227:45–52.e5.

28. Licciardi F, Pruccoli G, Denina M, et al. SARS-CoV-2-induced Kawasaki-like hyperinflammatory syndrome: A novel COVID phenotype in children. Pediatrics 2020;146(2). https://doi.org/10.1542/peds.2020-1711.

29. Young TK, Shaw KS, Shah JK, et al. Mucocutaneous manifestations of multisystem inflammatory syndrome in children during the COVID-19 Pandemic. JAMA Dermatol 2021;157(2):207–12.

30. Godfred-Cato S, Bryant B, Leung J, et al. COVID-19–associated multisystem inflammatory syndrome in children — United States, March–July 2020. MMWR Morb Mortal Wkly Rep 2020;69(32):1074–80.

31. Rowley AH, Shulman ST, Arditi M. Immune pathogenesis of COVID-19–related multisystem inflammatory syndrome in children. J Clin Invest 2020;130(11):5619–21.

32. Multisystem inflammatory syndrome in children in the United States. N Engl J Med 2020;383(18):1793–6.

33. Cheng MH, Zhang S, Porritt RA, et al. An insertion unique to SARS-CoV-2 exhibits superantigenic character strengthened by recent mutations. bioRxiv 2020. https://doi.org/10.1101/2020.05.21.109272.

34. Roe K. A viral infection explanation for Kawasaki disease in general and for COVID-19 virus-related Kawasaki disease symptoms. Inflammopharmacology 2020;28(5):1219–22.

35. Lima R, Gootkind EF, De La Flor D, et al. Establishment of a pediatric COVID-19 biorepository: Unique considerations and opportunities for studying the impact of the COVID-19 pandemic on children. BMC Med Res Methodol 2020;20(1). https://doi.org/10.1186/s12874-020-01110-y.

36. Grimaud M, Starck J, Levy M, et al. Acute myocarditis and multisystem inflammatory emerging disease following SARS-CoV-2 infection in critically ill children. Ann Intensive Care 2020;10(1). https://doi.org/10.1186/s13613-020-00690-8.

37. Blatz AM, Oboite M, Chiotos K, et al. Cutaneous findings in SARS-CoV-2-associated multisystem inflammatory disease in children. Open Forum Infect Dis 2021;8(3). https://doi.org/10.1093/ofid/ofab074.

38. Dolinger MT, Person H, Smith R, et al. Pediatric crohn disease and multisystem inflammatory syndrome in children (MIS-C) and COVID-19 treated with infliximab. J Pediatr Gastroenterol Nutr 2020;71(2):153–5.

39. Yozgat CY, Uzuner S, Bursal Duramaz B, et al. Dermatological manifestation of pediatrics multisystem inflammatory syndrome associated with COVID-19 in a 3-year-old girl. Dermatol Ther 2020;33(4). https://doi.org/10.1111/dth.13770.

40. Mazori DR, Derrick KM, Kapoor U, et al. Perineal desquamation: An early sign of the Kawasaki disease phenotype of MIS-C. Pediatr Dermatol 2020;pde:14462. https://doi.org/10.1111/pde.14462.

41. Rekhtman S, Tannenbaum R, Strunk A, et al. Mucocutaneous disease and related clinical characteristics in hospitalized children and adolescents with COVID-19 and multisystem inflammatory syndrome in children. J Am Acad Dermatol 2020;84(2):408–14.

42. Al Ameer HH, AlKadhem SM, Busaleh F, et al. Multisystem inflammatory syndrome in children temporally related to COVID-19: A case report from Saudi Arabia. Cureus 2020;12(9). https://doi.org/10.7759/cureus.10589.

43. Andina-Martinez D, Nieto-Moro M, Alonso-Cadenas JA, et al. Mucocutaneous manifestations in hospitalized children with COVID-19. J Am Acad Dermatol 2021. https://doi.org/10.1016/j.jaad.2021.03.083.

44. Yasuhara J, Watanabe K, Takagi H, et al. COVID-19 and multisystem inflammatory syndrome in children: A systematic review and meta-analysis. Pediatr Pulmonol 2021;ppul:25245.

45. Nathan N, Prevost B, Sileo C, et al. The wide spectrum of COVID-19 clinical presentation in children. J Clin Med 2020;9(9):2950.

46. Morris SB, Belay E, Levin M, et al. Multisysttem inflammatory syndrome in children (MIS-C) associated with coronavirus disease 2019 (COVID-19). Center for Disease Control and Prevention; 2020. Available at: https://emergency.cdc.gov/coca/calls/2020/callinfo_051920.asp?deliveryName=USCDC_1052-DM28623. Accessed February 23, 2021.

47. Mamishi S, Movahedi Z, Mohammadi M, et al. Multisystem inflammatory syndrome associated with SARS-CoV-2 infection in 45 children: A first report from Iran. Epidemiol Infect 2020;148. https://doi.org/10.1017/S095026882000196X.

48. Feldstein LR, Tenforde MW, Friedman KG, et al. Characteristics and outcomes of US children and adolescents with multisystem inflammatory syndrome in children (MIS-C) compared with severe acute COVID-19. JAMA 2021. https://doi.org/10.1001/jama.2021.2091.

49. Gkoutzourelas A, Bogdanos DP, Sakkas LI. Kawasaki disease and COVID-19. Mediterr J Rheumatol 2020;31(Suppl 2):268. https://doi.org/10.31138/mjr.31.3.268.

50. Burgi Vieira C, Ferreira AT, Botelho Cardoso F, et al. Kawasaki-like syndrome as an emerging

complication of SARS-CoV-2 infection in young adults. Eur J Case Reports Intern Med 2020; 7(10):001886.

51. Hayran Y, Yorulmaz A, Gür G, et al. Different hair loss patterns in two pediatric patients with COVID-19-associated multisystem inflammatory syndrome in children. Dermatol Ther 2021. https://doi.org/10.1111/dth.14820.

52. Multisystem Inflammatory Syndrome in Children (MIS-C) Interim Guidance. Available at: https://services.aap.org/en/pages/2019-novel-coronavirus-covid-19-infections/clinical-guidance/multisystem-inflammatory-syndrome-in-children-mis-c-interim-guidance/. Accessed January 17, 2021.

53. Cappel JA, Wetter DA. Clinical characteristics, etiologic associations, laboratory findings, treatment, and proposal of diagnostic criteria of pernio (chilblains) in a series of 104 patients at Mayo Clinic, 2000 to 2011. Mayo Clin Proc 2014;89(2):207–15. https://doi.org/10.1016/j.mayocp.2013.09.020.

54. Perniosis - NORD (National Organization for Rare Disorders). Available at: https://rarediseases.org/rare-diseases/perniosis/. Accessed January 20, 2021.

55. Weston WL, Morelli JG. Childhood pernio and cryoproteins. Pediatr Dermatol 2000;17(2):97–9.

56. Tan SW, Tam YC, Oh CC. Skin manifestations of COVID-19: A worldwide review. JAAD Int 2021;2: 119–33.

57. Recalcati S, Barbagallo T, Frasin LA, et al. Acral cutaneous lesions in the time of COVID-19. J Eur Acad Dermatol Venereol 2020;34(8):e346–7.

58. Le Cleach L, Dousset L, Assier H, et al. Most chilblains observed during the COVID-19 outbreak occur in patients who are negative for COVID-19 on polymerase chain reaction and serology testing*. Br J Dermatol 2020;183(5):866–74.

59. Freeman EE, McMahon DE, Lipoff JB, et al. Pernio-like skin lesions associated with COVID-19: A case series of 318 patients from 8 countries. J Am Acad Dermatol 2020;83(2):486–92.

60. Huang Y, Dai H, Ke R. Principles of effective and robust innate immune response to viral infections: a multiplex network analysis. Front Immunol 2019; 10:1736.

61. Volpi S, Picco P, Caorsi R, et al. Type I interferonopathies in pediatric rheumatology. Pediatr Rheumatol 2016;14(1). https://doi.org/10.1186/s12969-016-0094-4.

62. Trouillet-Assant S, Viel S, Gaymard A, et al. Type I IFN immunoprofiling in COVID-19 patients. J Allergy Clin Immunol 2020;146(1):206–8.e2.

63. Kolivras A, Dehavay F, Delplace D, et al. Coronavirus (COVID-19) infection–induced chilblains: A case report with histopathologic findings. JAAD Case Rep 2020;6(6):489–92.

64. Damsky W, Peterson D, King B. When interferon tiptoes through COVID-19: Pernio-like lesions and their prognostic implications during SARS-CoV-2 infection. J Am Acad Dermatol 2020;83(3): e269–70.

65. Hubiche T, Cardot-Leccia N, Le Duff F, et al. Clinical, laboratory, and interferon-alpha response characteristics of patients with chilblain-like lesions during the COVID-19 pandemic. JAMA Dermatol 2020. https://doi.org/10.1001/jamadermatol.2020.4324.

66. Cordoro KM, Reynolds SD, Wattier R, et al. Clustered cases of acral perniosis: Clinical features, histopathology, and relationship to COVID-19. Pediatr Dermatol 2020;37(3):419–23.

67. Mastrolonardo M, Romita P, Bonifazi E, et al. The management of the outbreak of acral skin manifestations in asymptomatic children during COVID-19 era. Dermatol Ther 2020;33(4). https://doi.org/10.1111/dth.13617.

68. Roca-Ginés J, Torres-Navarro I, Sánchez-Arráez J, et al. Assessment of acute acral lesions in a case series of children and adolescents during the COVID-19 pandemic. JAMA Dermatol 2020; 156(9):992–7.

69. Docampo-Simón A, Sánchez-Pujol MJ, Juan-Carpena G, et al. Are chilblain-like acral skin lesions really indicative of COVID-19? A prospective study and literature review. J Eur Acad Dermatol Venereol 2020;34(9):e445–7.

70. Heymann WR. The Profound Dermatological Manifestations of COVID-19: Part IV - Cutaneous Feaures. American Academy of Dermatology Association; 2020. Available at: https://www.aad.org/dw/dw-insights-and-inquiries/2020-archive/april/dermatological-manifestations-covid-19-part-4. Accessed February 26, 2021.

71. Neri I, Virdi A, Corsini I, et al. Major cluster of paediatric 'true' primary chilblains during the COVID-19 pandemic: a consequence of lifestyle changes due to lockdown. J Eur Acad Dermatol Venereol 2020;34(11):2630–5.

72. Freeman EE, McMahon DE, Hruza GJ, et al. Timing of PCR and antibody testing in patients with COVID-19–associated dermatologic manifestations. J Am Acad Dermatol 2021;84(2):505–7.

73. El Hachem M, Diociaiuti A, Concato C, et al. A clinical, histopathological and laboratory study of 19 consecutive Italian paediatric patients with chilblain-like lesions: lights and shadows on the relationship with COVID-19 infection. J Eur Acad Dermatol Venereol 2020;34(11):2620–9.

74. Du Z, Zhu F, Guo F, et al. Detection of antibodies against SARS-CoV-2 in patients with COVID-19. J Med Virol 2020;92(10):1735–8.

75. Hu X, Xing Y, Jia J, et al. Factors associated with negative conversion of viral RNA in patients hospitalized with COVID-19. Sci Total Environ 2020;728.

76. COVID-19 Serology Surveillance Strategy|CDC. Available at: https://www.cdc.gov/coronavirus/2019-ncov/covid-data/serology-surveillance/index.html. Accessed January 28, 2021.

77. Freeman EE, McMahon DE, Fox LP. Emerging evidence of the direct association between COVID-19 and chilblains. JAMA Dermatol 2021;157(2). https://doi.org/10.1001/jamadermatol.2020.4937.

78. Anand S, Montez-Rath M, Han J, et al. Prevalence of SARS-CoV-2 antibodies in a large nationwide sample of patients on dialysis in the USA: a cross-sectional study. Lancet 2020;396(10259):1335–44.

79. Colmenero I, Santonja C, Alonso-Riaño M, et al. SARS-CoV-2 endothelial infection causes COVID-19 chilblains: histopathological, immunohistochemical and ultrastructural study of seven paediatric cases. Br J Dermatol 2020;183(4):729–37.

80. Colonna C, Genovese G, Monzani NA, et al. Outbreak of chilblain-like acral lesions in children in the metropolitan area of Milan, Italy, during the COVID-19 pandemic. J Am Acad Dermatol 2020;83(3):965–9.

81. Promenzio L, Arcangeli F, Cortis E, et al. Erythema pernio-like in four adolescents in the era of the Coronavirus-2 infection. Rev Recent Clin Trials 2020;15. https://doi.org/10.2174/1574887115666201016153031.

82. Piccolo V, Neri I, Filippeschi C, et al. Chilblain-like lesions during COVID-19 epidemic: a preliminary study on 63 patients. J Eur Acad Dermatol Venereol 2020;34(7):e291–3.

83. Garcia-Lara G, Linares-González L, Ródenas-Herranz T, et al. Chilblain-like lesions in pediatrics dermatological outpatients during the COVID-19 outbreak. Dermatol Ther 2020;33(5). https://doi.org/10.1111/dth.13516.

84. Papa A, Salzano AM, Di Dato MT, et al. Images in practice: painful cutaneous vasculitis in a SARS-Cov-2 IgG-positive child. Pain Ther 2020;9(2):805–7.

85. Recalcati S, Barbagallo T, Tonolo S, et al. Relapse of chilblain-like lesions during the second wave of COVID-19. J Eur Acad Dermatol Venereol 2021. https://doi.org/10.1111/jdv.17168.

86. Torrelo A, Andina D, Santonja C, et al. Erythema multiforme-like lesions in children and COVID-19. Pediatr Dermatol 2020;37(3):442–6.

87. García-Gil MF, García García M, Monte Serrano J, et al. Acral purpuric lesions (erythema multiforme type) associated with thrombotic vasculopathy in a child during the COVID-19 pandemic. J Eur Acad Dermatol Venereol 2020;34(9):e443–5.

88. Fernandez-Nieto D, Jimenez-Cauhe J, Suarez-Valle A, et al. Characterization of acute acral skin lesions in nonhospitalized patients: A case series of 132 patients during the COVID-19 outbreak. J Am Acad Dermatol 2020;83(1):e61–3.

89. Mastrolonardo M, Romita P, Bonifazi E, et al. The management of the outbreak of acral skin manifestations in asymptomatic children during <scp>COVID</scp> -19 era. Dermatol Ther 2020;33(4). https://doi.org/10.1111/dth.13617.

90. Andina D, Colmenero I, Santonja C, et al. Suspected COVID-19-related reticulated purpura of the soles in an infant. Pediatr Dermatol 2020;pde:14409.

91. García-Gil MF, Monte Serrano J, Lapeña-Casado A, et al. Livedo reticularis and acrocyanosis as late manifestations of COVID-19 in two cases with familial aggregation. Potential pathogenic role of complement (C4c). Int J Dermatol 2020;59(12):1549–51.

92. Recalcati S. Cutaneous manifestations in COVID-19: a first perspective. J Eur Acad Dermatol Venereol 2020;34(5):e212–3.

93. Fertitta L, Welfringer-Morin A, Ouedrani A, et al. Immunological and virological profile of children with chilblain-like lesions and SARS-CoV-2. J Eur Acad Dermatol Venereol 2020. https://doi.org/10.1111/jdv.16972.

94. Marzano AV, Genovese G, Fabbrocini G, et al. Varicella-like exanthem as a specific COVID-19–associated skin manifestation: Multicenter case series of 22 patients. J Am Acad Dermatol 2020;83(1):280–5.

95. Morey-Olivé M, Espiau M, Mercadal-Hally M, et al. Cutaneous manifestations in the current pandemic of coronavirus infection disease (COVID 2019). An Pediatría (Engl Ed) 2020;92(6):374–5.

96. Schneider H, Adams O, Weiss C, et al. Clinical characteristics of children with viral single- and co-infections and a petechial rash. Pediatr Infect Dis J 2013;32(5):186–91.

97. Olisova OY, Anpilogova EM, Shnakhova LM. Cutaneous manifestations in COVID -19: A skin rash in a child. Dermatol Ther 2020;33(6):e13712.

98. Olisova OY, Anpilogova EM, Shnakhova LM. Cutaneous manifestations in COVID-19: A skin rash in a child. Dermatol Ther 2020;33(6). https://doi.org/10.1111/dth.13712.

99. Aghazadeh N, Homayouni M, Sartori-Valinotti JC. Oral vesicles and acral erythema: report of a cutaneous manifestation of COVID-19. Int J Dermatol 2020;59(9):1153–4.

100. Bursal Duramaz B, Yozgat CY, Yozgat Y, et al. Appearance of skin rash in pediatric patients with COVID-19: Three case presentations. Dermatol Ther 2020;33(4). https://doi.org/10.1111/dth.13594.

101. Kamali Aghdam M, Jafari N, Eftekhari K. Novel coronavirus in a 15-day-old neonate with clinical signs of sepsis, a case report. Infect Dis (Auckl) 2020;52(6):427–9.

102. de Miranda Henriques-Souza AM, de Melo ACMG, de Aguiar Coelho Silva Madeiro B, et al. Acute

disseminated encephalomyelitis in a COVID-19 pediatric patient. Neuroradiology 2020;63(1). https://doi.org/10.1007/s00234-020-02571-0.

103. Cao Q, Chen YC, Chen CL, et al. SARS-CoV-2 infection in children: Transmission dynamics and clinical characteristics. J Formos Med Assoc 2020;119(3):670–3.

104. Wang J, Li Y, Musch DC, et al. Progression of myopia in school-aged children after COVID-19 home confinement. JAMA Ophthalmol 2021. https://doi.org/10.1001/jamaophthalmol.2020.6239.

105. Michigan.gov. Children and COVID-19: State Data Report. 2021. Available at: https://www.michigan.gov/coronavirus/0,9753,7-406-98163_98173—,00.html. Accessed April 26, 2021.

106. Mass.gov. COVID-19 Response Reporting. 2021. Available at: https://www.mass.gov/info-details/covid-19-response-reporting. Accessed April 26, 2021.

107. HopkinsMedicine.org. New Variants of Coronavirus: What You Should Know. 2021. Available at: https://www.hopkinsmedicine.org/health/conditions-and-diseases/coronavirus/a-new-strain-of-coronavirus-what-you-should-know. Accessed April 26, 2021.

108. Jenco M. AAP helps pediatricians prepare to vaccinate children, adolescents against COVID-19. AAP News; 2021. Available at: https://www.aappublications.org/news/2021/04/08/covid-vaccine-children-aap-guidance-040821. Accessed April 26, 2021.

109. Gupta A, Gill A, Sharma M, et al. Multi-system inflammatory syndrome in a child mimicking Kawasaki disease. J Trop Pediatr 2020. https://doi.org/10.1093/tropej/fmaa060.

110. Huang WC, Huang LM, Chang IS, et al. Epidemiologic features of Kawasaki disease in Taiwan, 2003

2006. Pediatrics 2009;123(3). https://doi.org/10.1542/peds.2008-2187.

111. Lin M-T, Wu M-H. The global epidemiology of Kawasaki disease: Review and future perspectives. Glob Cardiol Sci Pract 2018;2017(3). https://doi.org/10.21542/gcsp.2017.20.

112. Agarwal S, Agrawal DK. Kawasaki disease: etiopathogenesis and novel treatment strategies. Expert Rev Clin Immunol 2017;13(3):247–58.

113. Baker AL, Lu M, Minich LLA, et al. Associated symptoms in the ten days before diagnosis of Kawasaki disease. J Pediatr 2009;154(4). https://doi.org/10.1016/j.jpeds.2008.10.006.

114. Taddio A, Rossi ED, Monasta L, et al. Describing Kawasaki shock syndrome: results from a retrospective study and literature review. Clin Rheumatol 2017;36(1):223–8.

115. Rosés-Gibert P, Gimeno Castillo J, Saenz Aguirre A, et al. Acral lesions in a pediatric population during the COVID-19 pandemic: a case series of 36 patients from a single hospital in Spain. World J Pediatr 2020;16(6):629–32.

116. Gallizzi R, Sutera D, Spagnolo A, et al. Management of pernio-like cutaneous manifestations in children during the outbreak of COVID-19. Dermatol Ther 2020;33(6). https://doi.org/10.1111/dth.14312.

117. Andina D, Noguera-Morel L, Bascuas-Arribas M, et al. Chilblains in children in the setting of COVID-19 pandemic. Pediatr Dermatol 2020;37(3):406–11.

118. Maniaci A, Iannella G, Vicini C, et al. A case of covid-19 with late-onset rash and transient loss of taste and smell in a 15-year-old boy. Am J Case Rep 2020;21:1–6.

119. Ahmed M, Advani S, Moreira A, et al. Multisystem inflammatory syndrome in children: A systematic review. EClinicalMedicine 2020;26. https://doi.org/10.1016/j.eclinm.2020.100527.

Cutaneous Manifestations of COVID-19 in the Inpatient Setting

Mytrang H. Do, PhD[a,†], Claire R. Stewart, BA[a,†], Joanna Harp, MD[b,*]

KEYWORDS

• COVID-19 • Cutaneous • Inpatient • Vasculopathy • Viral exanthem • Complement • MIS-C

KEY POINTS

- COVID-19 is associated with polymorphic cutaneous manifestations of varying reported prevalence; the diversity of mucocutaneous findings is likely secondary to varying immune responses in response to SARS-CoV-2 infection.
- Cutaneous manifestations of COVID-19 in hospitalized patients can be broadly divided into 2 categories: vasculopathy-related cutaneous lesions and viral exanthem/inflammatory eruptions.
- Among patients hospitalized with COVID-19, patients with vasculopathy-related cutaneous lesions had more severe disease and higher mortality rates.
- Many viral exanthem/inflammatory eruptions are reported more frequently in hospitalized patients; however, these eruptions are associated with less severe COVID-19 than vasculopathy-related findings.
- Prompt recognition of these cutaneous manifestations is paramount to facilitate diagnosis and treatment of COVID-19.

INTRODUCTION

Since December 2019, coronavirus disease 2019 (COVID-19) has spread globally and caused significant morbidity and mortality worldwide. Cutaneous manifestations have been observed in patients with COVID-19 with varying prevalence ranging from 0.2% to 24%.[1–4] However, the true prevalence of cutaneous lesions is difficult to assess. Many studies included patients with both suspected and confirmed cases of COVID-19, and the lack of adequate personal protective equipment, especially at the beginning of the pandemic, may have precluded a thorough skin examination in many patients. A recent publication showed that 35 of 396 patients (11.8%) hospitalized with COVID-19 had dermatologic findings.[5]

Similar to the heterogeneity of systemic symptoms of COVID-19, cutaneous manifestations of COVID-19 are wide-ranging. In addition to varying morphologies, the eruptions affect disparate age groups and exhibit varying time courses; although some portend serious disease, others are associated with milder illness.[6,7] Certain dermatologic conditions are more prevalent in the inpatient compared with the outpatient setting—an important distinction when reviewing the mucocutaneous eruptions associated with COVID-19.[5] It is thought that the varying clinical manifestations are due to patients' differing immune response to the Severe Acute Respiratory Syndrome Coronavirus 2 (SARS-CoV-2).[8] For example, those who successfully clear SARS-CoV-2 infection due to a robust or even exaggerated type I interferon

The authors have no relevant disclosures, commercial or financial conflicts, or funding sources.
[a] Weill Cornell Medicine, New York, NY, USA; [b] Weill Cornell Medicine, New York Presbyterian Hospital, New York, NY, USA
[†] These authors contributed equally to this work.
* Corresponding author. Department of Dermatology, 1305 York Ave, 9th Fl, New York, NY 10021.
E-mail address: joh9090@med.cornell.edu

Dermatol Clin 39 (2021) 521–532
https://doi.org/10.1016/j.det.2021.05.011
0733-8635/21/© 2021 Elsevier Inc. All rights reserved.

response before humoral immunity occurs are more likely to develop pernio-like lesions ("COVID toes"). Alternatively, those with severe COVID-19 requiring hospitalization are more likely to develop dermatologic manifestations associated with an increased clotting tendency (possibly related to excessive complement activation) resulting in retiform purpura—a condition occurring almost exclusively in the inpatient setting.[9,10]

The pathophysiology of these eruptions is not yet fully elucidated. SARS-CoV-2 can bind to angiotensin-converting enzyme 2 (ACE2) receptors expressed in the subcutaneous fat and epithelial cells,[11] and thus, direct viral invasion has been proposed to contribute to the development of cutaneous manifestations in patients with COVID-19.[9] The roles of a cytokine storm and complement activation have also been implicated.[9,12–14] Recent work has demonstrated the importance of varying type I interferon responses in clinical severity of COVID-19 as well as associated dermatologic findings; higher levels of interferon-alpha, a type I interferon crucial to the early immune response to viral infection, was found to be associated with less severe COVID-19 infection as well as the development of pernio-like lesions.[8]

In this review, we cover common and uncommon skin lesions in patients hospitalized with COVID-19. These skin findings can be broadly divided into 2 categories: vasculopathy-related cutaneous eruptions secondary to systemic dysregulation caused by COVID-19 and eruptions related to virally triggered inflammatory responses similar to skin manifestations from other viral triggers.[14] We review demographic and clinical characteristics associated with each morphology.

VASCULOPATHY-RELATED CUTANEOUS LESIONS

COVID-19 is associated with a hypercoagulable state resulting in arterial and venous thrombosis.[15] In the skin, manifestations of coagulopathy range from transient livedoid reticularis to fixed livedo racemosa, retiform purpura, ulcerations, and necrosis.

Livedo Reticularis

Livedo reticularis is characterized by nonfixed, dusky patches forming complete rings, reflecting the underlying dermal and subcutaneous vasculature, and is caused by partial or intermittent blood flow reduction to the skin.[16] Livedo reticularis was observed in 5.3% of confirmed COVID-19 patients with dermatologic manifestations included in the American Academy of Dermatology's (AAD) COVID-19 registry.[6] However, livedo reticularis was not reported in several other case series that included large numbers of patients[1,3,4] (Table 1). Given the scarcity of this morphology, full clinical characterization of livedo reticularis in patients with COVID-19 is not currently possible. However, cases of fluctuating or transient livedo reticularis on the trunk and thigh have been reported.[17,18] Pauci-inflammatory thrombotic vasculopathy was seen in a biopsy of livedo reticularis.[6] Most reported cases were mild, not associated with thromboembolic complications, and resolved without dermatologic treatment; however, one death was reported in a patient with livedo reticularis.[6] The presence of microthromboses or low-grade vascular inflammation and vasodilation resulting from endothelial cell damage due to SARS-CoV-2 infection has been proposed as an etiology.[17,18]

Livedo Racemosa/Retiform Purpura/ Cutaneous Necrosis

Livedo racemosa presents with persistent erythematous to violaceous broken rings that are rarely necrotic or ulcerative, indicating a significant reduction in blood flow to the skin (Fig. 1). Livedo racemosa was observed in 2.3% of patients with confirmed COVID-19 in the AAD's COVID-19 registry.[6] Retiform purpura exists on a spectrum with livedo racemosa but is a more severe variant caused by full blockage of cutaneous blood flow leading to persistent purpuric and reticular patches or plaques with frank or impending necrosis and/or ulceration (Fig. 2).[16] Retiform purpura was observed in 6.4% of patients with confirmed COVID-19 in the AAD's COVID-19 registry and in 9 of 35 hospitalized COVID-19 patients (25.7%) who developed dermatologic findings.[5,6]

Galvan-Casas et al. observed livedo (type not specified) and necrosis in 6% of patients with suspected and confirmed COVID-19[7] (see Table 1). Patients who developed retiform purpura were older, with a median age of 66 years, and sicker, with 91% requiring mechanical ventilation and 82% developing acute respiratory distress syndrome (ARDS).[6,7] Systemic thrombotic events such as deep venous thrombosis or pulmonary embolism occurred in 66% of the patients. With a 10% to 18% mortality rate, livedo racemosa and retiform purpura were among the highest mortality of COVID-19–associated cutaneous manifestations.[6,7]

Livedoid and necrotic skin lesions were also reported in case reports and case series with similarly poor prognosis.[19–22] Patients had varying degrees of alterations in coagulation parameters,

Table 1
Summary of clinical characteristics of COVID-19 patients with cutaneous manifestations

Cutaneous Manifestation	Frequency Among COVID-19 Cutaneous Manifestations (%)	Typical Age Range (years)	Relationship to Noncutaneous Symptoms	Hospitalization (%)[a]	COVID-19 Severity	Mortality Rate (%)[a]	Prominent Histologic Findings
Livedo reticularis[b]	At least 3 reported cases	40's to 60's	After	2/3 reported cases	Mild	0/3 reported cases	Pauci-inflammatory thrombotic vasculopathy
Livedo racemosa/retiform purpura/livedo and necrosis	2.3/6.4/6	60's	Concurrent or after	86–100	Severe	10–18	Pauci-inflammatory thrombotic vasculopathy
Pressure-associated ulceration and necrosis[b]	At least 25 reported cases	30's to 70's	After	11/25 reported cases	Severe	4/25 reported cases	Thrombotic vasculopathy and pressure necrosis
Multisystem Inflammatory Syndrome in Children	0.3	Children	Concurrent	100	Severe	1.8	Varied
Morbilliform eruptions	21–23	50's to 60's	Concurrent or after	45–80	Moderate	2.6–3.7	Spongiosis, basal cell vacuolation, and perivascular lymphocytic infiltrate
Urticarial eruptions	13.5–26	40's	Concurrent or after	33–44	Mild	1	Lichenoid and vacuolar interface dermatitis

(continued on next page)

Table 1
(continued)

Cutaneous Manifestation	Frequency Among COVID-19 Cutaneous Manifestations (%)	Typical Age Range (years)	Relationship to Noncutaneous Symptoms	Hospitalization (%)[a]	COVID-19 Severity	Mortality Rate (%)[a]	Prominent Histologic Findings
Vesicular eruptions	7.2	Middle age	Concurrent (though 15% before)	32	Moderate	0	Nonballooning acantholysis leading to intraepidermal unilocular vesicle; epidermal dyskeratosis
Erythema multiforme-like eruptions[b]	3.7	Children – Young Adults	Concurrent or after	NR	Mild	NR	Interface dermatitis with superficial and deep perivascular inflammation
Sweet's syndrome[b]	At least 1 case reported	60's	After	1/1 reported case	Moderate	0/1 reported case	Neutrophilic infiltration with vascular proliferation
Petechiae and purpuric eruptions[b]	At least 14 reported cases	30's to 70's	After	14/14 reported cases	Moderate-severe	0/14 reported cases	NR

Abbreviation: NR, not reported.

[a] Small sample size. Numbers reflect number of cases/reports instead of percentage.
[b] Information based on limited numbers of case reports.

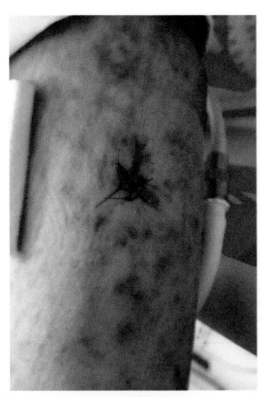

Fig. 1. Livedo racemosa on the arm with biopsy site in a patient with COVID-19 complicated by ARDS. Biopsy revealed pauci-inflammatory thrombotic vasculopathy. From Magro C, Mulvey JJ, Berlin D, et al. Complement associated microvascular injury and thrombosis in the pathogenesis of severe COVID-19 infection: A report of five cases. Transl Res. 2020;220:1-13.

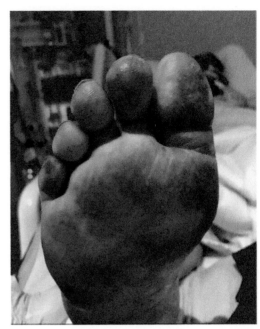

Fig. 2. Early retiform purpura on the right foot in a patient with COVID-19 complicated by ARDS and ischemic stroke. Biopsy revealed pauci-inflammatory thrombotic vasculopathy. From Magro C, Mulvey JJ, Berlin D, et al. Complement associated microvascular injury and thrombosis in the pathogenesis of severe COVID-19 infection: A report of five cases. Transl Res. 2020;220:1-13.

most notably elevated d-dimer, and many also had systemic thromboembolic complications. Although disseminated intravascular coagulation (DIC) has been implicated in patients with COVID-19, some patients with livedo racemosa or retiform purpura did not develop classic DIC laboratory parameters.[21,23,24] The presence of antiphospholipid antibodies was variable, as some COVID-19 patients with acro-ischemia were found to have antiphospholipid antibodies though others did not.[19,20,22] Nevertheless, antiphospholipid antibodies can arise transiently in patients with critical illness and infection.[25]

It is rare for these findings to precede the onset of COVID-19 symptoms. Freeman and colleagues described retiform purpura as often occurring after COVID-19 symptoms (91%). In contrast, Galvan-Casas et al., which was published early in the pandemic in April 2020, showed that livedo (type not specified) and necrosis paralleled the onset of COVID-19 symptoms (86%). Given that the constellation of COVID-19 symptoms was not well-characterized early during the pandemic, this discrepancy may reflect differences in perception of symptom onset by clinicians and patients. Livedoid eruptions occur more often on the acral areas and last approximately 10 days, whereas retiform purpura has been described on the extremities and the buttocks. Although a pressure component may contribute to the development of retiform purpura, these lesions were also present in patients who were intermittently proned.[26,27] Many patients were started on therapeutic anticoagulation during their hospital course due to increasing d-dimer and suspected or confirmed thrombotic events.[20,28] Although anticoagulation in severe cases of COVID-19 has been shown to reduce mortality, both the exact dosing and the timing of anticoagulation initiation in these patients remain to be determined.[29,30] It is critical to consider the overall clinical picture and the patient's comorbidities, particularly bleeding risk, when determining the best course of treatment.

The pathophysiology of this coagulopathy is an area of active research. Complement-mediated microvascular injury appears to play an essential role in some cases. Exaggerated complement

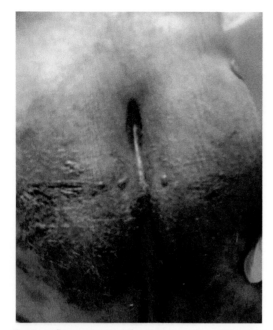

Fig. 3. Inflammatory retiform purpura in a COVID-19 patient complicated by ARDS. Biopsy revealed thrombotic. From Magro C, Mulvey JJ, Berlin D, et al. Complement associated microvascular injury and thrombosis in the pathogenesis of severe COVID-19 infection: A report of five cases. Transl Res. 2020;220:1-13.

activation has been implicated in severe COVID-19.[9,10] As the complement system links innate immunity to coagulation,[31] its overactivation could promote a thrombotic state in patients with severe COVID-19. Skin biopsies from patients with livedo racemosa and retiform purpura showed a pauci-inflammatory thrombogenic vasculopathy affecting capillaries, venules, and arteries with microvascular deposition of C3d, C4d, C5b-9, and MASP-2.[12,13,20] Excessive inflammation caused by a cytokine storm and the subsequent recruitment of immune cells has also been proposed as a potential cause of thrombophilic states in these patients.[32]

Pressure-Associated Ulceration and Necrosis

Critically ill hospitalized patients, including patients with COVID-19, are at an increased risk for sacral/buttock ulcerations caused by hospital-acquired pressure injuries (see **Table 1**). Ulcers described were often covered with black eschar with surrounding erythema and violaceous discoloration.[33] Livedoid plaques and retiform purpura, with biopsy showing thrombotic vasculopathy and evidence of pressure necrosis, were noted in some patients (**Fig. 3**).[12,33] Notably, patients with

COVID-19 were found to develop these lesions earlier than other patient populations.

In addition, acrofacial purpura and necrosis associated with minor pressure injuries due to direct contact with medical devices, such as nasal cannulas, endotracheal tubes, or pulse oximeters, have been reported in patients with COVID-19.[26,27] Importantly, given that many patients with COVID-19 are placed in a prone position to improve oxygenation status, pressure-associated ulceration and necrosis can occur in a unique distribution such as the bilateral cheeks compared to the usual locations such as the sacrum and heels. As ulcerations can serve as portals of entry for microbes leading to infection, it is critical to monitor patients closely to prevent additional morbidity and mortality.

VIRAL EXANTHEM/INFLAMMATORY ERUPTIONS
Multisystem Inflammatory Syndrome in Children

In the early months of the pandemic, a novel pediatric illness characterized by a hyperinflammatory syndrome and hemodynamic shock was reported in children with SARS-CoV-2 infection.[34] This illness, now termed Multisystem Inflammatory Syndrome in Children (MIS-C), is characterized by fever, multiorgan dysfunction, and known or suspected exposure to SARS-CoV-2.[35] Many symptoms of MIS-C, including fever, mucocutaneous findings, and cardiovascular involvement, are similar to Kawasaki Disease (KD), a medium-vessel vasculitis presenting in children typically younger than 5 years.[32–34] However, unlike KD, MIS-C predominantly affects older children, with a median age of 10 years.[36] Furthermore, MIS-C has been associated with gastrointestinal symptoms, such as nausea and diarrhea—symptoms uncommon in KD.[37] Cardiovascular involvement in MIS-C manifests as left ventricular dysfunction, often necessitating pressure support and even extracorporeal membrane oxygenation in some cases. Coronary artery dilations, which are the cardiac hallmark of KD, are less common in MIS-C.[37,38]

Mucocutaneous findings are seen in most patients with MIS-C. Skin lesions include morbilliform, scarlatiniform, urticarial, and reticulated morphologies; patients with localized, acrofacial lesions and more widespread eruptions have been reported. Patients may also present with conjunctival injection, palmoplantar erythema, periorbital erythema and edema, and strawberry tongue, which is notably similar to the mucocutaneous examination in patients with KD, necessitating a high index of suspicion for COVID-19–induced MIS-C in these patients.

Although COVID-19 infection in children is generally associated with a mild course with minimal or no symptoms, up to 68% of children with MIS-C required admission to a critical care unit, and 15% required ventilation[39] (see **Table 1**). In a prospective study of pediatric patients hospitalized with acute SARS-CoV-2 and MIS-C, lower absolute lymphocyte count and higher C-reactive protein were predictive of more severe MIS-C.[40] Although race/ethnicity was not predictive of disease severity, more than 75% of the cases reported to the Centers for Disease Control and Prevention have occurred in Hispanic/Latino or Black children.[40]

Treatment primarily consists of supportive care and intravenous immunoglobulin (IVIG) (2 gm/kg, based on ideal body weight), with low-moderate dose glucocorticoids (1–2 mg/kg/d) added for patients who have not developed shock or severe end-organ involvement.[41] Both interventions have been associated with shorter intensive care stays and hospitalizations.[42] Some guidelines have also recommended the use of immunosuppressive drugs like anakinra and tocilizumab.[43]

Morbilliform Eruptions

Morbilliform eruptions are characterized by pink to erythematous, blanching macules and papules caused by viral infections or drug hypersensitivity reactions. Morbilliform eruptions represent 21% to 23% of skin manifestations associated with COVID-19, making them among the most common rashes seen in patients with COVID-19[3,6,7,44] (see **Table 1**). Hospitalization rates for patients with morbilliform eruptions ranged from 45% to 80%, higher than the 30% to 38% seen in COVID-19 patients with nonmorbilliform cutaneous manifestations.[6,7] Morbilliform eruptions were shown to occur in 4 of 35 hospitalized COVID-19 patients (11.4%) who developed dermatologic findings.[5]

In both hospitalized and nonhospitalized patients, eruptions can occur concurrently or after other COVID-19 symptoms and last for an average of 1 week.[6,44,45] Truncal regions were the most commonly affected areas, followed by extremities. The most commonly reported symptom was pruritis. Patients who developed morbilliform eruptions were often in their fifties and sixties.[6,44,45] The overall rate for thrombotic events was 8% and for ARDS was 11%; 35% required ventilator support. The overall mortality of COVID-19 patients who developed morbilliform eruptions ranged from 2.6% to 3.7%.[6,44] Topical corticosteroids

and antihistamines may be helpful in controlling morbilliform eruptions and associated pruritus in patients with COVID-19.[46,47] Systemic corticosteroids may also be considered in certain cases.[46,47]

Morbilliform eruptions are likely secondary to the immune response to viral infection. Skin biopsies show spongiosis, basal cell vacuolation, and perivascular lymphocytic infiltrate,[6,48] which are typically seen in other viral-induced skin lesions. However, a biopsy showing fibrin microthrombi within the small vessels has also been reported, suggesting a more complex pathophysiology may be operational in some cases.[49]

Drug hypersensitivity reactions are another cause of morbilliform eruptions and are likely implicated in some cases of morbilliform eruptions reported in patients with COVID-19. Indeed, 81.3% of patients with morbilliform eruptions were shown to have concomitant drug intake.[44] The most common culprit medications were chloroquine/hydroxychloroquine, lopinavir/ritonavir, and azithromycin. Similarly, patients who developed pruritic papular exanthems on receiving new medications for COVID-19 have been reported. In these cases, skin biopsies were compatible with drug reactions, and all cases improved with discontinuation of medication and use of systemic or topical corticosteroids.[50,51] Therefore, a strong suspicion of drug hypersensitivity should be considered in the evaluation of COVID-19–associated morbilliform eruptions.

Urticarial Eruptions

Urticarial eruptions are transient erythematous and edematous plaques of varying sizes mediated by mast cell histamine release in the superficial dermis.[52] Urticarial eruptions account for 13.5% to 26% of cases of COVID-19 cutaneous manifestations[1,3,4,6,7] (see **Table 1**). Hospitalization rates were 33% to 44%, similar to COVID-19 patients with non-urticarial cutaneous manifestations (34%–48%).[6,7] Most of the hospitalized patients needed only supplemental oxygen and did not develop ARDS or thrombotic events; only one fatality was recorded in the total 27 urticarial cases reported in this series.[6]

Urticarial eruptions most commonly occurred in adults in their forties. Urticarial eruptions often occurred on the trunk and extremities, with pruritis being the most common symptom and duration averaging 1 week.[6,7] Urticarial eruptions were rare before the onset of COVID-19 symptoms but have been observed concurrently (22%–61%) and after (35%–67%) the onset of symptoms. Of note, urticaria with or without angioedema has also been reported as the presenting feature or as the only symptom of COVID-19, highlighting the importance of early recognition of urticarial rash in the diagnosis of COVID-19 as a means for limiting disease spread.[53–57] Some urticarial eruptions resolved without specific treatment, whereas others required antihistamine and/or low-dose systemic corticosteroids.[56,57]

Biopsy of a case of an urticarial plaque associated with COVID-19 revealed lymphocytic infiltrate with edema, spongiosis, lichenoid, and vacuolar interface dermatitis, consistent with viral exanthem.[58] Like morbilliform eruptions, the causes of urticarial eruptions in patients with COVID-19 must be interpreted with caution as some may represent reactions to medications. Viral infection can elicit a robust immune response and elevated proinflammatory cytokines. IL-6 level is notably elevated in patients with COVID-19.[59] As IL-6 can directly stimulate mast cell degranulation, elevated levels of proinflammatory cytokine could contribute to the development of urticaria in these patients. Also, as colocalization of SARS-CoV-2 glycoprotein with complement components has been demonstrated, it has been hypothesized that deposition of antigen-antibody complexes leading to complement activation and mast cell degradation could also cause urticaria in patients with COVID-19.[60,61]

Vesicular Eruptions

In a large cohort study, 7.2% of patients presenting with COVID-19–associated cutaneous manifestations were reported to have a vesicular eruption[5] (see **Table 1**). Two vesicular forms have been documented: a localized, monomorphic form found on the trunk and limbs and a diffuse, polymorphic form.[7,62] Most patients report minimal itching, which may help distinguish this eruption from the often very pruritic eruption of varicella.[63,64] Vesicular lesions associated with COVID-19 are most commonly seen in middle-aged men, with an average age of 45.6 ± 20 years.[6] The eruption is believed to be associated with early infection. The average latency time from onset of symptoms to rash is only 3 days (range -2 to 12 days); 15% of patients present with the lesions before any other COVID-19 symptoms.[6,45] In a cohort of Spanish patients, 32% with vesicular eruptions were admitted to a hospital, although only 6% required intensive care.[6] In a study comparing 24 COVID-19 patients with vesicular eruptions, of 6 patients with the localized pattern, 83.3% had concomitant COVID-19 pneumonia, compared to only 27.8% of those with the 18 patients who presented with the diffuse pattern; however, this was not

statistically significant, likely due to small sample size.[62] Further research is required to fully elucidate the differences in the vesicular eruptions of those with severe COVID-19 requiring hospitalization compared with those with milder or asymptomatic disease. Lesions resolved in an average of 8 to 10 days without scarring.[62,64]

It has been proposed that the direct pathogenic effect of the SARS-CoV-2 virus on basal layer keratinocytes may lead to acantholysis and dyskeratosis.[63] To date, there has not been a report of the SARS-CoV-2 virus inside vesicles, identified by PCR assay or other methods, indicating that the infective potential via vesicles is likely minimal.

Erythema Multiforme-Like Eruptions

In April, a new pattern of erythema multiforme (EM)-like lesions in four adults hospitalized with COVID-19 was first described; since then, there have been numerous reports of EM-like lesions in children and young adults associated with SARS-CoV-2 infection[65] (see **Table 1**). Lesions appear as erythematous macules, papules, and plaques with crusted centers consisting of two (atypical targets) or three (typical targets) rings often observed on the extremities.[65–67] Lesions may be pruritic or painful.[51] Some patients present with oral mucosal involvement, including palatal macules and petechiae, and erosive cheilitis.[68,69] The mean age of patients with EM-like eruptions is 12.2 years with a male predominance (59.5%).[45] Latency of EM-life eruptions has been reported to range from only a few days to 3 weeks after the onset of initial COVID-19 symptoms.[44,65,66,68] A review of the literature found that EM-like eruptions have been described in up to 3.7% of patients hospitalized with COVID-19.[45] Of note, the incidence of EM-like eruptions may be under-reported as some studies group unspecific rashes of annular appearance into an "other rash" category.[70] Many patients were treated with systemic corticosteroids with the resolution of lesions.[71]

The pathogenesis of EM-like eruptions is not fully understood. Still, it is likely viral in etiology, although exposure to certain medications received in the treatment of other COVID-19 symptoms may play a role.

MISCELLANEOUS CUTANEOUS MANIFESTATIONS OF COVID-19 IN HOSPITALIZED PATIENTS
Sweet's Syndrome

Sweet's syndrome, also known as acute febrile neutrophilic dermatosis, is a nonvasculitic sterile neutrophilic dermatosis syndrome often presenting with fever, arthralgias, and neutrophilia. Sweet's syndrome may be idiopathic, malignancy-associated, or drug-induced, and cases associated with viral infections have been reported.[72] There exists at least one case of a patient hospitalized with COVID-19 who developed Sweet's syndrome[73] (see **Table 1**). The patient developed numerous erythematous painful nodules on the scalp, extremities, trunk, and oral ulcers and fever; the lesions regressed without specific treatment as the patient recovered from COVID-19. Skin biopsy showed diffuse neutrophilic infiltration in the upper dermis with vascular proliferation. The elevated neutrophil count is a consistent finding in patients with COVID-19,[74] and this exaggerated neutrophilic response may have contributed to the development of Sweet's syndrome in this case.[73]

Petechiae and Purpuric Eruptions

Petechiae are nonblanching, nonpalpable pinpoint macules resulting from red blood cell extravasation; multiple petechiae coalesce to become purpura. Cases of petechiae and purpuric eruptions associated with thrombocytopenia have been reported in patients with COVID-19[75–79] (see **Table 1**). These eruptions often occurred after noncutaneous symptoms in hospitalized patients who were older and had had moderate to severe COVID-19. No deaths have been reported. IVIG, corticosteroids, thrombopoietin receptor agonists, and platelet transfusions have been used to manage these patients.[75–79] Although cases of thrombocytopenia secondary to DIC have been reported in COVID-19,[21] reported patients who developed petechiae and purpuric eruptions did not have DIC. Several mechanisms of thrombocytopenia have been proposed, including reduced platelet production due to cytokine storm, increased platelet destruction secondary to increased antibodies and immune complexes, and platelet aggregation resulting in microthrombi and platelet consumption.[80,81]

Perniosis ("COVID Toe")

Many cases of pernio or pernio-like lesions (red-purple tender papules typically affecting toes and fingers) have been reported typically as a late manifestation of confirmed or suspected COVID-19 infection. Although "COVID toe" is typically noted in young, healthy patients with mild or even asymptomatic COVID-19 infections, 16% of patients with "COVID toe" in one large international registry were hospitalized.[5] It should be noted, however, that misclassification of acral livedo or retiform purpura as "COVID toe" could occur given similar presenting locations and some overlap clinically (both present with purpura), especially if being evaluated and classified by nondermatologists. In one author's experience (J.H.), no cases of "COVID toe" or perniosis have been diagnosed in the inpatient setting of a large, academic hospital setting in New York City throughout the pandemic.

SUMMARY

Adults and children hospitalized with COVID-19 display a range of mucocutaneous eruptions, the diversity of which is likely due to the varying immune response generated in response to SARS-CoV-2 infection. In the hospitalized patient, livedo racemosa and retiform purpura were associated with more severe disease course, poorer prognosis, prolonged hospitalization, and higher mortality. In contrast, most viral exanthem and inflammatory lesions, such as urticarial and vesicular eruptions, were associated with a less severe COVID-19 disease course, although were nevertheless reported more frequently in the inpatient setting. One exception, however, is the presence of an inflammatory rash associated with MIS-C in the inpatient pediatric population, which has been associated with more severe COVID-19 disease and disease sequelae. Prompt recognition of the mucocutaneous manifestations presented in this article is paramount to facilitate timely diagnosis, proper treatment, and accurate prognostication of clinical course.

CLINICS CARE POINTS

- The two main categories of skin findings in patients with COVID-19 in the inpatient setting include vasculopathy -related (acral livedoid eruptions and retiform purpura) and inflammatory (vesicular, urticarial, erythema multiforme-like).

- Acral livedoid eruptions and retiform purpura in severe COVID-19 infections are often cutaneous manifestations of a systemic hypercoaguable state; and thus differ pathophysiologically and histopathologically from "COVID toe."

- Multisystem Inflammatory Syndrome in Children can prevent with a variety of mucocutaneous manifestations including variable rashes, conjunctival injection, palmoplantar erythema, and strawberry tongue.

REFERENCES

1. Recalcati S. Cutaneous manifestations in COVID-19: a first perspective. J Eur Acad Dermatol Venereol 2020;34(5):e212–3.
2. Guan WJ, Liang WH, Zhao Y, et al. Comorbidity and its impact on 1590 patients with COVID-19 in China: a nationwide analysis. Eur Respir J 2020;55(5).
3. Askin O, Altunkalem RN, Altinisik DD, et al. Cutaneous manifestations in hospitalized patients diagnosed as COVID-19. Dermatol Ther 2020;e13896.
4. De Giorgi V, Recalcati S, Jia Z, et al. Cutaneous manifestations related to coronavirus disease 2019 (COVID-19): A prospective study from China and Italy. J Am Acad Dermatol 2020;83(2):674–5.
5. Rekhtman S, Tannenbaum R, Strunk A, et al. Eruptions and related clinical course among 296 hospitalized adults with confirmed COVID-19. J Am Acad Dermatol 2021;84(4):946–52.
6. Freeman EE, McMahon DE, Lipoff JB, et al. The spectrum of COVID-19-associated dermatologic manifestations: An international registry of 716 patients from 31 countries. J Am Acad Dermatol 2020;83(4):1118–29.
7. Galvan Casas C, Catala A, Carretero Hernandez G, et al. Classification of the cutaneous manifestations of COVID-19: a rapid prospective nationwide consensus study in Spain with 375 cases. Br J Dermatol 2020;183(1):71–7.
8. Hubiche T, Cardot-Leccia N, Le Duff F, et al. Clinical, laboratory, and interferon-alpha response characteristics of patients with chilblain-like lesions during the COVID-19 pandemic. JAMA Dermatol 2021;157(2):202–6.
9. Magro CM, Mulvey JJ, Laurence J, et al. Docked severe acute respiratory syndrome coronavirus 2 proteins within the cutaneous and subcutaneous microvasculature and their role in the pathogenesis of severe coronavirus disease 2019. Hum Pathol 2020;106:106–16.
10. Carvelli J, Demaria O, Vely F, et al. Association of COVID-19 inflammation with activation of the C5a-C5aR1 axis. Nature 2020;588(7836):146–50.
11. Li MY, Li L, Zhang Y, et al. Expression of the SARS-CoV-2 cell receptor gene ACE2 in a wide variety of human tissues. Infect Dis Poverty 2020;9(1):45.
12. Magro C, Mulvey JJ, Berlin D, et al. Complement associated microvascular injury and thrombosis in the pathogenesis of severe COVID-19 infection: A report of five cases. Transl Res 2020;220:1–13.
13. Magro C, Mulvey JJ, Laurence J, et al. The differing pathophysiologies that underlie COVID-19 associated perniosis and thrombotic retiform purpura: a case series. Br J Dermatol 2021;184(1):141–50.
14. Suchonwanit P, Leerunyakul K, Kositkuljorn C. Cutaneous manifestations in COVID-19: Lessons learned from current evidence. J Am Acad Dermatol 2020;83(1):e57–60.
15. Abou-Ismail MY, Diamond A, Kapoor S, et al. The hypercoagulable state in COVID-19: Incidence, pathophysiology, and management. Thromb Res 2020;194:101–15.
16. Georgesen C, Fox LP, Harp J. Retiform purpura: A diagnostic approach. J Am Acad Dermatol 2020;82(4):783–96.
17. Manalo IF, Smith MK, Cheeley J, et al. A dermatologic manifestation of COVID-19: Transient livedo reticularis. J Am Acad Dermatol 2020;83(2):700.
18. Verheyden M, Grosber M, Gutermuth J, et al. Relapsing symmetric livedo reticularis in a patient with COVID-19 infection. J Eur Acad Dermatol Venereol 2020;34(11):e684–6.
19. Llamas-Velasco M, Munoz-Hernandez P, Lazaro-Gonzalez J, et al. Thrombotic occlusive vasculopathy in a skin biopsy from a livedoid lesion of a patient with COVID-19. Br J Dermatol 2020;183(3):591–3.
20. Droesch C, Do MH, DeSancho M, et al. Livedoid and purpuric skin eruptions associated with coagulopathy in severe COVID-19. JAMA Dermatol 2020;156(9):1–3.
21. Zhang Y, Cao W, Xiao M, et al. [Clinical and coagulation characteristics in 7 patients with critical COVID-2019 pneumonia and acro-ischemia]. Zhonghua Xue Ye Xue Za Zhi 2020;41(4):302–7.
22. Zhang Y, Xiao M, Zhang S, et al. Coagulopathy and antiphospholipid antibodies in patients with Covid-19. N Engl J Med 2020;382(17):e38.
23. Novara E, Molinaro E, Benedetti I, et al. Severe acute dried gangrene in COVID-19 infection: a case report. Eur Rev Med Pharmacol Sci 2020;24(10):5769–71.
24. Tang N, Li D, Wang X, et al. Abnormal coagulation parameters are associated with poor prognosis in patients with novel coronavirus pneumonia. J Thromb Haemost 2020;18(4):844–7.
25. Uthman IW, Gharavi AE. Viral infections and antiphospholipid antibodies. Semin Arthritis Rheum 2002;31(4):256–63.
26. Karagounis TK, Shaw KS, Caplan A, et al. Acrofacial purpura and necrotic ulcerations in COVID-19: a case series from New York City. Int J Dermatol 2020;59(11):1419–22.
27. Le MQ, Rosales R, Shapiro LT, et al. The down side of prone positioning: the case of a coronavirus 2019 survivor. Am J Phys Med Rehabil 2020;99(10):870–2.
28. Bosch-Amate X, Giavedoni P, Podlipnik S, et al. Retiform purpura as a dermatological sign of coronavirus disease 2019 (COVID-19) coagulopathy. J Eur Acad Dermatol Venereol 2020;34(10):e548–9.
29. Tang N, Bai H, Chen X, et al. Anticoagulant treatment is associated with decreased mortality in

severe coronavirus disease 2019 patients with coagulopathy. J Thromb Haemost 2020;18(5):1094–9.

30. Chowdhury JF, Moores LK, Connors JM. Anticoagulation in hospitalized patients with Covid-19. N Engl J Med 2020;383(17):1675–8.

31. Foley JH. Examining coagulation-complement crosstalk: complement activation and thrombosis. Thromb Res 2016;141(Suppl 2):S50–4.

32. Castelnovo L, Capelli F, Tamburello A, et al. Symmetric cutaneous vasculitis in COVID-19 pneumonia. J Eur Acad Dermatol Venereol 2020;34(8):e362–3.

33. Young S, Narang J, Kumar S, et al. Large sacral/buttocks ulcerations in the setting of coagulopathy: A case series establishing the skin as a target organ of significant damage and potential morbidity in patients with severe COVID-19. Int Wound J 2020; 17(6):2033–7.

34. Riphagen S, Gomez X, Gonzalez-Martinez C, et al. Hyperinflammatory shock in children during COVID-19 pandemic. Lancet 2020;395(10237): 1607–8.

35. Prevention CfDCa. Multisystem inflammatory syndrome in children (MIS-C) associated with coronavirus disease 2019 (COVID-19). 2020. Available at: https://www.emergency.cdc.gov/han/2020/han0043 2.asp. Accessed December 14, 2020.

36. Belhadjer Z, Meot M, Bajolle F, et al. Acute heart failure in multisystem inflammatory syndrome in children in the context of global SARS-CoV-2 pandemic. Circulation 2020;142(5):429–36.

37. Feldstein LR, Rose EB, Horwitz SM, et al. Multisystem inflammatory syndrome in U.S. children and adolescents. N Engl J Med 2020;383(4): 334–46.

38. Rodriguez-Gonzalez M, Castellano-Martinez A, Cascales-Poyatos HM, et al. Cardiovascular impact of COVID-19 with a focus on children: A systematic review. World J Clin Cases 2020;8(21):5250–83.

39. Kaushik A, Gupta S, Sood M, et al. A systematic review of multisystem inflammatory syndrome in children associated with SARS-CoV-2 infection. Pediatr Infect Dis J 2020;39(11):e340–6.

40. Fernandes DM, Oliveira CR, Guerguis S, et al. Severe acute respiratory syndrome coronavirus 2 clinical syndromes and predictors of disease severity in hospitalized children and youth. J Pediatr 2021;230:23–31.e10.

41. Henderson LA, Canna SW, Friedman KG, et al. American College of Rheumatology Clinical Guidance for Pediatric Patients with Multisystem Inflammatory Syndrome in Children (MIS-C) associated with SARS-CoV-2 and hyperinflammation in COVID-19. Version 2. Arthritis Rheumatol 2021; 73(4):e13–29.

42. Belhadjer Z, Auriau J, Meot M, et al. Addition of corticosteroids to immunoglobulins is associated with recovery of cardiac function in multi-inflammatory

syndrome in children. Circulation 2020;142(23): 2282–4.

43. Tabaac S, Kothari P, Cassidy-Smith T. Multisystem inflammatory syndrome in children. J Emerg Med 2021;60(4):531–5.

44. Catala A, Galvan-Casas C, Carretero-Hernandez G, et al. Maculopapular eruptions associated to COVID-19: A subanalysis of the COVID-Piel study. Dermatol Ther 2020;e14170.

45. Daneshgaran G, Dubin DP, Gould DJ. Cutaneous manifestations of COVID-19: An evidence-based review. Am J Clin Dermatol 2020;21(5):627–39.

46. Avellana Moreno R, Estela Villa LM, Avellana Moreno V, et al. Cutaneous manifestation of COVID-19 in images: a case report. J Eur Acad Dermatol Venereol 2020;34(7):e307–9.

47. Najarian DJ. Morbilliform exanthem associated with COVID-19. JAAD Case Rep 2020;6(6):493–4.

48. Ahouach B, Harent S, Ullmer A, et al. Cutaneous lesions in a patient with COVID-19: are they related? Br J Dermatol 2020;183(2):e31.

49. Shehi E, Chilimuri S, Shin D, et al. Microthrombi in skin biopsy of a patient with COVID-19. JAAD Case Rep 2020;6(12):1327–9.

50. Reymundo A, Fernaldez-Bernaldez A, Reolid A, et al. Clinical and histological characterization of late appearance maculopapular eruptions in association with the coronavirus disease 2019. A case series of seven patients. J Eur Acad Dermatol Venereol 2020;34(12):e755–7.

51. Rosell-Diaz AM, Mateos-Mayo A, Nieto-Benito LM, et al. Exanthema and eosinophilia in COVID-19 patients: has viral infection a role in drug induced exanthemas? J Eur Acad Dermatol Venereol 2020; 34(10):e561–3.

52. Peroni A, Colato C, Schena D, et al. Urticarial lesions: if not urticaria, what else? The differential diagnosis of urticaria: part I. Cutaneous diseases. J Am Acad Dermatol 2010;62(4):541–55. quiz 555-546.

53. Lu S, Lin J, Zhang Z, et al. Alert for non-respiratory symptoms of coronavirus disease 2019 patients in epidemic period: A case report of familial cluster with three asymptomatic COVID-19 patients. J Med Virol 2021;93(1):518–21.

54. Henry D, Ackerman M, Sancelme E, et al. Urticarial eruption in COVID-19 infection. J Eur Acad Dermatol Venereol 2020;34(6):e244–5.

55. Hassan K. Urticaria and angioedema as a prodromal cutaneous manifestation of SARS-CoV-2 (COVID-19) infection. BMJ Case Rep 2020;13(7).

56. Shanshal M. Low- dose systemic steroids, an emerging therapeutic option for COVID-19 related urticaria. J Dermatolog Treat 2020;1–2.

57. Quintana-Castanedo L, Feito-Rodriguez M, Valero-Lopez I, et al. Urticarial exanthem as early diagnostic clue for COVID-19 infection. JAAD Case Rep 2020;6(6):498–9.

58. Amatore F, Macagno N, Mailhe M, et al. SARS-CoV-2 infection presenting as a febrile rash. J Eur Acad Dermatol Venereol 2020;34(7):e304–6.

59. Lucas C, Wong P, Klein J, et al. Longitudinal analyses reveal immunological misfiring in severe COVID-19. Nature 2020;584(7821):463–9.

60. Criado PR, Abdalla BMZ, de Assis IC, et al. Are the cutaneous manifestations during or due to SARS-CoV-2 infection/COVID-19 frequent or not? Revision of possible pathophysiologic mechanisms. Inflamm Res 2020;69(8):745–56.

61. Kaushik A, Parsad D, Kumaran MS. Urticaria in the times of COVID-19. Dermatol Ther 2020;e13817.

62. Fernandez-Nieto D, Ortega-Quijano D, Jimenez-Cauhe J, et al. Clinical and histological characterization of vesicular COVID-19 rashes: a prospective study in a tertiary care hospital. Clin Exp Dermatol 2020;45(7):872–5.

63. Mahe A, Birckel E, Merklen C, et al. Histology of skin lesions establishes that the vesicular rash associated with COVID-19 is not 'varicella-like'. J Eur Acad Dermatol Venereol 2020;34(10):e559–61.

64. Marzano AV, Genovese G, Fabbrocini G, et al. Varicella-like exanthem as a specific COVID-19-associated skin manifestation: Multicenter case series of 22 patients. J Am Acad Dermatol 2020; 83(1):280–5.

65. Jimenez-Cauhe J, Ortega-Quijano D, Carretero-Barrio I, et al. Erythema multiforme-like eruption in patients with COVID-19 infection: clinical and histological findings. Clin Exp Dermatol 2020;45(7): 892–5.

66. Janah H, Zinebi A, Elbenaye J. Atypical erythema multiforme palmar plaques lesions due to Sars-Cov-2. J Eur Acad Dermatol Venereol 2020;34(8): e373–5.

67. Garcia-Gil MF, Garcia Garcia M, Monte Serrano J, et al. Acral purpuric lesions (erythema multiforme type) associated with thrombotic vasculopathy in a child during the COVID-19 pandemic. J Eur Acad Dermatol Venereol 2020;34(9):e443–5.

68. Khalili M, Iranmanesh B, Mohammadi S, et al. Cutaneous and histopathological features of coronavirus disease 2019 in pediatrics: A review article. Dermatol Ther 2020;e14554.

69. Labe P, Ly A, Sin C, et al. Erythema multiforme and Kawasaki disease associated with COVID-19 infection in children. J Eur Acad Dermatol Venereol 2020;34(10):e539–41.

70. de Masson A, Bouaziz JD, Sulimovic L, et al. Chilblains is a common cutaneous finding during the COVID-19 pandemic: A retrospective nationwide study from France. J Am Acad Dermatol 2020; 83(2):667–70.

71. Torrelo A, Andina D, Santonja C, et al. Erythema multiforme-like lesions in children and COVID-19. Pediatr Dermatol 2020;37(3):442–6.

72. Cohen PR. Sweet's syndrome–a comprehensive review of an acute febrile neutrophilic dermatosis. Orphanet J Rare Dis 2007;2:34.

73. Taskin B, Vural S, Altug E, et al. Coronavirus 19 presenting with atypical Sweet's syndrome. J Eur Acad Dermatol Venereol 2020;34(10):e534–5.

74. Wang J, Li Q, Yin Y, et al. Excessive neutrophils and neutrophil extracellular traps in COVID-19. Front Immunol 2020;11:2063.

75. Bomhof G, Mutsaers P, Leebeek FWG, et al. COVID-19-associated immune thrombocytopenia. Br J Haematol 2020;190(2):e61–4.

76. Mahevas M, Moulis G, Andres E, et al. Clinical characteristics, management and outcome of COVID-19-associated immune thrombocytopenia: a French multicentre series. Br J Haematol 2020;190(4): e224–9.

77. Murt A, Eskazan AE, Yilmaz U, et al. COVID-19 presenting with immune thrombocytopenia: A case report and review of the literature. J Med Virol 2021;93(1):43–5.

78. Zulfiqar AA, Lorenzo-Villalba N, Hassler P, et al. Immune thrombocytopenic purpura in a patient with Covid-19. N Engl J Med 2020;382(18):e43.

79. Yang Y, Zhao J, Wu J, et al. A rare case of immune thrombocytopenic purpura, secondary to COVID-19. J Med Virol 2020;92(11):2358–60.

80. Xu P, Zhou Q, Xu J. Mechanism of thrombocytopenia in COVID-19 patients. Ann Hematol 2020;99(6): 1205–8.

81. Yang X, Yang Q, Wang Y, et al. Thrombocytopenia and its association with mortality in patients with COVID-19. J Thromb Haemost 2020;18(6):1469–72.

Cutaneous Pathology of COVID-19 as a Window into Immunologic Mechanisms of Disease

Antonia E. Gallman, PhD[a,b], Marlys S. Fassett, MD, PhD[a,c],*

KEYWORDS

- COVID-19 • SARS-CoV-2 • Immunology • Autoantibody • Type I interferon • Chilblains • Livedo

KEY POINTS

- Both protective and autoreactive antibodies are produced during coronavirus disease 2019 (COVID-19) infection.
- Autoreactive antibody (autoantibody) targets detected in patients with COVID-19 include phospholipids as well as proteins expressed in skin, connective tissue, and vasculature.
- Autoantibodies likely contribute to the pathogenesis of multisystem inflammatory syndrome in children.
- Viral nucleotide sensing by the innate immune system may provide a mechanistic basis for the chilblains–COVID-19 association.
- Chilblains and severe COVID-19 lie at 2 ends of a type I interferon spectrum.

INTRODUCTION

Collaborative efforts among the international dermatology community have facilitated significant progress over the last year toward delineating the constellation of skin manifestations of severe acute respiratory syndrome coronavirus-2 (SARS-CoV-2) infection.[1,2] These cutaneous manifestations range from early viral exanthems to vasculopathy or vasculitis-associated–like skin lesions that typically appear weeks after systemic symptom onset (eg, livedo, acral cyanosis, chilblains, purpura).[3–11] Like fever, malaise, cough, and other common signs of viral infection, skin manifestations of coronavirus disease 2019 (COVID-19) reflect activation of both localized and systemic immune responses to the pathogen. Similar to other viruses, SARS-CoV-2 triggers both innate and adaptive immune responses, including complement, antibody-mediated, T cell–mediated, and cytokine-mediated inflammatory pathways.[12] This article discusses the ways in which dysregulation of the immune response contributes to COVID-19 pathology, with an emphasis on cutaneous manifestations of disease, as well as insights from genetic and autoimmune disease pathology. Elucidating the protective and pathologic features of the anti–SARS-CoV-2 immune response is directly relevant to clinical dermatologists because understanding mechanisms of disease is always an important first step toward optimizing skin-directed and systemic treatment.

Disclosure: The authors have no conflicts of interest to disclose.
[a] Department of Microbiology and Immunology, University of California, San Francisco, San Francisco, CA, USA; [b] Medical Scientist Training Program, University of California, San Francisco, 513 Parnassus Avenue, Room HSE1001A, San Francisco, CA 94143, USA; [c] Department of Dermatology, University of California, San Francisco, 513 Parnassus Avenue, Room HSE1001E, San Francisco, CA 94143, USA
* Corresponding author. 513 Parnassus Avenue, Room HSE1001E, San Francisco, CA 94143.
E-mail address: marlys.fassett@ucsf.edu

Dermatol Clin 39 (2021) 533–543
https://doi.org/10.1016/j.det.2021.05.008
0733-8635/21/© 2021 Elsevier Inc. All rights reserved.

Evidence of Intravascular Complement Activation in the Presence of Severe Acute Respiratory Syndrome Coronavirus-2 Proteins Highlights Contributions of Innate Immunity to Coronavirus Disease 2019–Associated Skin Conditions

Early clinical reports of critically ill patients with COVID-19 described skin findings suggestive of underlying vasculitis or vasculopathy, including livedo reticularis or racemosa, retiform purpura, and even acroischemia evolving to cyanosis and dry gangrene.[4–8,13] These observations supported the hypothesis that COVID-19 infection induces a hypercoagulable state in skin as in other organs.[14] When skin from patients with retiform purpura was biopsied, SARS-CoV-2 envelope and spike proteins were found deposited near vascular endothelial cells, along with striking amounts of complement.[4,8,13,15] Detected components of the complement cascade included elements of the lectin pathway as well as the terminal effector molecules of the membrane attack complex, proteins C5b to C9. Detection of complement deposition in situ in skin was informative because it suggested that this fundamental component of the innate immune system could trigger an overly vigorous immune response to the perceived threat and act as an inciting event to drive changes that ultimately result in immune disorder and harm to the host. The complement cascade is capable of activating the coagulation cascade,[16] and patients with COVID-19 with evidence of severe cutaneous vascular disorder also showed increased serum D-dimer levels and fibrin thrombi within cutaneous vessels.[4–8,13] Therefore, detection of complement in these early case reports from critically ill patients highlighted the important possibility that the immune response to SARS-CoV-2 proteins could play a central role in initiating this cutaneous vascular disorder, and COVID-19–associated skin disorder generally.

Humoral Immune Responses

Severe acute respiratory syndrome coronavirus-2 infection leads to activation of a humoral immune response and protective antibody production

The immune response to SARS-CoV-2 features the same fundamental building blocks that are used by the immune system to respond to all pathogens (Fig. 1). Epithelial and mucosal surfaces form a physical and chemical barrier to invasion. Breach of these defenses leads to immediate activation of the innate arm of the immune system. The innate immune system is able to recognize common molecular patterns unique to pathogens, including viruses such as SARS-CoV-2, allowing rapid mobilization of defensive cells and molecules

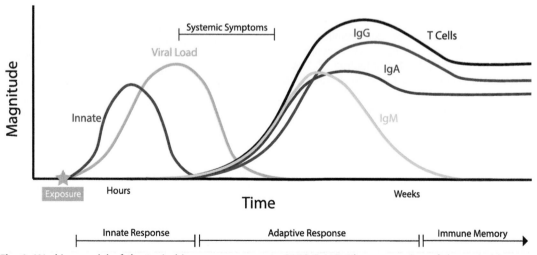

Fig. 1. Working model of the typical immune response to SARS-CoV-2. The progression of the typical immune response to SARS-CoV-2 in a patient with nonsevere disease.[12,17,18,20,22,82] The innate immune response is triggered immediately following viral exposure and acts to instruct the adaptive immune system. The adaptive immune response, consisting of lymphocyte activation and antibody production, takes several days to weeks to manifest. Although an increase in pathogen-specific immunoglobulin (Ig) M level usually precedes the appearance of other antibody isotypes, available data for patients with COVID-19 do not support a significantly earlier appearance of IgM compared with IgA and IgG.[18,22] IgA is found in serum as well as in saliva and respiratory tract secretions, and the magnitude and timing of its appearance in these two fluids may differ (not depicted).[22] T cells and B cells secreting IgG and IgA are maintained following infection, leading to immunologic memory.[24,25]

within hours of infection, such as activation of the complement cascade and production of type I interferons (IFNs), as discussed in this article. Often the actions of the innate immune system are sufficiently efficacious to dispel the threat to the host. However, a second essential function of the innate immune system is to instruct the adaptive immune system on the presence and nature of a pathogenic challenge. Although it takes weeks for an adaptive immune response by B and T lymphocytes to develop, these cells are capable of iteratively adapting their antigen receptor DNA sequences to evolve exquisitely specific capacities for recognition of individual pathogens. On recognition of pathogen-derived antigens, B and T lymphocytes target those pathogens with several effector mechanisms, one of which is the production of antibodies by B cell–derived plasma cells.[17]

The fundamental elements of the immune response to SARS-CoV-2 have been reviewed elsewhere,[12] but for the purposes of this review it is worth noting that the human adaptive immune system contains both T and B cells that can recognize the virus. Antibodies against SARS-CoV-2 viral components are detected in the serum and nasopharynx of infected patients.[18–22] Multiple classes of antibodies called isotypes are produced in the course of SARS-CoV-2 infection, including immunoglobulin (Ig) M, IgA, and IgG.[18,22] IgG is found in the bloodstream and in the extracellular spaces in tissues, and is the main isotype associated with disease protection. However, because SARS-CoV-2 is a respiratory virus that first encounters the immune system at mucosal surfaces, IgA also plays an important role. An initial large wave of IgA+ antibody-secreting B cells is in seen in the blood of patients, peaking between 10 and 15 days after symptom onset, followed by a wave of IgG+ antibody-secreting B cells that become dominant by day 22.[22] IgA+ cells express receptors for homing to mucosal tissues such as the respiratory tract, where they secrete IgA in a dimeric form. Studies on patients with COVID-19 have shown that dimeric IgA antibodies from the respiratory tract were many-fold more potent at SARS-CoV-2 neutralization compared with IgG, and remained detectable in saliva for several months after infection.[21,22]

Although severe cases of COVID-19 tend to generate higher titers of antibodies, some patients develop antibody responses even with mild or asymptomatic disease,[19] including skin-only presentations.[23] Low-titer to moderate-titer antibody production after mild infection has been shown to be sufficient for neutralizing viral entry,[19] and the antibodies generated seem to be long lived, having been measured up to 8 months following infection.[24,25]

The exquisite specificity of T and B lymphocytes is a powerful weapon in the arsenal of the immune system, but dysregulation of the adaptive response can lead these effector cells to become misguided, targeting host-derived self-antigens instead of foreign pathogen–derived antigens, in a process called autoreactivity. It is well established that viral infections can trigger autoreactive antibody production in susceptible individuals.[26] This article discusses growing evidence that dysregulation of the humoral immune response is a hallmark of SARS-CoV-2 infection, and may contribute to skin manifestations of COVID-19–associated disease.

Coronavirus disease 2019 infection can trigger autoreactive antibody formation

Antiphospholipid antibodies One mechanism by which autoantibody generation is thought to occur after infection is molecular mimicry, a naturally occurring phenomenon wherein T cells or antibody-producing B cells generated against pathogen-specific antigens also, by chance, bind host tissue because of structural similarity between pathogen-encoded proteins and host proteins.[27] A well-defined example of molecular mimicry occurs in rheumatic fever, in which antibodies generated during *Streptococcus pyogenes* infection react not only against *S pyogenes* but also against normal cardiac proteins.[28] Another group of autoantibodies thought to arise as a result of molecular mimicry are antiphospholipid antibodies; that is, antibodies that bind phospholipids and phospholipid-binding proteins present in cell membranes.[29] Intriguingly, 2 case series reported detection of antiphospholipid autoantibodies in approximately half of critically ill patients with COVID-19.[30,31] Other viral infections have been shown to increase the risk of developing antiphospholipid autoantibodies, and although in most cases these autoantibodies are present only transiently, persistent serum antiphospholipid antibodies have been reported in some patients and have been linked to thromboembolic events.[27] The presence of antiphospholipid antibodies in patients with COVID-19 is of note when considering skin manifestations of SARS-CoV-2. The intense deposition of complement appreciable in cutaneous biopsies from patients with COVID-19 with retiform purpura is reminiscent of what can be seen in antiphospholipid syndrome (APS),[29] a condition that can also manifest with retiform purpura and livedo reticularis.[32] In APS, the binding of antiphospholipid autoantibodies to endothelial cell membranes can tip the vasculature toward a prothrombotic state.[29]

Given the association between postviral or APS-associated antiphospholipid antibody production and thromboembolus formulation, it can be hypothesized that antiphospholipid autoantibodies may also contribute to late-onset vascular skin findings in patients with COVID-19. The time period between COVID-19 symptom onset and presentation of respiratory distress and livedo[8] roughly corresponds to the minimum window required for B-cell activation and antibody production. Furthermore, mouse models of APS also show deposition of C5b to C9 on the endothelial vasculature, as seen in patients with COVID-19, with the complement cascade in these mouse models playing a critical role in triggering the characteristic thromboses.[29] When researchers injected purified IgG from patients with COVID-19 into mouse models of thrombosis, the immunoglobulin from patients with COVID-19 accelerated thrombus formation in vivo, at levels comparable with immunoglobulin from patients with catastrophic APS.[31] Taken together, these data allow us to speculate that local immune stimulation, as shown by SARS-CoV-2 spike protein staining in the cutaneous vasculature,[4,8,13,15] may synergize with antiphospholipid autoantibodies found in patients with severe COVID-19 to jointly trigger the complement cascade and stimulate thrombosis. This thrombosis may result in rashes associated with underlying vascular insults: livedo reticularis/racemosa, retiform purpura, and acroischemia.

Multisystem inflammatory syndrome in children
Another COVID-19 disease process that may result from a dysregulated immune response leading to autoantibody production is the rare multisystem inflammatory syndrome in children (MIS-C). MIS-C presents weeks after mild or asymptomatic infection with SARS-CoV-2 and is marked by high fever, increased levels of inflammatory markers, end-organ damage, and mucocutaneous findings.[33–36] This clinical presentation is similar to that seen in Kawasaki disease, a medium-sized vessel vasculitis that commonly presents in children and is thought to result from the production of autoantibodies in response to acute viral infection.[37] Children with MIS-C show an altered immune profile compared with those with uncomplicated acute COVID-19 infection,[34–36] and several lines of evidence support the hypothesis that, like Kawasaki disease, MIS-C may represent a postinfectious inflammatory episode driven by SARS-CoV-2. First, MIS-C presents 4 to 6 weeks after confirmed SARS-CoV-2 expression, and it responds well to immunomodulatory therapies such as intravenous immunoglobulin, suggesting the involvement of circulating factors produced during the adaptive immune response.[34–36,38] Second, profiling of plasma from patients with MIS-C revealed the presence of autoantibodies that react to known autoantigens Jo-1 and La; to proteins involved in immune signaling pathways; and to factors expressed in normal endothelial, cardiac, and mucosal tissues.[34,35] Strikingly, these autoantibody targets mirror many organ system manifestations of MIS-C disease.[34,35] Children with MIS-C were shown to have increased numbers of proliferating antibody-secreting cells weeks after clearance of the virus, suggesting these cells may potentially be autoreactive, autoantibody-producing clones.[36] Furthermore, circulating neutrophils and monocytes in affected children showed increased expression of CD64, an Fc receptor that can engage autoantibodies and immune complexes, triggering tissue injury.[39,40] In addition, serum IgG from severely ill patients with MIS-C was shown to bind more tightly to cardiac endothelial cells in culture compared with serum from children with moderate MIS-C.[36] Although the pathophysiology behind this disease is just beginning to be elucidated, it can be posited that the severe inflammation, end-organ damage, and mucocutaneous responses seen in MIS-C are a result of an autoantibody-directed or immune-complex–directed attack against the host.

Broad autoreactivity found in coronavirus disease 2019 patient sera The broad spectrum of autoantibody tissue reactivity observed in case studies of children with MIS-C[34] suggests that molecular mimicry is insufficient to explain the large number of autoreactive lymphocytes that target such a wide variety of host antigens in multiple tissues. A recent article describes efforts to profile autoantibody-antigen specificities in adults with acute COVID-19 disease, allowing an exploration of the hypothesis that misguided antibody production could contribute to the wide spectrum of clinical presentations seen not only in MIS-C but in acute SARS-CoV-2 infection as well.[41] Remarkably, patients with COVID-19 show a dramatic increase in circulating autoantibodies compared with healthy controls, with the number of distinct autoantibody targets increasing with disease severity. For at least 10% of the autoreactivities identified, the autoreactive clones developed over the course of disease progression, implying that these 10% of autoreactivities are newly acquired, presumably as a result of COVID-19 infection. Many of these autoantibodies targeted various cells and tissues, including components of the immune system. The investigators were able to show that the autoantibodies corresponded to downstream alterations in their targeted immune signaling pathways or leukocyte frequencies. In some cases, there was dramatic depletion of autoantibody target cells, such as monocytes and B cells, which could contribute to impaired viral clearance.

Wang and colleagues[41] also reported a notable number of acutely ill patients with COVID-19 with circulating autoantibodies whose target antigens mirror the variety of organ systems known to be involved in the disease course. For example, more than 20 autoantibodies were identified as reactive to proteins of the central nervous system, an interesting finding considering the population of severe patients with COVID-19 who develop neurologic symptoms.[42] Of interest to the dermatology community, 26 of the identified autoantibodies were found to target the vasculature, connective tissue, and skin. Whether and how these autoantibodies contribute to the range of cutaneous findings of COVID-19 has yet to be established, but it seems plausible that they may augment the immune response that has been shown to be ongoing in the skin.

The breadth of targets across different patients is surprising and, as noted earlier, it suggests that self-reactive B-cell clones are unlikely to arise solely as a result of molecular mimicry. Instead it can be posited that the intense inflammatory milieu that has been described for COVID-19 is capable of disrupting fundamental tolerance checkpoints traditionally engaged by the adaptive immune system. Immunologists have described a phenomenon termed bystander activation in which an exaggerated immune response against a pathogenic challenge, such as a virus, leads to tissue damage and an increase in the exposure to self-antigens.[43] These antigens can activate local autoreactive B and T cells, manifesting as autoimmunity.[43] Autoreactivity may be an intrinsic part of the immunopathogenesis of COVID-19, but it remains to be seen whether this dysregulated host response is unique to SARS-CoV-2 or common to many other infections that have not been similarly investigated.

Chilblains as a Cutaneous Manifestation of Severe Acute Respiratory Syndrome Coronavirus-2

Evidence of an immune basis for severe acute respiratory syndrome coronavirus-2 association
Early in the COVID-19 pandemic, several case reports described children and adults with new-onset acral lesions closely resembling chilblains.[44–47] A definitive link between chilblains and COVID-19 has remained elusive because most patients in the gathered cohorts tested negative for serum antibodies against SARS-CoV-2,

and many reported no respiratory or systemic symptoms of COVID-19 infection. This finding led some investigators to propose that these lesions are not caused by SARS-CoV-2 but instead represent an epiphenomenon.[48–52] However, several studies provide histopathologic evidence that SARS-CoV-2 contributes to the pathogenesis of chilblains occurring during the pandemic. Two groups detected SARS-CoV-2 viral presence in skin biopsies from chilblains lesions. In a series of 7 pediatric cases, 1 group observed cytoplasmic granular positivity for the SARS-CoV-2 spike protein within vascular endothelial cells as well as in eccrine epithelial cells. Using electron microscopy, they were able to visualize spiked structures within the endothelial cells, which they interpreted as coronavirus particles.[53] A second group detected SARS-CoV-2 RNA as well as viral envelope and spike proteins within biopsy tissue from chilblains lesions, with well-described reagent controls.[13] In the latter case series, there was 1 patient with chilblains who tested negative for serum antibodies against SARS-CoV-2, but whose biopsy tissue contained detectable SARS-CoV-2 RNA and COVID-19 proteins, confirming presence of infection.[13]

These results highlight the potential for false-negative serum COVID-19 antibody testing in patients with true COVID-infected chilblains. Patients who present with chilblains but are otherwise asymptomatic are likely to evade polymerase chain reaction (PCR) and serology-based diagnostic testing for COVID-19 infection for multiple reasons. The authors hypothesize that a primary reason for the low sensitivity of COVID-19 PCR testing in patients with chilblains is one of test timing; the delayed onset of chilblains (ranging from 9 days to 1–2 months after onset of systemic symptoms, when present[9–11]) may occur after the window of nasopharyngeal viral particle shedding has closed. The low rate of COVID-19 seropositivity is more difficult to understand. Although many studies have reported cohorts with no seropositivity, 2 studies of 40 French and 19 Italian children detected serologic evidence of infection in 30% and 53% of children, respectively.[9,11] One hypothesis to explain low rates of seropositivity posits that an initial, highly robust innate immune system response in these patients facilitates viral clearance such that little antigen remains to stimulate a robust adaptive immune response.[11] Interestingly, IgA was revealed to be the most commonly detected antibody isotype in these groups, and several of the IgA+ patients were IgM and IgG negative. This finding is consistent with our unpublished case series of 7 adults in San Francisco, California, who developed chilblains during the first wave of infection; their blood was examined using an established enzyme-linked immunosorbent assay assay[54] for the presence of anti–SARS-CoV-2 IgA. In our cohort, 1 patient was IgA+IgM+IgG− and another was IgA+IgG+IgM−; 3 others were borderline positive for IgA and negative for the other isotypes. The development of anti-COVID serum IgA reactivity may reflect a strong initial mucosal immune response in patients infected with SARS-CoV-2 who go on to develop chilblains lesions. This article is working under the assumption that many chilblains cases arising during the COVID-19 pandemic represent cutaneous pathology caused by SARS-CoV-2 infection.

Numerous studies have examined the histology of COVID-associated chilblains lesions, with a consensus emerging regarding the typical features. They are characterized by superficial and deep perivascular inflammation that extends in many cases to the eccrine glands.[9,11,13,48–51,53,55–60] The inflammatory infiltrate is composed of mostly T cells, with a slight predominance of CD4+ rather than CD8+, and practically absent B cells. Interestingly, many studies have reported the presence of clusters of plasmacytoid dendritic cells (pDCs), cells of the innate immune system that are characterized by their strong production of the antiviral molecules, type I IFNs.[12,55,57,58] Endothelial cells are often found to be edematous or damaged, and vessels in many cases feature intraluminal microthrombi.[9,48,53] Although not noted in all cases, several reports highlight the findings of fibrinoid necrosis in the walls of the vessels and/or direct immunofluorescence staining for C3, IgM, and/or IgA.[9,11,48,58]

Familial chilblains pathogenesis provides clues to the inflammatory basis of coronavirus disease 2019–associated chilblains

Chilblains associated with COVID-19 is grossly and histologically similar to both idiopathic chilblains and familial chilblains, and this congruence may provide clues as to the pathophysiology of COVID-19–associated chilblains.[13,55] Familial chilblains is an inherited condition known to flare in colder temperatures, similar to recurrent chilblains associated with SARS-CoV-2 infection.[61,62] Familial chilblains is caused by specific mutations in intracellular exonucleases, which lead to inefficient nucleotide breakdown and thus intracellular nucleotide buildup.[63] Innate immune receptors whose responsibility is to sense the presence of pathogen-derived nucleotides within the cell can also detect this pathologic increase in nucleotides, mistake it for a sign of viral infection, and trigger activation of the type I IFN system. Patients with familial chilblains show broad granular deposits of C3 and IgM along the basement membrane in

cutaneous biopsies, as do mouse models of the disease, suggesting chilblain disorder involves not just the innate immune response but the adaptive immune response as well.[63,64] Skin biopsies from familial chilblains have increased expression of type I IFN–induced genes,[63] and the type I IFN response is central to the disease pathology, because genetic ablation of type I IFN signaling rescues mice from the development of autoimmunity.[65] Several studies have proposed that COVID-19–associated chilblains may be the result of an overactive type I IFN response,[13,55,57,59,60,66] a proposition that is supported by the presence of type I IFN–producing pDCs in COVID-19 chilblain biopsies, and by strong staining for the IFN-induced protein MxA in these biopsies.[13,55]

Type I Interferon Is Central to Coronavirus Disease 2019 Pathology

Increasing evidence suggests that activation of type I IFN pathways is essential for successful immune-mediated clearance of SARS-CoV-2. A critical arm of the immune response to many pathogens, the type I IFN family includes 3 secreted cytokines: IFN-α, IFN-β, and IFN-ω. These type I IFNs are produced toll-like receptor–mediated sensing of viral nucleotides. Type I IFNs are secreted and then sensed by other cells in the tissue environment, which respond by transcribing a large suite of antiviral genes. The system thus acts as an alarm, putting local cells on alert and bolstering the innate immune system in its initial response against viruses.[17] However, when type I IFNs are activated inappropriately in response to self-antigens or the buildup of nucleic acids, this same pathway can contribute to the development of autoimmune disease, as described earlier for familial chilblains, and as seen in other autoimmune diseases, including lupus.[67] Studies published in the summer of 2020 established that severe COVID-19 infections were correlated with low blood levels of type I IFN and low white blood cell expression of type I IFN–stimulated genes.[68,69] Two complementary studies subsequently showed that deficiencies in the type I IFN pathway, either through inherited mutations or the development of autoantibodies, predispose patients to developing severe COVID-19. In the first, Zhang and colleagues[70] show that 3.5% of patients with severe COVID-19 had inherited loss-of-function mutations in 8 genes involved in the pathway responsible for sensing viral nucleotides and leading to type I IFN production. In the accompanying study, Bastard and colleagues[71] examined whether autoantibodies specific for elements of the type I IFN pathway might predispose to severe COVID-19. Astonishingly, the investigators found that, of 937 people tested with severe COVID-19, 135 (or 13.5%) had autoantibodies against type I IFN, versus 0% of patients with mild or asymptomatic COVID-19 and 0.3% of healthy controls, in agreement with subsequent publications.[41] Three-fourths of these autoantibody-positive patients possessed autoantibodies capable of neutralizing downstream signaling of type I IFNs, which led to vastly reduced blood levels of type I IFN.

This article has discussed how inflammation induced by SARS-CoV-2 may lead to the development of autoantibodies. However, Bastard and colleagues[71] argue that the autoantibodies they detect against the type I IFN pathway in patients with COVID-19 may predate SARS-CoV-2 infection because they were detected at an early time point, within 1 to 2 weeks of symptom onset. In their study profiling broad autoreactivities, Wang and colleagues[41] also noted that 50% of the autoantibodies detected by their platform were present within 10 days of symptom onset, suggesting that many of these antibodies could have been preexisting in patients. Thus it can be hypothesized that preexisting autoantibodies may predispose patients to developing severe COVID-19. Intriguingly, these autoantibodies and genetic mutations against the type I IFN pathway were clinically silent before COVID-19 diagnosis, meaning that patients in the studies from Bastard and colleagues[71] and Zhang and colleagues[70] did not report any previous life-threatening infections. This finding suggests that although alternative mechanisms may protect these individuals against other viral pathogens, a successful type I IFN response may lie at the crux of successful immune defense against SARS-CoV-2.[72]

Chilblains and severe coronavirus disease 2019 lie at 2 ends of a type I interferon spectrum

Viruses are well known to use immunoevasive strategies to promote survival within their hosts.[73] SARS-CoV-2 uses many mechanisms to avoid triggering type I IFN responses.[74] Together with the observation that patients with severe COVID-19 are more likely to have disruptions in their type I IFN pathway,[70,71] this suggests that this axis is one of the major determinants of how an individual's immune system interacts with SARS-CoV-2. There may exist a spectrum of possible type I IFN responses, with strong or even overactive IFN responses at one end, and severe IFN impairment from inherited mutations or preexisting autoantibodies at the other. An individual's genetics and environment may dictate where they are on this spectrum, with severe COVID-19 disease as one outcome, and asymptomatic or mild SARS-CoV-2 infection as the polar opposite outcome. Chilblains may be one of the few

clinically apparent signs of a robust type I IFN response. When blood cells from hospitalized, ambulatory, and chilblains-only patients with COVID-19 were stimulated to examine their ability to produce type I IFN, the patients with chilblains produced significantly more IFN-a than the other 2 groups, even when the patients were age matched.[11] Type I IFNs have been shown directly to drive thrombotic microangiopathy in mouse models,[75] and recombinant IFN given therapeutically to patients with multiple sclerosis has also been associated with thrombotic events in several patients.[76,77] Thus SARS-CoV-2 infection may trigger a robust type I IFN response in young, genetically predisposed individuals that leads to the cutaneous disorder directly observed in COVID-19–associated chilblains.

Coronavirus Disease 2019 Longhaulers

Cutaneous disorder resulting from SARS-CoV-2 infection is intimately linked with the immune response to infection. Recent studies have underscored the role of the innate and adaptive immune systems in directing successful viral clearance but also the role these systems play in immune-mediated disorders.

With the epidemic ongoing, the number of patients with COVID-19 cared for by dermatologists will grow. Although most of these cutaneous manifestations are self-limited, there have been reports of so-called COVID-19 longhaulers, even in dermatology.[23] These patients include some with persistent chilblains and some with alopecia.[78] One commonly reported nondermatologic COVID longhauler symptom is postural tachycardia syndrome (POTS), in which patients develop an exaggerated orthostatic tachycardia. Recent research into POTS cases that predate the COVID-19 pandemic revealed that patients with this condition show autoantibodies against various receptors important in blood pressure regulation.[79–81] Some of the persistent cutaneous manifestations of COVID-19 may be similarly mediated by self-directed immune responses, a hypothesis that would be consistent with the number of autoreactivities that have been described against immune targets, phospholipids, and molecules expressed in vascular, connective, and mucosal tissues, and skin.[30,31,34,41] Further research is needed to examine the persistence and disease relevance of SARS-CoV-2–associated autoreactive T-cell and B-cell clones and the antibodies they produce.

SUMMARY

The immune system is intricately linked with the increasing number and variety of skin findings being reported by dermatologists over the course of this pandemic. Significant opportunities remain for additional research into the epidemiologic and biological relationships between immune pathways activated or dysregulated by SARS-CoV-2 and cutaneous manifestations of COVID-19 infection. This mechanistic understanding has the potential to highlight therapeutic opportunities to restore immune homeostasis in the skin.

CLINICS CARE POINTS

- It is possible to detect histopathologic evidence of SARS-CoV-2 infection in some patients who test negative for serum antibodies; consistent with Centers for Disease Control and Prevention guidelines, remember that a negative antibody test result cannot rule out infection in an individual patient.

- Because patients with COVID-19 are at increased risk of carrying autoantibodies and the long-term clinical consequences of this are unknown, it may be prudent to include COVID-19 antibody testing in the work-up for patients who develop new autoimmune disease manifestations after infection.

- The inverse relationship between type I interferons and COVID-19 disease severity suggests that therapeutically modulating this pathway may benefit patients with COVID-19 in the future.

ACKNOWLEDGMENTS

The authors wish to acknowledge Dr Jason Cyster, PhD, for helpful discussions. In addition, we wish to thank the patients and Dr Michael Wilson, MD; Kanishka Koshal; and Dr Jason Cyster, PhD, for their support in serology testing of patients with COVID-19 chilblains. This work was supported by NIAID F30AI150061 (AEG), NIAMS K08AR074556(MSF), and the Dermatology Foundation (MSF).

REFERENCES

1. Freeman EE, McMahon DE, Lipoff JB, et al. The spectrum of COVID-19–associated dermatologic manifestations: An international registry of 716 patients from 31 countries. J Am Acad Dermatol 2020;83(4):1118–29.

2. Jia JL, Kamceva M, Rao SA, et al. Cutaneous manifestations of COVID-19: A preliminary review. J Am Acad Dermatol 2020;83(2):687–90.

3. Naderi-Azad S, Vender R. Lessons From the First Wave of the Pandemic: Skin Features of COVID-19 can be Divided Into Inflammatory and Vascular Patterns. J Cutan Med Surg 2020;7(1). 120347542097234-120347542097238.

4. Droesch C, Do MH, DeSancho M, et al. Livedoid and Purpuric Skin Eruptions Associated With Coagulopathy in Severe COVID-19. JAMA Dermatol 2020; 156(9):1–3.

5. Zhang Y, Cao W, Xiao M, et al. Clinical and coagulation characteristics in 7 patients with critical COVID-2019 pneumonia and acro-ischemia. Chin J Hematol 2020;41(4):302–7.

6. Zhang Y, Xiao M, Zhang Z, et al. Coagulopathy and Antiphospholipid Antibodies in Patients with Covid-19. N Engl J Med 2020;382(17):1–3.

7. Del Giudice P, Boudoumi D, Le Guen B, et al. Catastrophic acute bilateral lower limbs necrosis associated with COVID-19 as a likely consequence of both vasculitis and coagulopathy. J Eur Acad Dermatol Venereol 2020;34(11):e679–80.

8. Magro C, Mulvey JJ, Berlin D, et al. Complement associated microvascular injury and thrombosis in the pathogenesis of severe COVID-19 infection: A report of five cases. Translational Res 2020;220:1–13.

9. Hachem El M, Diociaiuti A, Concato C, et al. A clinical, histopathological and laboratory study of 19 consecutive Italian paediatric patients with chilblain-like lesions: lights and shadows on the relationship with COVID-19 infection. J Eur Acad Dermatol Venereol 2020;34(11):2620–9.

10. Fernandez-Nieto D, Jimenez-Cauhe J, Suarez-Valle A, et al. Characterization of acute acral skin lesions in nonhospitalized patients: A case series of 132 patients during the COVID-19 outbreak. J Am Acad Dermatol 2020;83(1):e61–3.

11. Hubiche T, Cardot-Leccia N, Le Duff F, et al. Clinical, Laboratory, and Interferon-Alpha Response Characteristics of Patients With Chilblain-like Lesions During the COVID-19 Pandemic. JAMA Dermatol 2020;1–12. https://doi.org/10.1001/jamadermatol.2020.4324.

12. Sette A, Crotty S. Adaptive immunity to SARS-CoV-2 and COVID-19. Cell 2021;1–31. https://doi.org/10.1016/j.cell.2021.01.007.

13. Magro CM, Mulvey JJ, Laurence J, et al. The differing pathophysiologies that underlie COVID-19-associated perniosis and thrombotic retiform purpura: a case series. Br J Dermatol 2021;184(1):141–50.

14. Levi M, Thachil J, Iba T, et al. Coagulation abnormalities and thrombosis in patients with COVID-19. Lancet Haematol 2020;7(6):e438–40.

15. Magro CM, Mulvey J, Kubiak J, et al. Severe COVID-19: A multifaceted viral vasculopathy syndrome. Ann Diagn Pathol 2021;50:151645.

16. Foley JH, Conway EM. Cross Talk Pathways Between Coagulation and Inflammation. Circ Res 2016;118(9):1392–408.

17. Murphy K, Travers P, Walport M, et al. Janeway's immunobiology. 8th edition. New York, NY: Garland Science; 2012.

18. Long Q-X, Liu B-Z, Deng H-J, et al. Antibody responses to SARS-CoV-2 in patients with COVID-19. Nat Med 2020;1–15. https://doi.org/10.1038/s41591-020-0897-1.

19. Robbiani DF, Gaebler C, Muecksch F, et al. Convergent antibody responses to SARS-CoV-2 in convalescent individuals. Nature 2020;1–23. https://doi.org/10.1038/s41586-020-2456-9.

20. Rodda LB, Netland J, Shehata L, et al. Functional SARS-CoV-2-Specific Immune Memory Persists after Mild COVID-19. Cell 2021;184(1):169–83.e17.

21. Wang Z, Lorenzi JCC, Muecksch F, et al. Enhanced SARS-CoV-2 neutralization by dimeric IgA. Sci Translational Med 2021;13(577):1–13.

22. Sterlin D, Mathian A, Miyara M, et al. IgA dominates the early neutralizing antibody response to SARS-CoV-2. Sci Translational Med 2021;13(577):eabd2223.

23. McMahon DE, Gallman AE, Hruza GJ, et al. Comment Long COVID in the skin: a registry analysis of COVID-19 dermatological duration. Lancet Infect Dis 2021;1–2. https://doi.org/10.1016/S1473-3099(20)30986-5.

24. Dan JM, Mateus J, Kato Y, et al. Immunological memory to SARS-CoV-2 assessed for up to 8 months after infection. Science 2021. https://doi.org/10.1126/science.abf4063. eabf4063–23.

25. Gaebler C, Wang Z, Lorenzi JCC, et al. Evolution of antibody immunity to SARS-CoV-2. Nature 2021;1–33. https://doi.org/10.1038/s41586-021-03207-w.

26. Novelli L, Motta F, De Santis M, et al. The JANUS of chronic inflammatory and autoimmune diseases onset during COVID-19 – A systematic review of the literature. J Autoimmun 2021;117:102592.

27. Mendoza-Pinto C, García-Carrasco M, Cervera R. Role of Infectious Diseases in the Antiphospholipid Syndrome (Including Its Catastrophic Variant). Curr Rheumatol Rep 2018;1–7. https://doi.org/10.1007/s11926-018-0773-x.

28. Cunningham MW. Rheumatic Fever, Autoimmunity, and Molecular Mimicry: The Streptococcal Connection. Int Rev Immunol 2014;33(4):314–29.

29. Chaturvedi S, Brodsky RA, McCrae KR. Complement in the Pathophysiology of the Antiphospholipid Syndrome. Front Immunol 2019;10:295–9.

30. Xiao M, Zhang Y, Zhang S, et al. Antiphospholipid Antibodies in Critically Ill Patients With COVID-19. Arthritis Rheumatol 2020;72(12):1998–2004.

31. Zuo Y. Prothrombotic autoantibodies in serum from patients hospitalized with COVID-19. Sci Translational Med 2020;12(570):1–12.

32. Toubi E, Shoenfeld Y. Livedo Reticularis as a Criterion for Antiphospholipid Syndrome. Clinic Rev Allerg Immunol 2007;32(2):138–44.

33. Young TK, Shaw KS, Shah JK, et al. Mucocutaneous Manifestations of Multisystem Inflammatory Syndrome in Children During the COVID-19 Pandemic. JAMA Dermatol 2020;1–6. https://doi.org/10.1001/jamadermatol.2020.4779.

34. Gruber CN, Patel RS, Trachtman R, et al. Mapping Systemic Inflammation and Antibody Responses in Multisystem Inflammatory Syndrome in Children (MIS-C). Cell 2020;183(4):982–95.e14.

35. Consiglio CR, Cotugno N, Sardh F, et al. The Immunology of Multisystem Inflammatory Syndrome in Children with COVID-19. Cell 2020;183(4):968–81.e7.

36. Ramaswamy A, Brodsky NN, Sumida TS, et al. Immune dysregulation and autoreactivity correlate with disease severity in SARS-CoV-2-associated multisystem inflammatory syndrome in children. Immunity 2021;54(5):1083–95. e7.

37. Sakurai Y. Autoimmune Aspects of Kawasaki Disease. J Investig Allergol Clin Immunol 2019;29(4):251–61.

38. Kazatchkine MD, Kaveri SV. Immunomodulation of autoimmune and inflammatory diseases with intravenous immune globulin. N Engl J Med 2001;345(10):1–9.

39. van der Poel CE, Spaapen RM, van de Winkel JGJ, et al. Functional Characteristics of the High Affinity IgG Receptor, FcγRI. J Immunol 2011;186(5):2699–704.

40. Tanaka M, Krutzik SR, Sieling PA, et al. Activation of FcγRI on Monocytes Triggers Differentiation into Immature Dendritic Cells That Induce Autoreactive T Cell Responses. J Immunol 2009;183(4):2349–55.

41. Wang EY, Mao T, Klein J, et al. Diverse Functional Autoantibodies in Patients with COVID-19. Nature 2021.

42. Mao L, Jin H, Wang M, et al. Neurologic Manifestations of Hospitalized Patients With Coronavirus Disease 2019 in Wuhan, China. JAMA Neurol 2020;77(6):683–8.

43. Getts DR, Chastain EML, Terry RL, et al. Virus infection, antiviral immunity, and autoimmunity. Immunol Rev 2013;255(1):197–209.

44. Mazzotta F, Troccoli T. Acute acro-ischemia in the child at the time of COVID-19. Eur J Pediat Dermatol 2020;30:71–4.

45. Romaní J, Baselga E, Mitjà O, et al. Chilblain and Acral Purpuric Lesions in Spain during Covid Confinement: Retrospective Analysis of 12 Cases. Actas Dermosifiliogr 2020;111(5):426–9.

46. Alramthan A, Aldaraji W. Two cases of COVID-19 presenting with a clinical picture resembling chilblains: first report from the Middle East. Clin Exp Dermatol 2020;45(6):746–8.

47. Galván Casas C, Català A, Carretero Hernández G, et al. Classification of the cutaneous manifestations of COVID-19: a rapid prospective nationwide consensus study in Spain with 375 cases. Br J Dermatol 2020;183(1):71–7.

48. Herman A, Peeters C, Verroken A, et al. Evaluation of Chilblains as a Manifestation of the COVID-19 Pandemic. JAMA Dermatol 2020;156(9):998–1003.

49. Roca-Ginés J, Torres-Navarro I, Sánchez-Arráez J, et al. Assessment of Acute Acral Lesions in a Case Series of Children and Adolescents During the COVID-19 Pandemic. JAMA Dermatol 2020;156(9): 992–6.

50. Hébert V, Duval-Modeste A-B, Joly P, et al. Lack of association between chilblains outbreak and severe acute respiratory syndrome coronavirus 2: Histologic and serologic findings from a new immunoassay. J Am Acad Dermatol 2020;83(5):1434–6.

51. Denina M, Pellegrino F, Morotti F, et al. All that glisters is not COVID: Low prevalence of seroconversion against SARS-CoV-2 in a pediatric cohort of patients with chilblain-like lesions. J Am Acad Dermatol 2020;183(4):729–37. https://doi.org/10.1016/j.jaad.2020.08.021.

52. Stavert R. Evaluation of SARS-CoV-2 antibodies in 24 patients presenting with chilblains-like lesions during the COVID-19 pandemic. J Am Acad Dermatol 2020;34(7):1–4.

53. Colmenero I, Santonja C, Alonso Riaño M, et al. SARS-CoV-2 endothelial infection causes COVID-19 chilblains: histopathological, immunohistochemical and ultrastructural study of seven paediatric cases. Br J Dermatol 2020;183(4):729–37.

54. Whitman JD, Hiatt J, Mowery CT, et al. Evaluation of SARS-CoV-2 serology assays reveals a range of test performance. Nat Biotechnol 2020;1–15. https://doi.org/10.1038/s41587-020-0659-0.

55. Battesti G, Khalifa El J, Abdelhedi N, et al. New insights in COVID-19 associated chilblains: A comparative study with chilblain lupus erythematosus. J Am Acad Dermatol 2020;83(4):1219–22.

56. de Masson A, Bouaziz J-D, Sulimovic L, et al. Chilblains is a common cutaneous finding during the COVID-19 pandemic: A retrospective nationwide study from France. J Am Acad Dermatol 2020; 83(2):667–70.

57. Sohier P, Matar S, Meritet J-F, et al. Histopathological features of Chilblain-like lesions developing in the setting of the COVID-19 pandemic. Arch Pathol Lab Med 2020;1–29. https://doi.org/10.5858/arpa.2020-0613-SA.

58. Kanitakis J, Lesort C, Danset M, et al. Chilblain-like acral lesions during the COVID-19 pandemic ("COVID toes"): Histologic, immunofluorescence, and immunohistochemical study of 17 cases. J Am Acad Dermatol 2020;83(3):870–5.

59. Cordoro KM, Reynolds SD, Wattier R, et al. Clustered cases of acral perniosis: Clinical features, histopathology, and relationship to COVID-19. Pediatr Dermatol 2020;37(3):419–23.

60. Kolivras A, Dehavay F, Delplace D, et al. Coronavirus (COVID-19) infection-induced chilblains: A case report with histopathologic findings. JAAD Case Rep 2020;6(6):489–92.

61. Orcesi S, La Piana R, Fazzi E. Aicardi-Goutieres syndrome. Br Med Bull 2009;89:183–201.

62. Freeman EE, McMahon DE, Lipoff JB, et al. Cold and COVID: Recurrent Pernio during the COVID-19 Pandemic. Br J Dermatol 2021. https://doi.org/10.1111/bjd.19894.

63. Peschke K, Friebe F, Zimmermann N, et al. Deregulated Type I IFN Response in TREX1-Associated Familial Chilblain. Lupus 2010;1–4. https://doi.org/10.1038/jid.2013.496.

64. Günther C, Berndt N, Wolf C, et al. Familial Chilblain Lupus Due to a Novel Mutation in the Exonuclease III Domain of 3′ Repair Exonuclease 1 (TREX1). JAMA Dermatol 2015;151(4):426.

65. Stetson DB, Ko JS, Heidmann T, et al. Trex1 Prevents Cell-Intrinsic Initiation of Autoimmunity. Cell 2008;134(4):587–98.

66. Damsky W, Peterson D, King B. When interferon tiptoes through COVID-19: Pernio-like lesions and their prognostic implications during SARS-CoV-2 infection. J Am Acad Dermatol 2020;83(3): e269–70.

67. Crow MK. Type I Interferon in the Pathogenesis of Lupus. J Immunol 2014;192(12):5459–68.

68. Trouillet-Assant S, Viel S, Gaymard A, et al. Type I IFN immunoprofiling in COVID-19 patients. J Allergy Clin Immunol 2020;146(1):206–8.e2.

69. Hadjadj J, Yatim N, Barnabei L, et al. Impaired type I interferon activity and inflammatory responses in severe COVID-19 patients. Science 2020; 369(6504):718.

70. Zhang Q, Bastard P, Liu Z, et al. Inborn errors of type I IFN immunity in patients with life-threatening COVID-19. Science 2020;370(6515). eabd4570–16.

71. Bastard P, Rosen LB, Zhang Q, et al. Autoantibodies against type I IFNs in patients with life-threatening COVID-19. Science 2020;370(6515). eabd4585–15.

72. Meffre E, Iwasaki A. Interferon deficiency can lead to severe COVID. Nature 2020;587(7834):374–6.

73. Ploegh HL. Viral Strategies of Immune Evasion. Science 1998;280(5361):248–53.

74. Blanco-Melo D, Nilsson-Payant BE, Liu W-C, et al. Imbalanced Host Response to SARS-CoV-2 Drives Development of COVID-19. Cell 2020;181(5): 1036–45.e9.

75. Kavanagh D, McGlasson S, Jury A, et al. Type I interferon causes thrombotic microangiopathy by a dose-dependent toxic effect on the microvasculature. Blood 2016;128(24):2824–33.

76. Larochelle C, Grand'maison F, Bernier GP, et al. Thrombotic thrombocytopenic purpura-hemolytic uremic syndrome in relapsing-remitting multiple sclerosis patients on high-dose interferon β. Mult Scler 2014;20(13):1783–7.

77. Hunt D, Kavanagh D, Drummond I, et al. Thrombotic Microangiopathy Associated with Interferon Beta. N Engl J Med 2014;370(13):1268–70.

78. Xiong Q, Xu M, Li J, et al. Clinical sequelae of COVID-19 survivors in Wuhan, China: a single-centre longitudinal study. Clin Microbiol Infect 2021;27(1):89–95.

79. Li H, Yu X, Liles C, et al. Autoimmune basis for postural tachycardia syndrome. JAHA 2014;3(1): e000755.

80. Fedorowski A, Li H, Yu X, et al. Antiadrenergic auto-immunity in postural tachycardia syndrome. EP Europace 2016;19(7):1211–9.

81. Yu X, Li H, Murphy TA, et al. Angiotensin II Type 1 Receptor Autoantibodies in Postural Tachycardia Syndrome. JAHA 2018;7(8):e008351.

82. Wu KJ, Corum J. Charting a Covid-19 Immune Response. The New York Times 2020. Available at: https://www.nytimes.com/interactive/2020/10/05/science/charting-a-covid-immune-response.html.

The Use of Biologics During the COVID-19 Pandemic

Madison E. Jones, BA[a], Alison H. Kohn, BS[b], Sarah P. Pourali, BS[c],
Jeffrey R. Rajkumar, BS[d], Yasmin Gutierrez, BS[e], Rebecca M. Yim, BA[a],
April W. Armstrong, MD, MPH[a],*

KEYWORDS

- COVID-19 • Biologics • Psoriasis • Atopic dermatitis • Hidradenitis suppurativa • TNF-Inhibitor
- IL inhibitor • Dupilumab

KEY POINTS

- For biologics used in psoriasis, such as tumor necrosis factor inhibitors, interleukin (IL)-12/23 inhibitors, IL-17 inhibitors, and IL-23 inhibitors, current data suggest that they do not seem to increase the risk of coronavirus disease 2019 (COVID-19) infection or worsened COVID-19 outcomes. It is generally recommended that patients with psoriasis not actively infected with severe acute respiratory syndrome coronavirus-2 (SARS-CoV-2) initiate or continue their biologics to treat moderate to severe psoriasis.
- Adalimumab is the only biologic currently US Food and Drug Administration (FDA) approved to treat hidradenitis suppurativa. In patients on adalimumab to treat hidradenitis suppurativa, current data suggest that adalimumab does not seem to increase the risk of COVID-19 infection or worsened COVID-19 outcomes. It is generally recommended that patients with hidradenitis suppurativa not actively infected with SARS-CoV-2 initiate or continue adalimumab to treat moderate to severe hidradenitis suppurativa.
- Dupilumab is the only biologic currently FDA approved to treat moderate to severe atopic dermatitis. In patients on dupilumab to treat atopic dermatitis, current data suggest that dupilumab does not seem to increase the risk of COVID-19 infection or worsened COVID-19 outcomes. It is generally recommended that patients with atopic dermatitis not actively infected with SARS-CoV-2 initiate or continue dupilumab to treat moderate to severe atopic dermatitis.

INTRODUCTION

The coronavirus disease 2019 (COVID-19) pandemic has prompted questions regarding the use of biologics in patients with inflammatory skin conditions. Infection with COVID-19 incites an initial antiviral response, followed by a systemic inflammatory response.[1] The multiphasic immune response involves numerous cytokines, few of which serve as biologic therapy targets. Note that the cytokines involved in the antiviral and systemic hyperinflammatory responses differ. Viral

All hard copies of the journal edition may be mailed to the USC Dermatology Research Office: 1441 Eastlake Ave, Norris Topping Tower Suite 3427, Los Angeles, CA 90033.

[a] University of Southern California Keck School of Medicine, Los Angeles, CA, USA; [b] Florida Atlantic University Charles E Schmidt College of Science, 777 Glades Road BC-71, Boca Raton, FL 33431, USA; [c] Vanderbilt University School of Medicine, 1161 21st Ave S # D3300, Nashville, TN 37232, USA; [d] Univeristy of Illinois College of Medicine at Chicago, 1853 W Polk St, Chicago, IL 60612, USA; [e] University of California Riverside School of Medicine, 92521 Botanic Gardens Dr, Riverside, CA 92507, USA

* Corresponding author. University of Southern California, 1975 Zonal Avenue, KAM 510, MC 9034, Los Angeles, CA 90089.

E-mail address: armstrongpublication@gmail.com

Dermatol Clin 39 (2021) 545–553
https://doi.org/10.1016/j.det.2021.05.010

clearance primarily involves interleukin (IL)-15, interferon alpha (IFN-α)/IFN-β, and IFNγ, whereas the systemic hyperinflammatory response primarily involves tumor necrosis factor (TNF), IL-6, IL-17A, granulocyte-macrophage colony-stimulating factor, and granulocyte colony-stimulating factor.[2] Many biologics target the proinflammatory cytokines involved in the systemic hyperinflammatory phase, but they often do not target key antiviral cytokines, and thereby leave the antiviral response unaffected.[2] In addition, because biologics target specific mediators of the immune system, they do not cause broad immunosuppression. In certain circumstances, biologics may even exert beneficial effects by attenuating the hyperinflammatory state seen in severe COVID-19; several are being studied for their therapeutic effects in COVID-19.[2] This article discusses the latest guidance on biologic use during the COVID-19 pandemic for inflammatory skin conditions, including psoriasis, hidradenitis suppurativa, and atopic dermatitis (AD).

PSORIASIS

Among inflammatory skin conditions, moderate to severe plaque psoriasis currently has the most biologics US Food and Drug Administration (FDA) approved for its treatment. The latest guidance for each biologic class FDA approved to treat psoriasis is discussed here, including TNF-α inhibitors, IL-12/23 inhibitors, IL-17 inhibitors, and IL-23 inhibitors in the context of the COVID-19 pandemic.

Tumor Necrosis Factor Alpha Inhibitors (Adalimumab, Certolizumab, Etanercept, and Infliximab)

The TNF-α inhibitors currently FDA approved to treat psoriasis and psoriatic arthritis (PsA) include adalimumab, certolizumab, etanercept, and infliximab. These biologics work by inhibiting TNF-α, a proinflammatory cytokine, effectively reducing the downstream surge in inflammation seen in psoriasis.[3]

Several studies have investigated the effect of TNF-inhibitors on COVID-19 susceptibility. In order to assess this effect, a meta-analysis used data from previous clinical trials to extrapolate the potential risk of a medication based on its respiratory tract infection (RTI) rate compared with placebo.[4] The data included reported findings from phase 3 pivotal trials for adalimumab, infliximab, etanercept, and certolizumab.[4] The meta-analysis found that there was no significant risk of RTI in TNF inhibitors compared with placebo (odds ratio [OR], 1.06; 95% confidence interval [CI], 0.81–1.40; $P = .55$).[4]

Observational studies have gathered real-world data to assess the effect of TNF inhibitors on COVID-19. A prospective case series in New York assessed 86 patients with known immune-mediated inflammatory disease (IMID) who were receiving biologics or other immunomodulatory therapies when they contracted COVID-19.[5] The level of patient care required to treat COVID-19 was then characterized by capturing whether the patients were hospitalized or received only outpatient care. Importantly, this study found that the incidence rate for COVID-19 hospitalization among patients with IMID was consistent with the general population.[5] Furthermore, TNF inhibitors were not associated with increased odds of COVID-19 hospitalization (OR, 0.15; 95% CI, 0.02–1.12).[5] Similarly, a retrospective cohort study based in Detroit, Michigan, assessed 213 patients with IMID who were receiving treatment with immunosuppressive therapies during the COVID-19 pandemic.[6] The IMID cohort receiving immunosuppressive treatment had similar odds of COVID-19 infection, hospitalization, need for invasive ventilation, and mortality compared with the general population.[6] Furthermore, biologics predicted a decreased rate of hospitalization (OR, 0.26; 95% CI, 0.066–0.95), which was driven by anti-TNF monotherapy (OR, 0.16; 95% CI, 0.032–0.72).[6]

Together, the current clinical trial and real-world data suggest that being on TNF inhibitors does not seem to increase patients' risk of contracting severe acute respiratory syndrome coronavirus-2 (SARS-CoV-2), and, when infected, patients do not seem to experience worsened COVID-19 outcomes compared with the general population. Additional recommendations by US and international organizations for biologics used in psoriasis are provided later and are outlined in **Table 1**. The American Academy of Dermatology (AAD) also provides non–disease-specific guidance for the use of systemic medications in dermatology.[7]

interleukin -12/23 Inhibitors (Ustekinumab)

There is currently only 1 FDA-approved biologic for psoriasis and PsA that inhibits IL-12/23, which is ustekinumab. Ustekinumab works by binding to the p40 protein subunit used by both IL-23 and IL-12.[3] Ustekinumab disrupts IL-23–mediated and IL-12–mediated signaling of T-helper (Th) 17 and Th1 pathways, thereby reducing the feed-forward inflammatory mechanism in psoriasis.[3]

To help inform the impact of IL-12/23 inhibitors on COVID-19 susceptibility, a meta-analysis using phase 3 clinical trial data evaluated the risk of RTIs in patients with autoimmune disease on IL-12/23 and IL-23 inhibitors compared with those on

Table 1
Summary of recommendations on psoriasis management by international and US organizations during the coronavirus disease 2019 pandemic, as of April 1, 2021[a]

Status of Infection	International Recommendation: IPC and the EADV Psoriasis Task Force/SPIN	US Recommendation: NPF
No active COVID-19 infection, on systemic therapy (ie, biologics or oral medications)	Continue taking systemic therapy (EADV)	Continue taking systemic therapy
High-risk group, on immunomodulatory agents	Consult a health care provider regarding these risk factors[b] (EADV)	Consult a health care provider regarding these risk factors[c]
No active COVID-19 infection, being considered to initiate immunomodulatory agents	No statement at the time of writing	Consult a health care provider
COVID-19 infection, on systemic therapy (ie, biologics or oral medications)	Discontinue or postpone taking immunosuppressant treatment (IPC, EADV)	Consult a health care provider
Recovered from COVID-19	No statement at the time of writing	Consult a health care provider

Professional Organization	Resource
IPC	https://www.psoriasiscouncil.org/blog/Statement-on-COVID-19-and-Psoriasis.htm
EADV Psoriasis Task Force/SPIN	https://www.eadv.org/cms-admin/showfile/7_PSORIASIS-SPIN%20TF%20Recommandations_Covid-Corner.pdf
NPF	https://www.psoriasis.org/advance/coronavirus

Abbreviations: EADV, European Association of Dermatology and Venereology; IPC, International Psoriasis Council; NPF, National Psoriasis Foundation.

[a] The American Academy of Dermatology (AAD) also issued recommendations for biologics, but they are not specific to a particular disease state. They are recommendations for all patients with dermatologic diseases on immunosuppressive agents during the COVID-19 pandemic.

[b] For EADV, high-risk is defined as advanced age (60 or older), have underlying health conditions (ie, obesity, diabetes, hypertension, cardiovascular disease, chronic lung disease, asthma), and those who live in an area of high incidence of COVID-19 or those who have close contacts of confirmed persons with COVID-19.

[c] For NPF, high risk is defined as advanced age (65 years or older) and having comorbidities such as chronic lung, heart, or kidney disease and metabolic disorders such as diabetes and obesity.

placebo.[8] The analysis distinguished between upper RTIs (URTIs) and viral URTIs; viral URTI served as the model for coronavirus infection comparison. IL-12/23 and IL-23 antagonists were found to increase risk of URTIs (Mantel-Haenszel risk difference [MHRD], 0.019; 95% CI, 0.005–0.033; $P = .007$), but not viral URTIs (MHRD, 0.001; 95% CI, -0.002–0.003; $P = .60$).[8] When examined alone, ustekinumab did not increase the risk of viral URTIs (MHRD, 0.001; 95% CI, -0.002–0.004; $P = .42$).[8]

Real-world data also suggest that IL-12/23 inhibitors may be used safely during the COVID-19 pandemic.[5] In the New York–based case series examining patients with IMID, ustekinumab was not associated with increased rates of COVID-19 hospitalization (OR, 0.86; 95% CI, 0.65–1.15).[5]

Together, the current clinical trial and real-world data suggest that being on IL-12/23 inhibitors does not seem to increase patients' risk of contracting SARS-CoV-2, and, when infected, patients do not seem to experience worsened COVID-19 outcomes compared with the general population. Additional recommendations are provided later and outlined in **Table 1**.

Interleukin -17 Inhibitors (Secukinumab, Ixekizumab, and Brodalumab)

The IL-17 inhibitors currently FDA approved to treat psoriasis and PsA include secukinumab and ixekizumab. Brodalumab is FDA approved for psoriasis, and it is also approved in other countries for PsA. By inhibiting IL-17, these medications mitigate the downstream inflammatory response in psoriasis.[3] Although IL-17 is not a key contributor to viral clearance, it is important to understand the impact of IL-17 inhibition in the context of COVID-19.[9]

A meta-analysis using pivotal clinical trial data for secukinumab, ixekizumab, and brodalumab assessed the risk of RTIs in patients on IL-17 inhibitors compared with placebo.[9] The study found an increased risk of RTIs in patients receiving IL-17 inhibitors compared with placebo (OR, 1.56; 95% CI, 1.04–2.33).[9] However, this study noted that evaluating the risk of RTI in clinical trials is difficult because the diagnosis of RTI is made clinically, without objective testing.[9] Therefore, the cause of RTI symptoms is unknown and could be viral, bacterial, or allergic. This study suggested that further evaluation is needed to understand the impact of IL-17 on RTIs in the setting of the COVID-19 pandemic.[9]

Real-world data suggest that patients on IL-17 inhibitors do not experience worsened COVID-19 disease severity compared with the general population.[5] For example, the New York–based case series found that patients with IMID taking IL-17 inhibitors do not have increased odds of COVID-19 hospitalization compared with the general population (OR, 0.48; 95% CI, 0.03–1.23).[5]

Together, the current clinical trial and real-world data suggest that being on IL-17 inhibitors does not seem to increase patients' risk of contracting SARS-CoV-2, and, when infected, patients do not seem to experience worsened COVID-19 outcomes compared with the general population. Additional recommendations are provided later and outlined in **Table 1**.

Interleukin-23 Inhibitors (Guselkumab, Tildrakizumab, and Risankizumab)

The IL-23 inhibitors currently FDA approved to treat psoriasis include guselkumab, tildrakizumab, and risankizumab. Guselkumab is also FDA approved for PsA. IL-23 plays a central role in maintaining Th17 cells. Although IL-23 is not a key contributor to antiviral response, because of its effect on mucosal immunity, it is important to understand IL-23 inhibition in the context of COVID-19 infection.[8]

As previously mentioned, a meta-analysis of pivotal clinical trial data investigated the impact of IL-12/23 and IL-23 antagonists on COVID-19 susceptibility. This meta-analysis found that IL-12/23 and IL-23 antagonists increased the risk of

URTIs, but they did not increase the risk of viral URTIs.[8] When evaluated alone, IL-23 antagonists did not increase the risk of viral URTIs (OR, 1.15; 95% CI, 0.88–1.49).[8]

Real-world data corroborate the safe usage of IL-23 inhibitors during the pandemic. In the New York prospective case series of patients with IMID, IL-23 blockers were not associated with increased hospitalization compared with the general population (OR, 0.75; 95% CI, 0.50–1.12).[5]

Together, the current clinical trial and real-world data suggest that being on IL-23 inhibitors does not seem to increase patients' risk of contracting SARS-CoV-2, and, when infected, patients do not seem to experience worsened COVID-19 outcomes compared with the general population. Additional recommendations are provided later and outlined in **Table 1**.

Additional Real-world Data of Psoriasis Biologics in Coronavirus Disease 2019

Several studies investigating the impact of psoriasis biologics on COVID-19 do not delineate results by the different biologic classes, and instead group the results of biologics together as a whole. In 1 study, 2 Italian provinces collected data from telemedicine visits in 246 patients with psoriasis on biologic or small-molecule therapy.[10] Only 1 patient tested positive for COVID-19, and this patient remained asymptomatic.[10] The study concluded that psoriasis (whether treated by biologic or small-molecule therapy or not) does not confer a higher risk of COVID-19 infection.[10] A separate study in Verona, Italy, compared the risk of hospitalization or death caused by COVID-19 in 980 patients with psoriasis on biologics versus the general population of Verona.[11] Patients with psoriasis on biologics did not have increased rates of hospitalization and death compared with the general population.[11] A global registry-based study investigated the impact of biologics on COVID-19 outcomes in patients with psoriasis.[12] Out of 374 patients with psoriasis with confirmed or suspected COVID-19, 71% were receiving a biologic, 18% were receiving a nonbiologic, and 10% were not receiving any systemic treatment of psoriasis.[12] The study found that hospitalization was more frequent in patients using nonbiological therapy than in those using biologics (OR, 2.84; 95% CI, 1.31–6.18).[12]

Summary of Recommendations for the Use of Psoriasis Biologics in Coronavirus Disease 2019

In order to provide evidence-based guidelines on psoriasis management during the pandemic, the

National Psoriasis Foundation (NPF) in the United States established a COVID-19 Task Force. This task force issued guidelines that are a so-called living resource and are amended when necessary by the rapidly evolving science of COVID-19.[13] This article provides a summary of these guidelines (see **Table 1**). The NPF guidelines state that existing data generally suggest that psoriatic therapies do not meaningfully alter the risk of acquiring COVID-19 infection or having worse COVID-19 outcomes. For patients with psoriasis who are not infected with COVID-19, the NPF recommends continuing biologic therapies. In addition, patients and physicians are encouraged to undergo shared decision making to guide discussions about biologic use during the pandemic. If patients with psoriasis become infected with COVID-19, the NPF recommends that they monitor their symptoms and discuss treatment management with their physicians. If the decision is made to hold biologics during infection, the resumption of biologics should be decided on a case-by-case basis. In general, most patients can resume their psoriasis biologics after complete resolution of COVID-19 symptoms.[13]

The International Psoriasis Council (IPC) provides similar guidelines as the NPF (see **Table 1**).[14] However, for patients who have active COVID-19 infection, the IPC recommends discontinuing biologics.[14]

HIDRADENITIS SUPPURATIVA

The only biologic currently FDA approved to treat hidradenitis suppurativa (HS) is adalimumab. When the TNF-α inhibitor, adalimumab, is used to treat HS, it is administered every week, compared with the frequency of once every 2 weeks for psoriasis indication in adults.

Based on data from phase 3 pivotal trials in HS, the rates of respiratory infection in patients with HS on adalimumab were similar to those of patients on placebo.[15,16]

Observational studies have also investigated the impact of adalimumab on patients with HS during the COVID-19 pandemic. In northern Italy, a retrospective study of 96 patients with HS on systemic therapy was conducted; 48% of these patients were on adalimumab.[17] There were no cases of hospitalization or deaths from COVID-19 in patients with HS.[17] This finding was particularly significant, given that patients with HS are generally burdened by metabolic and cardiovascular comorbidities. Similarly, a retrospective study in southern Italy observed 93 patients with HS on systemic therapy; 80% of these patients were on adalimumab.[18] There were no formally reported

COVID-19 cases; only 1 patient reported COVID-19 symptoms, which spontaneously resolved.[18] In addition to these completed observational studies, an ongoing global registry has been developed to monitor and report outcomes of COVID-19 in patients with HS.[19]

Using the most recent COVID-19 data, the North America–based Hidradenitis Suppurativa Foundation (HSF) assembled recommendations to guide HS clinical management during the pandemic.[20] A summary of these important guidelines is provided in **Table 2**. The guidelines state that existing data suggest that biologics are not associated with an increased risk of COVID-19 in patients with HS. Therefore, if patients with HS are well controlled on biologics, they should continue their current regimens. Discontinuing biologics is not recommended because this could lead to skin symptom flare, which could lead patients with HS to seek care at a health care facility and have potential exposure. If patients with HS develop symptoms of COVID-19, the HSF recommends that patients consult their health care providers, who may recommend delaying a dose of the biologic. For patients with HS recovered from COVID-19, there is currently no recommendation statement issued by the HSF.[20]

International guidelines developed by European Academy of Dermatology and Venereology (EADV) and European Hidradenitis Suppurativa Foundation (EHSF) are similar to the North America–based HSF guidelines (see **Table 2**).[21] For patients infected with COVID-19, the international guidelines recommend discontinuing biologics.[21]

ATOPIC DERMATITIS

For the treatment of AD, dupilumab is the only biologic currently FDA approved. Dupilumab is an IL-4α receptor antagonist that inhibits IL-4 and IL-13 signaling. IL-4 is critical in mediating type 2 Th2 cell polarization and humoral immunity.[22]

A clinical trial meta-analysis investigated infection rates with dupilumab in pivotal phase 3 trials for AD.[22] This study examined rates of overall infection, URTI, and nasopharyngitis. Across these 3 infection categories, the rate of infection was not increased in dupilumab-treated patients compared with placebo.[22]

Several case reports have examined the effect of dupilumab on the clinical course and outcomes of patients with AD with COVID-19. In 2 of these cases, the patients who tested COVID-19 positive became symptomatic and were continued on dupilumab.[23] One patient experienced a mild course of the disease and recovered without complications.[23] The other patient developed

Table 2
Summary of recommendations on hidradenitis suppurativa management by international and North American organizations during the coronavirus disease 2019 pandemic, as of April 1, 2021[a]

Status of Infection	International Recommendation: EADV Acne, Rosacea, HS Task Force, and the EHSF	North American Recommendation: HSF
Without symptoms of COVID-19, on biologic therapy	Take extra precaution with TNF-alpha inhibitors	Continue current biologic regimen
No active COVID-19 infection, not on immunomodulatory agents, but being considered to initiate immunomodulatory agents	No statement at the time of writing	No statement at the time of writing
With symptoms suspicious of COVID-19, on systemic therapies (ie, biologics or oral medications)	Consult a health care provider and/or postpone or discontinue systemic therapy	Consult a health care provider, may recommend delaying a dose of the immunomodulator[b]
Active COVID-19 infection, on systemic therapies (ie, biologics or oral medications)	Discontinue taking immunomodulatory agent and consult a doctor	Consult a health care provider
Recovered from COVID-19	No statement at the time of writing	No statement at the time of writing
Professional Organization:		**Resource**
EADV Acne, Rosacea, HS Task Force, and the EHSF		https://eadv.org/cms-admin/showfile/_HS%20TF%20Recommandations_COVID%20Corner.pdf
HSF		https://www.hs-foundation.org/hidradenitis-suppurativa-treatment-and-covid-19-coronavirus/

[a] The AAD also issued recommendations for biologics, but they are not specific to a particular disease state. They are recommendations for all patients with dermatologic diseases on immunosuppressive agents during the COVID-19 pandemic.
[b] For HSF, the recommendation for this cohort also includes persons with known COVID-19 exposure.

interstitial pneumonia, but recovered after 10 days; this patient's spouse (who was not on dupilumab) also contracted COVID-19 and developed interstitial pneumonia, but passed away.[23] A third case report features a high-risk patient (aged >65 years) who tested positive for 9 consecutive weeks, but remained asymptomatic. This patient was continued on dupilumab during the period he tested positive.[24]

Researchers have theorized about the potential benefits of using dupilumab in patients with COVID-19. In patients who died of COVID-19, excess Th2 cytokines have been observed.[25] The increase in IL-4 level, and thus Th2 level, during COVID-19 illness could worsen the hyperinflammatory response.[25] Therefore, IL-4 inhibition might be beneficial. In addition, IL-6 plays a large role in the cytokine storm, which causes lung damage in patients with COVID-19.[26] IL-6 shifts the Th1/Th2

balance toward the Th2 direction.[26] Differentiation of Th2 by IL-6 depends on production of IL-4, whose activity is reduced by dupilumab.[26] However, this theoretic advantage is not yet supported by robust clinical data. Thus, physicians treating patients with AD should remain informed about developing data.

Although no explicit guidelines are currently offered by the National Eczema Association (NEA) in the United States, a record of expert panel discussion is available on their Web site. The AAD issued recommendations regarding systemic immunomodulatory therapies for skin conditions; however, these recommendations are not specific to AD.[7]

The International Eczema Association (IEC) has issued guidelines specific for AD management during the COVID-19 pandemic (**Table 3**).[27] For patients with no infection, or who are asymptomatic or mildly symptomatic, the IEC recommends continuing biologic treatment. For patients with

Table 3
Summary of recommendations on atopic dermatitis management by international organizations during the coronavirus disease 2019 pandemic, as of April 1, 2021[a]

Status of Infection	International Recommendation: IEC
No active COVID-19 infection or asymptomatic/mildly symptomatic of COVID-19, on systemic therapy (ie, on biologics or oral medications)	Continue systemic immunosuppressant treatment
No active COVID-19 infection, not on immunomodulatory agents, but being considered to initiate immunomodulatory agents	No statement at the time of writing
Active COVID-19 infection or symptomatic of COVID-19, on systemic therapy (ie, on biologics or oral medications)	Discontinue or dose-reduced systemic therapy
Recovered from COVID-19	No statement at the time of writing

Professional Organization:	Resource:
IEC	https://iecc.memberclicks.net/iec-statement-on-covid-19

[a] The AAD also issued recommendations for biologics, but they are not specific to a particular disease state. They are recommendations for all patients with dermatologic diseases on immunosuppressive agents during the COVID-19 pandemic.

active COVID-19 infection, the IEC recommends discontinuing or reducing the dose of biologics; however, patients with comorbid asthma should continue systemic therapy because asthma is a risk factor for severe COVID-19 infection.[27]

SUMMARY

Across inflammatory skin conditions, current data suggest that biologics used for psoriasis, HS, and AD do not seem to increase the risk of COVID-19 infection or lead to worsened COVID-19 outcomes, likely because the existing biologics for these dermatologic conditions target cytokines involved in the systemic hyperinflammatory response but often do not substantially affect cytokines involved in viral clearance.[2] Of note, some biologics may even be beneficial by mitigating the hyperinflammatory state seen in patients with severe COVID-19.[2,25,26] Data on this topic are currently evolving, and the guidelines continue to be updated accordingly. Clinicians should remain vigilant for the evolution of scientific evidence and closely follow their patients with dermatologic diseases on biologics.

CLINICS CARE POINTS

- For biologics used in psoriasis, including TNF-inhibitors, IL-12/23 inhibitors, IL-17 inhibitors, and IL-23 inhibitors, current data suggest that they do not increase the risk of COVID-19

infection or worsened COVID-19 outcomes. It is generally recommended that psoriasis patients not actively infected with SARS-CoV-2 initiate or continue their biologics to treat moderate-to-severe psoriasis.

- Adalimumab is currently the only biologic FDA-approved to treat HS. In patients with on adalimumab to treat HS, adalimumab does not increase the risk of COVID-19 infection or worsened COVID-19 outcomes. It is generally recommended that HS patients not actively infected with SARS-CoV-2 initiate or continue adalimumab to treat moderate-to-severe HS.

- Dupilumab is the currently the only biologic FDA-approved to treat moderate-to-severe AD. In patients on dupilumab to treat AD, current data suggest that dupilumab does not appear to increase the risk of COVID-19 infection or worsened COVID-19 outcomes. It is generally recommended that AD patients not actively infected with SARS-CoV-2 initiate or continue dupilumab to treat moderate-to-severe AD.

DISCLOSURE

Dr A.W. Armstrong has served as a research investigator and/or scientific advisor to AbbVie, BMS, Incyte, Leo, UCB, Janssen, Lilly, Novartis, Ortho Dermatologics, Sun, Dermavant, Dermira, Sanofi, Regeneron, Pfizer, and Modmed. Madison Jones, Alison Kohn, Sarah Pourali, Jeffrey Rajkumar, Yasmin Gutierrez, and Rebecca Yim have nothing to disclose.

REFERENCES

1. Damiani G, Pacifico A, Bragazzi NL, et al. Biologics increase the risk of SARS-CoV-2 infection and hospitalization, but not ICU admission and death: real-life data from a large cohort during RED-ZONE declaration. Dermatol Ther 2020;e13475.

2. Schett G, Sticherling M, Neurath MF. COVID-19: risk for cytokine targeting in chronic inflammatory diseases? Nat Rev Immunol 2020;20(5):271–2.

3. Armstrong AW, Read C. Pathophysiology, clinical presentation, and treatment of psoriasis: A review. JAMA 2020;323(19):1945–60.

4. Syed MN, Shah M, Shin DB, et al. Effect of anti–tumor necrosis factor therapy on the risk of respiratory tract infections and related symptoms in patients with psoriasis—A meta-estimate of pivotal phase 3 trials relevant to decision making during the COVID-19 pandemic. J Am Acad Dermatol 2020;84(1):161–3.

5. Haberman R, Axelrad J, Chen A, et al. Covid-19 in immune-mediated inflammatory diseases—case series from New York. N Engl J Med 2020;383(1):85–8.

6. Veenstra J, Buechler CR, Robinson G, et al. Antecedent immunosuppressive therapy for immune-mediated inflammatory diseases in the setting of a COVID-19 outbreak. J Am Acad Dermatol 2020;83(6):1696–703.

7. American Academy of Dermatology. Guidance on the use of immunosuppressive agents. 2020. Available at: https://www.aad.org/member/practice/coronavirus/clinical-guidance/biologics. Accessed January 2021.

8. Akiyama S, Yamada A, Micic D, et al. The risk of respiratory tract infections and interstitial lung disease with IL-12/23 and IL-23 antagonists in patients with autoimmune diseases: a systematic review and meta-analysis. J Am Acad Dermatol 2021;84(3):676–90.

9. Wan MT, Shin DB, Winthrop KL, et al. The risk of respiratory tract infections and symptoms in psoriasis patients treated with IL-17-pathway inhibiting biologics: A meta-estimate of pivotal trials relevant to decision-making during the COVID-19 pandemic. J Am Acad Dermatol 2020;83(2):677–9.

10. Vispi M, Corradin T, Peccianti C, et al. Psoriasis, biological drugs and Coronavirus Disease 2019: Real life experience of two Italian provinces. Dermatol Rep 2020;12(1).

11. Gisondi P, Zaza G, Del Giglio M, et al. Risk of hospitalization and death from COVID-19 infection in patients with chronic plaque psoriasis receiving a biologic treatment and renal transplant recipients in maintenance immunosuppressive treatment. J Am Acad Dermatol 2020;83(1):285–7.

12. Mahil SK, Dand N, Mason KJ, et al. Factors associated with adverse COVID-19 outcomes in patients with psoriasis-insights from a global registry-based study. J Allergy Clin Immunol 2021;147(1):60–71.

13. Gelfand JM, Armstrong AW, Bell S, et al. National psoriasis foundation COVID-19 task force guidance for management of psoriatic disease during the pandemic: Version 1. J Am Acad Dermatol 2020;83(6):1704–16.

14. International Psoriasis Foundation. IPC Statement on the Coronavirus (COVID-19) Outbreak. 2020. Available at: https://www.psoriasiscouncil.org/blog/Statement-on-COVID-19-and-Psoriasis.htm. Accessed January 16, 2021.

15. Blaszczak A, Trinidad JCL, Cartron AM. Adalimumab for treatment of hidradenitis suppurativa during the COVID-19 pandemic: Safety considerations. J Am Acad Dermatol 2020;83(1):e31.

16. Kimball AB, Okun MM, Williams DA, et al. Two phase 3 trials of adalimumab for hidradenitis suppurativa. N Engl J Med 2016;375(5):422–34.

17. Giulia R, Alice R, Teresa FM, et al. Moderate to severe hidradenitis suppurativa under systemic therapy during the COVID-19 outbreak. Dermatol Ther 2020;33(4):e13680.

18. Marasca C, Ruggiero A, Megna M, et al. Biologics for patients affected by Hidradenitis suppurativa in the COVID-19 era: data from a referral centre of Southern Italy. J Dermatol Treat 2020;1–3 (just-accepted).

19. University of California San Francisco. Global Hidradenitis Suppurativa COVID-19 Registry. Available at: https://hscovid.ucsf.edu/.

20. Hidradenitis Suppurativa Foundation. Frequently Asked Questions about Hidradenitis Suppurativa (HS) and COVID-19. 2020. Available at: https://www.hs-foundation.org/hidradenitis-suppurativa-treatment-and-covid-19-coronavirus/. Accessed January 16, 2021.

21. European Academy of Dermatology and Venereology. Systemic Therapy for Patients with Hidradenitis suppurativa/Acne inversa during the pandemic phase of SARS-CoV-2 (Coronavirus). 2020. Available at: https://eadv.org/cms-admin/showfile/_HS%20TF%20Recommandations_COVID%20Corner.pdf. Accessed January 16, 2021.

22. Kearns DG, Uppal S, Chat VS, et al. Assessing the risk of dupilumab use for atopic dermatitis during the COVID-19 pandemic. J Am Acad Dermatol 2020;83(3):e251–2.

23. Ferrucci S, Romagnuolo M, Angileri L, et al. Safety of dupilumab in severe atopic dermatitis and infection of Covid-19: two case reports. J Eur Acad Dermatol Venereol 2020;34(7):e303–4.

24. Caroppo F, Biolo G, Belloni Fortina A. SARS-CoV-2 asymptomatic infection in a patient under treatment

with dupilumab. J Eur Acad Dermatol Venereol 2020;
34(8):e368.

25. Förster-Ruhrmann U, Szczepek AJ, Bachert C,
et al. COVID-19 in a patient with severe chronic rhi-
nosinusitis with nasal polyps during therapy with
dupilumab. J Allergy Clin Immunol 2020;146(1):
218–20.

26. Patruno C, Stingeni L, Fabbrocini G, et al. Dupilumab and COVID-19: what should we expect? Dermatol Ther 2020;33(4):e13502.

27. International Eczema Foundation. IEC Statement on
COVID-19. 2020. Available at: https://iecc.
memberclicks.net/iec-statement-on-covid-19. Accessed January 16, 2021.

Occupational Dermatoses Related to Personal Protective Equipment Used During the COVID-19 Pandemic

Selli Abdali, MS[a], JiaDe Yu, MD[b],*

KEYWORDS

- COVID-19 • Personal protective equipment • Allergic contact dermatitis • Irritant contact dermatitis
- Seborrheic dermatitis • Rosacea • Acne • Mask dermatitis

KEY POINTS

- There has been a significant increase in prevalence of reported occupational dermatoses due to the enhanced infection prevention measures adopted by both health care workers and the general public in response to the COVID-19 pandemic.
- Irritant contact dermatitis is the most common occupational dermatitis reported and most often due to excessive hand washing and wearing of facial personal protective equipment such as masks and respirators.
- Gentle skin care, adequate moisturizing, and strategies to alleviate pressure are important preventative strategies for occupational dermatoses related to personal protective equipment.

INTRODUCTION

The outbreak of Coronavirus disease of 2019 (COVID-19) began in December 2019 in Wuhan, China[1] due to the severe acute respiratory syndrome coronavirus 2 (SARS-CoV2).[2,3] The first confirmed case in the United States (US) was reported on January 20th, 2020,[2] and on March 11th, 2020 the World Health Organization declared COVID-19 as a global pandemic.[4] By the end of 2020, there were 2 million reported cases and 345,000 deaths in the US due to COVID-19.[5]

SARS-CoV2 spread quickly due to its multiple modes of transmission: contact, droplet, and airborne transmission.[6] The Centers for Disease Control (CDC) released guidelines emphasizing the importance of wearing a facemask, handwashing, and disinfecting surfaces,[7] which led consumers and hospitals to stock facemasks, gloves, disinfectants, detergents, soaps, and hand sanitizers. In addition, the CDC guidelines for proper use of personal protective equipment (PPE) to protect health care workers (HCWs) recommended the routine use of N95 respirators, surgical masks, isolation gowns, eye protection (goggles or face shields), and gloves.[8]

Prolonged wearing of PPE, frequent handwashing, and disinfecting of surfaces have resulted in an increased number of skin complaints in both HCWs and non-HCWs. One study surveyed 542 HCWs and 97% reported skin damage caused by enhanced infection-prevention during the COVID-19 outbreak.[9] The associated dermatoses include allergic contact dermatitis (ACD), irritant contact dermatitis (ICD), seborrheic dermatitis (SD), acne, and rosacea. In this review, the incidence and diagnosis of PPE-associated occupational dermatoses in both HCWs and non-HCWs as well as recommendations for the prevention and treatment of these dermatoses are also discussed.

[a] Philadelphia College of Osteopathic Medicine, Philadelphia, PA 19131, USA; [b] Department of Dermatology, Massachusetts General Hospital, Harvard Medical School, 50 Staniford St, Boston, MA 02114, USA
* Corresponding author.
E-mail address: jiade.yu@mgh.harvard.edu

Dermatol Clin 39 (2021) 555–568
https://doi.org/10.1016/j.det.2021.05.009

COMMON TYPES OF OCCUPATIONAL DERMATITIS

ACD and ICD are the 2 most common causes of occupational dermatitis. According to the American Academy of Dermatology, contact dermatitis (including both ACD and ICD) was the fifth most common diagnosis in the dermatology clinic and costs more than 1.54 billion health care dollars in 2016.[10]

ACD accounts for 20% of occupational contact dermatitis cases.[11] ACD is a biphasic type IV delayed type hypersensitivity reaction that develops in response to contact allergens such as preservatives (formaldehyde), dyes (disperse blue), and metals (nickel).[12] Acute episodes of ACD can present with edema, erythema, and vesiculation.[11] Chronic ACD can lead to lichenification and fissuring of the skin.[11] Epicutaneous patch testing is the gold standard for the diagnosis of ACD.[11] During the COVID-19 pandemic, ACD has been reported due to PPE and personal care products (soaps, moisturizers, etc.) for the hands, trunk, and face (**Table 1**).[13]

ICD is responsible for 80% of all cases of occupational contact dermatitis.[11] ICD occurs from direct cytotoxic injury to the skin induced by a physical or chemical irritant.[12] ICD may include ulcerations and fissuring at the affected site,[12] with symptoms of pruritis and burning sensation occurring immediately after exposure.[11] ICD has been reported as a result of prolonged wearing of PPE and rigorous and frequent hand washing in the setting of COVID-19 (**Table 2**). Common body areas affected by ICD include the hands and convex surfaces of the face including the nose, ears, and cheeks from facemasks, goggles, and face shields.[19]

SD is a chronic inflammatory skin condition that presents as erythematous patches with greasy, yellow scales most commonly in areas densely populated with sebaceous glands such as the face (nasolabial folds, ears, eyebrows, and central forehead), scalp, chest, back, axilla, and groin.[26] SD is likely due to an overgrowth of the *Malassezia* yeast and subsequent inflammatory reaction elicited by the yeast. It is thought that increased wear of facial PPE provides the ideal temperature and moist environment for *Malassezia* to grow and increases the risk to developing SD (**Table 3**).[27]

Acne vulgaris and rosacea (maskne) are the 2 types of papulopustular eruptions that have been associated with the prolonged use of facial PPE during the COVID-19 pandemic (see **Table 3**).[21,28,34] Acne has 4 pathogenetic factors: the production of excess sebum, follicular epithelial hyperproliferation and plugging, follicular colonization by *Propionibacterium acnes*, and the presence of inflammation.[35] The use of face masks allows for a warm, humid, and occlusive microclimate on the skin, which contributes to the development of acne.[34,36] Rosacea has been seen to a lesser degree in the recent COVID-19 pandemic, although this may be due to underreporting.

Table 1
Reported cases of allergic contact dermatitis due to personal protective equipment and hand hygiene during COVID-19

Authors (Alphabetical), Year Published	Country of Origin	HCWs or Non-HCWs	Number of Patients	Location of Dermatitis	Causative Agent
Aerts et al,[14] 2020	Belgium	HCWs	1	Nose Cheeks	Formaldehyde and 2-bromo-2-nitropropane-1,3-diol (bronopol)
Bothra et al,[15] 2020	India	Both	4	Periauricular	No patch testing—suspected thermoplastic elastomer, rubber, latex
Ferguson et al,[16] 2020	United Kingdom	HCWs	13	Face	Unknown
			30	Hands	Limited patch testing—"rubber accelerators"
Singh et al,[17] 2020	India	HCWs	3	Face	Unknown
Xie et al,[18] 2020	China	Non-HCWs	1	Nasal Bridge Cheeks	Toluene-2,4-diisocyanate, diaminodiphenylmethane, and hexamethylene diisocyanate

Table 2
Reported cases of irritant contact dermatitis due to personal protective equipment and hand hygiene during COVID-19

Authors (Alphabetical), Year Published	Country of Origin	HCWs or Non-HCWs	Number of Patients	Location of ICD	Cause of Irritant Contact Dermatitis
Alluhayyan et al,[20] 2020	Saudi Arabia	HCWs	Not specifically reported	Nasal bridge Cheeks Ears	Pressure from goggles and facemasks
			200	Hands Wrists Forearms	Chemicals from hand cleansers, disinfectants, and natural rubber/latex gloves
Bothra et al,[15] 2020	India	Both	5	Retroauricular	Mask straps (thermoelastic polymer, latex) Dyes and disinfectant use on masks
Chaiyabutr et al,[21] 2020	Thailand	Non-HCW	Not specifically reported	Face	Multilayer surgical masks leading to occlusion; N95 mask borders leading to abrasion
Ferguson et al,[16] 2020	United Kingdom	HCWs	69	Face	Pressure from fitted mask and length of mask worn
			110	Hands	Chemicals from Clinell wipes (GAMA Healthcare, Watford, UK), benzalkonium chloride
Hu et al,[22] 2020	China	HCWs	58	Face Nasal bridge Ears	Pressure from N95 respirators
			54	Hands	Latex gloves
			37	Body	Disposable gowns worn 10 h daily for 3.5 mo
Kiely et al,[23] 2020	Ireland	HCWs	26.28%	Forehead Nose Cheeks	Length of use of facial PPE
			76.43% *223 total HCW—some complained of facial and hand dermatitis	Hands	Excessive handwashing
Metin et al,[24] 2020	Turkey	HCWs	194	Face	Excessive face washing
			782	Hands	Excessive hand hygiene Excessive glove use
			200	Body	Excessive daily showering

(continued on next page)

Table 2
(continued)

Authors (Alphabetical), Year Published	Country of Origin	HCWs or Non-HCWs	Number of Patients	Location of ICD	Cause of Irritant Contact Dermatitis
Singh et al,[17] 2020	India	HCWs	28	Forehead Temple Ears Eyelids/canthus Cheeks and chin Nasal bridge Lips/mouth	Duration of wear and fitting of goggles, N95 respirators, and face shields
Techasatian et al,[25] 2020	Thailand	Both	454	Ears Face	Physical/frictional from ear straps and pressure from face masks

Rosacea can be clinically characterized as transient erythema, telangiectasias, and inflammatory papules/pustules.[37] Acne can be distinguished from rosacea due to the presence of comedones.

FACIAL PERSONAL PROTECTIVE EQUIPMENTS

Facial PPE are one of the most important methods to prevent the spread of COVID-19 in the hospitals and the community. Various forms of facial PPE are used, including respirators (eg, N-95), cloth masks, surgical/medical masks, goggles, and face shields that are used by both HCWs and non-HCWs. Previous studies have shown that increased wearing of facial PPE leads to an increased prevalence of ACD, ICD, pressure-related skin injury, and worsening of underlying dermatoses such as acne and rosacea.[9,12,38] Since March 2020, there has been an increase in reported cases of occupational dermatoses related to facial PPE.[32] The type of mask, composition of mask, duration of wear, and underlying skin conditions are all potential factors in the development of occupational dermatoses to facial PPE.

The composition of the facial PPE materials are important to consider in potential cases of occupational dermatitis.[19] ACD to facial PPE has been reported to textile dyes,[39] elastic bands,[12] metal wiring for nosepiece,[40] and formaldehyde[41] that may remain from the manufacturing process of the polypropylene shell. Wearing facial PPE for extended periods of time also increases risk of ICD, pressure-induced dermatitis, and worsening of preexisting skin conditions such as acne and rosacea.[34] In one survey of HCWs, 61.7% experienced worsening of their preexisting skin condition due to wearing facial PPE, and 90.5% of HCWs had reported developing new skin

problems related to PPE use.[32] One study showed that cloth facemasks resulted in less adverse skin reactions compared with surgical masks and N95 respirators.[21]

In addition to masks and respirators, goggles and face shields are other common forms of facial PPE used. Reported adverse skin reactions with the use of goggles and face shields include pressure injury, ICD, ACD, urticaria, xerosis, and worsening of preexisting facial dermatoses such as acne and rosacea.[13,42] In one survey, 28% of HCWs complained of eczema and xerosis from the use of masks, goggles, and face shields, most frequently involving the nasal bridge, ears, and periocular region.[24] In another study, the use of surgical masks and goggles for 8 hours or more had led to skin erosions on the forehead, nasal bridge, and zygoma.[43] Skin damage over the nasal bridge was also seen in 87.9% of HCWs who wore goggles for more than 6 hours.[9] Goggles led to 51.92% of facial occupational dermatoses in one study, followed by N95 respirators (30.77%) and face shields (17.31%).[17]

Allergic Contact Dermatitis to Facial Personal Protective Equipment

Cases of ACD to facial PPE reported during the current COVID-19 pandemic are summarized in **Table 1**. The most common causes of ACD due to facial PPE are additives and materials used in the manufacturing of respirators, surgical masks, face shields, and goggles.[40] ACD has been reported to rubber accelerators such as thiurams, carbamates, dialkyl thioureas, and N-isopropyl-N-phenyl-p- phenylendiamine in elastic bands[12] used to secure the facial PPE on the face.[40,44] Facial PPE also contain potentially allergenic metals such as nickel and cobalt in the nose piece

Table 3
Reported cases of seborrheic dermatitis, acne, and rosacea during COVID-19

Authors (Alphabetical), Year Published	Country of Origin	HCWs or Non-HCWs	Number of Patients	Type of Dermatitis	Location of Dermatitis	Treatment/Outcome
Chaiyabutr et al,[21] 2020	Thailand	Non-HCWs	248	Acne	Face	-
Chiriac et al,[28] 2020	Romania	HCWs	1	Papulopustular rosacea	Face	Slight improvement after 2 wk of metronidazole, 1 g/d, twice a day and pimecrolimus 1% 1 h after removal of facemask
Daye et al,[29] 2020	Turkey	HCWs	44	Acne	Face	-
Giacalone et al,[30] 2020	Italy	Non-HCWs	1	Seborrheic Dermatitis	Nose Cheeks Beard	Low-potency steroid for 5 d and pimecrolimus 1% daily for 10 d
			1	Acne	Jaw and chin	Adapalene gel 0.1% and benzoyl peroxide gel 2.5% for 8 wk, zinc gluconate, 175 mg, and nicotinamide, 27 mg, daily for 3 mo
			1	Rosacea	Cheeks	Doxycycline, 40 mg, for 12 wk. Treatments provided clinical benefit
Han et al,[31] 2020	China	Non-HCWs	5	Acne	Cheeks and nose	Good response to Adapalene gel 0.1%, +/− face peel with 20% α-hydroxy acid
Hu et al,[22] 2020	China	HCWs	1	Acne	Face	-
Ferguson et al,[16] 2020	United Kingdom	HCWs	16	Seborrheic Dermatitis	Face	-
			26	Acne		
			5	Rosacea		
Metin et al,[24] 2020	Turkey	HCWs	82	Seborrheic dermatitis	Face and scalp	-
			131	Acne/folliculitis	Face	
Singh et al,[17] 2020	India	HCWs	5	Acne	Face	-
Techasatian et al,[25] 2020	Thailand	Both	333	Acne	Face	-
Trepanowski et al,[32] 2020	USA	HCWs	11	Seborrheic dermatitis	Face	-
			79	Acne		
			31	Rosacea		
Veraldi and Angileri,[27] 2020	Italy	Both	20	Seborrheic dermatitis	Face	-
Zuo et al,[33] 2020	China	HCWs	9	Seborrheic dermatitis	Face	-
			44	Acne		
			14	Rosacea		

Abbreviation: HCW, healthcare workers

to mold the mask to the wearers' face.[12,40,44] Textile dyes in surgical or cloth masks have also been reported to lead to ACD.[39] Furthermore, formaldehyde used in the manufacturing of surgical masks and N95 respirators may still remain in the final product and have been reported to cause ACD.[14,18,41,45] Other preservatives with potential to induce ACD due to facial PPE include methyldibromoglutanitrile,[40] 2-bromo-2-nitropropane-1,3-diol,[14] toluene-2,4-diisocyanate,[18] diaminodiphenylmethane,[18] and hexamethylene diisocyanate.[18]

The only way to prevent and treat ACD is to avoid the causative allergen, which can be identified via epicutaneous patch testing.[19] Persistent exposure to the allergen can lead to worsening ACD resulting in inappropriate wear or fit of PPE, thereby increasing risk for contracting COVID-19. If avoidance is not possible or the relevant allergen is not identified, effort should be made to treat the cutaneous symptoms until a suitable alternative is found.

Irritant Contact Dermatitis to Facial Personal Protective Equipment

ICD is common with widespread use of facial PPE in both HCWs and non-HCWs. Reported cases of ICD due to facial PPE during the current COVID-19 pandemic is summarized in **Table 2**. One survey compared non-HCWs who wore cloth masks with those who wore surgical masks or N95 respirators.[21] Pruritis was the number one complaint among all facial PPE.[21] There were also more ICD in those who wore facial PPE for more than 8 hours daily.[21] The study revealed that surgical masks had a greater number of adverse skin reactions when compared with cloth masks.[21] A study in China surveyed HCWs who wore N95 respirators for an average of 12 hours a day for 3.5 months; 95.1% reported adverse skin reactions to N95s, including nasal bridge scarring (68.9%) due to pressure from the metal nose piece, facial itching (27.9%), skin damage (26.2%), dry skin (24.6%), and rash (16.4%).[22] These findings were also similar to a study conducted during the 2003 SARS outbreak in Singapore where 307 HCWs were surveyed and 35.5% of those wearing N95 respirators complained of adverse skin reactions, most commonly acne (59.6%), facial itch (51.4%), and rash (35.8%).[34] One group in India noticed an increase of cases in retroauricular dermatitis caused by wearing of cloth or surgical masks and N95 respirators with ear loops (composed of latex or thermoelastic polymer).[15] In 1 month, 14 patients complained of skin pruritis, scaling, and erythema.[15]

Prevention of ICD relies on strategies to alleviate friction and pressure and are outlined in **Table 4**.[19] Hydrocolloid dressings and barrier products made of acrylate, silicon, or dimethicone may be used on areas that are frequently irritated, such as the bridge of the nose, cheeks, and ears.[19] Application of a thin dressing (such as DuoDERM Extra Thin, ConvaTec, Deeside, UK) between the facial PPE and the skin can offer some barrier protection.[19] However, the effect on the seal of N95 is unknown. One recent small study analyzed the effect of 5 barrier protectants on the fit of 3M 1860 N95 respirator (St. Paul, MN). They found fit-testing pass rates ranged from 56% to 88% depending on the skin protectant used; only 36% of their cohort passed with all 5 protectants.[46] Therefore, it is imperative to make sure that these dressings or barrier products do not interfere with the fit and safety of the facial PPE, and refit testing is necessary especially with N95 respirators to ensure a tight seal. To avoid retroauricular pressure-related irritant dermatitis, surgical masks with ear loops can be alternated with masks that tie to the back of the head to limit possible ICD to the tight elastic bands.[19]

A recent study examining ways to maintain skin integrity and prevent skin irritation and injury after the use of N95 respirators found alcohol-free liquid acrylate film and hydrocolloid dressings to be the most effective.[47] A headband face mask may help limit retroauricular irritation and pressure when wearing a mask for a long time.[15] Another way to prevent irritation is to relieve the pressure on the skin by removing the mask for 5 to 15 minutes every 2 to 4 hours if it is safe to do so.[48–50]

Treatment of Facial Personal Protective Equipment–Induced Allergic Contact Dermatitis and Irritant Contact Dermatitis

For all cases of potential ACD or ICD due to facial PPE, avoidance of possible allergen or irritant is preferred. Gentle skin care management such as washing with a fragrance-free, hypoallergenic nonsoap cleanser and applying daily moisturizer are key foundations to prevent xerosis that may increase susceptibility to ACD and ICD.[19] Treatment of facial ACD and ICD include low-potency topical steroids for short periods of time,[11] as prolonged use of topical steroids can increase the risk of periorificial dermatitis, cutaneous atrophy, and striae formation. Nonsteroidal alternatives suitable for long-term use on the face include topical calcineurin inhibitors such as tacrolimus 0.03% or 0.1% ointment, pimecrolimus 1% cream, and crisaborole 2% ointment. Discontinuation of current PPE and switching to a suitable alternative may be necessary in recalcitrant cases.

Table 4
Clinical features and recommendations for the prevention and treatment of dermatoses associated with PPE wear and hand hygiene

	Allergic Contact Dermatitis	Irritant Contact Dermatitis	Seborrheic Dermatitis	Acne	Rosacea
Prevention	Avoidance of known allergen	Use of 100% cotton or less occlusive facemasks alone or under surgical masks (if not in health care setting) Schedule 15-min breaks every 2 h for HCWs wearing facial PPE[51] Use of hydrocolloid dressings, silicon or dimethicone barrier creams, acrylate film at pressure or irritated areas[19,47] Use of daily gentle skin cleansers and moisturizer throughout the day	Use of daily gentle skin cleansers and moisturizer throughout the day If recurrent, can use ketoconazole 2% as shampoo or face wash empirically 2-3x/wk as prevention	Daily gentle cleansing with salicylic acid or benzoyl peroxide Use of noncomedogenic facial products Use of cloth/less occlusive facemasks for the general public[25] Schedule 15-min breaks every 2 h for HCWs wearing facial PPE[51]	Use of daily gentle skin cleansers and moisturizer throughout the day Avoid triggers: extreme temperature, sunlight, spicy food, alcohol, strenuous exercise, acute psychological stressors[52]
Clinical Diagnostic Features	Well-demarcated, intensely pruritic eczematous eruptions; vesicular (acute) or lichenified (chronic)	Acute ICD presents as painful, pruritic, erythematous, edematous lesions with vesicles and bullae[11] Chronic ICD presents as lichenified and hyperkeratotic lesions[11]	Pink patches with greasy white/yellow scale in areas with high concentration of sebaceous glands (nasolabial folds, ears, eyebrows, scalp)[26]	Presence of open and/or closed comedones. Inflammatory lesions such as papules, pustules, nodules, or cysts may also be present[53]	Involvement of the nose, malar, and perioral areas. Involvement of at least one primary and secondary feature. Central facial erythema, flushing, telangiectasia, inflammatory papules/pustules, rhinophyma[54]

(continued on next page)

Table 4
(continued)

	Allergic Contact Dermatitis	Irritant Contact Dermatitis	Seborrheic Dermatitis	Acne	Rosacea
Diagnostic Tests	Patch testing is the gold standard Skin biopsy can be helpful to differentiate from other dermatoses	Skin biopsy if clinical diagnosis is not possible	Skin biopsy if clinical diagnosis is not possible	Skin biopsy if clinical diagnosis is not possible	Skin biopsy if clinical diagnosis is not possible Presence of *Demodex* mites in follicles[55]
Treatment	Avoid known allergen Localized: topical steroids or calcineurin inhibitors Widespread: systemic corticosteroids or other immunosuppressive therapies	Avoid known irritant Topical steroids or calcineurin inhibitors appropriate for body region	Ketoconazole 2% shampoo/body wash or antifungal cream as needed Low-potency topical corticosteroid or topical calcineurin inhibitors for itching and erythema	Mild - Wash daily with benzoyl peroxide or salicylic acid wash - Topical retinoid (tretinoin, adapalene, tazarotene) - Topical antibiotics such as clindamycin 1% lotion daily Moderate - Follow all recommendations for mild acne and add in oral antibiotics (eg, doxycycline) - For women, combined oral contraceptives and/or oral spironolactone are also appropriate Severe - Consider oral isotretinoin	Mild - Azelaic acid 15%, topical ivermectin 1%, topical metronidazole 0.75% cream or 1% gel, sodium sulfacetamide wash Moderate/severe - Follow all recommendations for mild rosacea and add in oral antibiotics (eg doxycycline) - Consider isotretinoin for severe cases For erythema - Topical brimonidine 0.33% gel - Topical oxymetazoline 1% cream

Seborrheic Dermatitis

Long-term use of facial PPE may increase the skin permeability and temperature, which causes a change in the microbiota allowing *Malassezia* to proliferate and thrive in these conditions leading to worsening SD.[27] During the COVID-19 pandemic, there have been several cases of SD exacerbated by facial PPE (see **Table 3**). A survey identified 37.5% of HCWs whose underlying SD had worsened due to facial PPE.[33] Another study showed 34 new cases of SD in HCWs after the first month of the pandemic and worsening of SD in 47% of HCWs.[24] Wearing facemasks for 6 to 10 hours per day exacerbated SD in 46.5% of patients in one series.[27] Of these patients with worsening symptoms, 75% were men and 35% of them worked in health care settings.[27]

The best method to prevent exacerbation of SD is to cleanse the face with gentle facial cleansers before and after prolonged mask wearing and limit the time of continuous contact with facial PPE if possible.[33] Treatment of underlying SD is also important with antifungal shampoos and creams such as ketoconazole 2% and low-potency topical steroids or calcineurin inhibitors.

Papulopustular Eruption (Acne and Rosacea)

New onset and exacerbation of acne and rosacea on the face occurs frequently due to facial PPE (see **Table 3**). Among HCWs and non-HCWs, acne flares were the biggest complaint with facial PPE (39.9%).[25] The use of facial PPE for extended periods leads to a warm and humid environment under the PPE that can increase the sebum secretion rate and occlude pores, leading to comedone formation predisposing to acne flare-ups.[31] During the 2003 SARS pandemic, 59.6% of HCWs complained of facial acne as one of the most difficult adverse skin reactions to wearing N95 respirators for many hours.[34] The pressure from the close-fitting facial PPE also leads to pilosebaceous duct occlusion, resulting in acne mechanica.[34,36] A survey of 390 HCWs reported that 61.7% had worsening of their skin since the start of COVID-19 pandemic with acne being the most frequently reported.[32] HCWs had more symptoms compared with non-HCWs due to the increased duration of facial PPE worn and the use of N95 respirators.[25] Another study in non-HCWs showed cloth masks led to fewer acne flares compared with surgical masks.[21] It was recommended to decrease the flare ups, non-HCWs should use cloth masks instead of surgical masks.[25] Because of the shortage of surgical masks, many HCWs and non-HCWs would reuse their disposable surgical masks. Compared with those who did not reuse their surgical masks, reusing surgical masks contributed to 1.5× increased risk of adverse skin reactions including acne.[25]

Practicing proper facial skin care is important to help prevent and treat acne and rosacea. Washing with gentle cleansers and, if tolerated, salicylic acid or benzoyl peroxide cleansers is an effective first step in treatment of acne and rosacea.[51] Limiting cosmetics and make up products on the days of extended mask wearing can also be helpful. Application of retinoids such as retinol, adapalene, and tretinoin nightly can aid in follicular turnover preventing acne formation. Moderate-to-severe cases can be treated with systemic antibiotics if necessary.[19,42] Prolong wearing of mask can aggravate existing acne vulgaris,[34,36,44] and taking breaks from the mask 15 minutes every 2 hours can be helpful, if it is safe to do so.[51]

GOWNS

Gowns in the hospital setting provide an additional barrier to protect HCWs from risk of contracting COVID-19 from patients. There are limited reports of occupational dermatoses associated with prolonged wearing of gowns.[45] Gowns that tightly adhere to the skin result in increased friction, moisture, and warmth can increase the risk of developing ICD especially in intertriginous areas such as the axilla, under the breasts, and in the skin folds.[45] In addition, chemicals and dyes used in the manufacturing of gowns including formaldehyde resins and textile dyes can contribute to the development of ICD and ACD.[45] During the SARS pandemic in Singapore, repeated wearing of disposable gowns led to increased complaints of pruritus and dermatitis at the wrists of HCWs.[34] One study found that protective clothing and gowns were the top nonglove PPE responsible for ICD.[44] A study conducted during the COVID-19 pandemic surveyed 61 HCWs who regularly wore disposable protective clothing for 10 hours a day for 3.5 months.[22] In that study, 60.7% of HCWs complained of adverse skin reactions such as dry skin (36.1%), pruritus (34.4%), rash (11.5%), and wheals (3.28%).[22]

HANDS

Because SARS-CoV2 can spread via contact and droplet transmission, proper hand hygiene is essential for decreasing viral transmission.[6] The CDC recommends wearing gloves, washing hands, and the routine use of disinfectant wipes on all contact surfaces to decrease the spread of COVID-19.[7] The US Environmental Protection Agency provides a database to search for effective surface disinfectants for SARS-CoV2.[56] Disinfectant wipes containing citric acid, ethyl alcohol, hydrogen peroxide, quaternary ammonium, or sodium hypochlorite as the active ingredients are said to have virucidal effects on surfaces.[56,57] Because of these enhanced hygiene practices, there is an increasing prevalence of occupational hand dermatitis.[58] Hands are affected in greater than 80% to 90% occupational contact dermatitis.[59] In HCWs, hand dermatitis is the most prevalent form of occupational dermatitis with greater than 30% of HCWs affected before the current pandemic.[60] The most commonly reported hand symptoms in HCWs during the COVID-19 pandemic were dryness (92.9%), itchiness (50%), and redness (46.4%) mostly due to hand cleansers followed by the use of disinfectants and gloves.[20] Cases of allergic hand dermatitis and irritant hand dermatitis are presented in **Tables 1** and **2**, respectively.

Hand Hygiene

Occupational dermatoses due to excessive hand washing are the most common complaint seen during the COVID-19 pandemic.[9] The CDC recommends frequent handwashing with soap and warm water for 20 seconds.[7] Repeated exposure to water with soaps, detergents, and antiseptic handwashes can affect the pH of the epidermis and negatively affect the skin's structural integrity and protection against the environment.[61] In addition, excessive handwashing can deplete the lipid barrier of the stratum corneum, leading to an increase in transepidermal water loss (TEWL). A damaged stratum corneum can allow irritants and allergens to penetrate the epidermis, ultimately leading to irritant and allergic hand dermatitis.[62] One study showed that handwashing during the COVID-19 pandemic increased the risk of xerosis and eczema by 3.57 times.[24] Another study showed that 74.5% of HCWs complained of skin symptoms, which included dryness, tenderness, itching, and burning due to excessive hand washing.[9] Soaps, detergents, and antiseptic handwashes contain fragrances, surfactants, and preservatives that are potential contact allergens that can also cause ACD.[58]

The CDC recommends the use of hand sanitizers containing at least 60% ethanol or 70% isopropyl alcohol for use by HCWs.[7] Alcohol-based hand sanitizers (ABHSs) are thought to be better in preventing ICD because they often contain emollients and moisturizers, thus resulting in less disruption to the lipid barrier on the skin than hot water, harsh soaps, and detergents.[63] ABHSs with moisturizers are a better alternative to traditional soaps because they have the least sensitizing and irritancy potential with fewer allergens.[64] However, ABHSs has also been implicated in causing skin dryness and subsequent ICD.[64] ABHSs often contain ingredients (fragrances, tocopherol, propylene glycol, benzoates, and cetyl stearyl alcohol) that can also cause ACD.[64,65]

Gloves

Rubber gloves provide an additional layer of protection for HCWs and non-HCWs in preventing viral transmission.[66] Excessive glove use can be harmful to the skin, causing xerosis and hand dermatitis.[34] One study showed that excessive use of gloves can lead to a 2.68 times increased risk of developing xerosis.[24] Long-term use of gloves can also paradoxically lead to overhydration of the stratum corneum, which may lead to maceration and erosion of the skin.[42] One study reported that 88.5% of HCWs wearing rubber latex gloves during the COVID-19 pandemic for an average of 10 hours a day for 3.5 months complained of skin reactions.[22] The symptoms most commonly reported were dry skin (55.7%), itching (31.2%), rash (24%), and chapped skin (21.3%).[22] Frequent moisturizing of the hands and using a cotton glove liner can also decrease the risk of developing irritant hand dermatitis.[20]

Most rubber gloves contain rubber accelerators, such as thiurams, carbamates, diphenylguanidine, mixed dialkyl thioureas, and benzothiazoles, that accelerate the process to synthesize rubber consumer products from its raw material but are leading causes of glove-related ACD.[60,64] The American Contact Dermatitis Society recommends the use of accelerator-free gloves for those with suspected or confirmed hand ACD.[58,67] One study provided HCWs suffering from hand ACD a 1-month supply of rubber accelerator-free gloves, and both disease severity and patient quality of life improved dramatically.[68]

Surface Disinfectants

Because of the indirect contact transmission of COVID-19, disinfecting surfaces multiple times throughout the day has become a habitual practice. Repeated cleaning and use of disinfectants may damage the skin surface and compromise the skin barrier leading to ICD.[69] This exposes harsh chemicals such as N-alkyl dimethyl benzyl ammonium chloride on the skin.[70] Exposure to fat soluble disinfectants such as 75% alcohol, chlorine-based disinfectants, and peroxyacetic acid can lead to ACD and can present with desquamation, rhagades, pruritis, and bleeding.[43] Disinfectant wipes for surface cleaning should not be used directly on the skin. When cleaning surfaces, proper skin protection such as the use of gloves when handling chemicals is recommended to protect the skin from any injury or direct chemical exposure. Rare cases of ACD have also been documented due to disinfectants. Cases of occupational airborne ACD have been seen from the use of a disinfectant spray containing linalyl acetate[71] and cleaning detergent containing N-alkyl dimethylbenzylammonium chloride and n-alkyl dimethylethylbenzyl ammonium chloride.[70]

If irritant hand dermatitis is suspected, the first step is to avoid the potential irritant whether it is in detergents, gloves, or harsh soaps. Switching to gentle cleansers and regularly moisturizing immediately after can alleviate most cases of hand dermatitis. Use of ABHSs with emollients can be helpful in select cases. Moisturizers that include petrolatum in the form of ointments can serve as a physical barrier and prevent further TEWL. Humectants such as urea and glycerin attract water and moisture to the epidermis.[72] It is recommended that patients apply a thick petrolatum-based emollient nightly to the hands and cover with white cotton gloves before bed, leaving the gloves on until the next morning. Treatment of acute, itchy, irritant dermatitis with potent topical steroids can also help alleviate symptoms through judicious use of potent topical steroids, given the thickness of the stratum corneum on the hands.[58]

Management of patients with allergic hand dermatitis includes identification of the allergen through patch testing and avoidance of the allergen. Potential allergens can be found in soaps, cleansers, gloves, and moisturizers. Avoidance of the allergen is curative in cases of ACD.

SUMMARY

In this review the authors discussed the common types of occupational dermatoses that have been reported due to increased use of PPE and enhanced hygiene practices used by both HCWs and non-HCWs to prevent the spread of COVID-19. They also discussed preventative, diagnostic, and treatment strategies for PPE-related occupational dermatoses. Until an effective vaccine and treatments become available worldwide, the authors will likely continue to see heightened prevalence of PPE-related dermatoses.

CLINICS CARE POINTS

- Irritant contact dermatitis is the most common dermatoses seen due to frequent use of PPE during the COVID-19 pandemic

- Allergic contact dermatitis has been reported to hand washing soaps, moisturizers, alcohol based cleansers, masks, rubber gloves, gowns, etc. Patch testing is key to diagnosis

- Acne, rosacea, and seborrheic dermatitis can occur due to chronic mask wearing as a result of friction, sweating, and perturbation of the microenvironment

- Avoidance of offending PPE and consideration of safe alternatives is essential

DISCLOSURE

The authors have no commercial or financial conflicts of interests relevant to this publication.

REFERENCES

1. Zhu N, Zhang D, Wang W, et al. A novel coronavirus from patients with pneumonia in China, 2019. N Engl J Med 2020;382(8):727–33.
2. Holshue ML, DeBolt C, Lindquist S, et al. First case of 2019 novel coronavirus in the United States. N Engl J Med 2020;382(10):929–36.
3. Gorbalenya AE, Baker SC, Baric RS, et al. The species severe acute respiratory syndrome-related coronavirus: classifying 2019-nCoV and naming it SARS-CoV-2. Nat Microbiol 2020;5(4):536–44.
4. WHO Director-General's opening remarks at the media briefing on COVID-19-11 March 2020. Available at: https://www.who.int/dg/speeches/detail/who-director-general-s-opening-remarks-at-the-media-briefing-on-covid-19. [Accessed 14 December 2020].
5. CDC COVID Data Tracker. Available at: https://covid.cdc.gov/covid-data-tracker/#trends_totalandratedeaths. [Accessed 2 January 2021].
6. Health WHO, Programme E, Panel EA. Transmission of SARS-CoV-2 : implications for infection prevention precautions. 2020 (July):1–10. Available at: https://www.who.int/publications/i/item/modes-of-transmission-of-virus-causing-covid-19-implications-for-ipc-precaution-recommendations. [Accessed 14 December 2020].
7. Protect yourself. Available at: https://www.cdc.gov/coronavirus/2019-ncov/prevent-getting-sick/prevention.html. [Accessed 14 December 2020].
8. General optimization strategies. Available at: https://www.cdc.gov/coronavirus/2019-ncov/hcp/ppe-strategy/general-optimization-strategies.html. [Accessed 15 December 2020].
9. Lan J, Song Z, Miao X, et al. Skin damage among health care workers managing coronavirus disease-2019. J Am Acad Dermatol 2020;82(5):1215–6.
10. Lim HW, Collins SAB, Resneck JS, et al. The burden of skin disease in the United States. J Am Acad Dermatol 2017;76(5):958–72.

11. Sasseville D. Occupational contact dermatitis. Allergy Asthma Clin Immunol 2008;4(2):59–65.

12. Yu J, Chen JK, Mowad CM, et al. Occupational dermatitis to facial personal protective equipment in health care workers: a systematic review. J Am Acad Dermatol 2021;84(2):486–94.

13. Gheisari M, Araghi F, Moravvej H, et al. Skin reactions to non-glove personal protective equipment: an emerging issue in the COVID-19 pandemic. J Eur Acad Dermatol Venereol 2020; 34(7):e297–8.

14. Aerts O, Dendooven E, Foubert K, et al. Surgical mask dermatitis caused by formaldehyde (releasers) during the COVID-19 pandemic. Contact Dermatitis 2020;83(2):172–3.

15. Bothra A, Das S, Singh M, et al. Retroauricular dermatitis with vehement use of ear loop face masks during COVID-19 pandemic. J Eur Acad Dermatol Venereol 2020;34(10):e549–52.

16. Ferguson FJ, Street G, Cunningham L, et al. Occupational dermatology in the time of the COVID-19 pandemic: a report of experience from London and Manchester, UK. Br J Dermatol 2020;2020–2.

17. Singh M, Pawar M, Bothra A, et al. Personal protective equipment induced facial dermatoses in healthcare workers managing coronavirus disease 2019. J Eur Acad Dermatol Venereol 2020;34(8):e378–80.

18. Xie Z, Yang YX, Zhang H. Mask-induced contact dermatitis in handling COVID-19 outbreak. Contact Dermatitis 2020;83(2):166–7.

19. Yu J, Goldminz A, Chisolm S, et al. Facial personal protective equipment: materials, resterilization methods, and management of occupation-related dermatoses. Dermatitis 2021;32(2):78–85.

20. Alluhayyan OB, Alshahri BK, Farhat AM, et al. Occupational-related contact dermatitis: prevalence and risk factors among healthcare workers in the Al'Qassim region, Saudi Arabia during the COVID-19 pandemic. Cureus 2020;12(10):e10975.

21. Chaiyabutr C, Sukakul T, Pruksaeakanan C, et al. Adverse skin reactions following different types of mask usage during the COVID-19 pandemic. J Eur Acad Dermatol Venereol 2020;95:1–3.

22. Hu K, Fan J, Li X, et al. The adverse skin reactions of health care workers using personal protective equipment for COVID-19. Medicine (Baltimore) 2020;99(24):e20603.

23. Kiely LF, Moloney E, O'Sullivan G, et al. Irritant contact dermatitis in healthcare workers as a result of the COVID-19 pandemic: a cross-sectional study. Clin Exp Dermatol 2020;46:142–4.

24. Metin N, Turan Ç, Utlu Z. Changes in dermatological complaints among healthcare professionals during the COVID-19 outbreak in Turkey. Acta Dermatovenerol Alp Pannonica Adriat 2020;29(3):115–22.

25. Techasatian L, Lebsing S, Uppala R, et al. The effects of the face mask on the skin underneath: a prospective survey during the COVID-19 pandemic. J Prim Care Community Heal 2020;11. 2150132720966167.

26. Clark GW, Pope SM, Jaboori KA. Diagnosis and treatment of seborrheic dermatitis. Am Fam Physician 2015;91(3):185–90.

27. Veraldi S, Angileri L, Barbareschi M. Seborrheic dermatitis and anti-COVID-19 masks. J Cosmet Dermatol 2020;19(10):2464–5.

28. Chiriac AE, Uwe W, Doina A. Flare-up of rosacea due to face mask in healthcare workers during COVID-19. Maedica 2020;15(16):416–7.

29. Daye M, Cihan FG, Durduran Y. Evaluation of skin problems and dermatology life quality index in health care workers who use personal protection measures during COVID-19 pandemic. Dermatol Ther 2020;33:e14346.

30. Giacalone S, Minuti A, Spigariolo CB, et al. Facial dermatoses in the general population due to wearing of personal protective masks during the COVID-19 pandemic: first observations after lockdown. Clin Exp Dermatol 2021;46(2): 368–9.

31. Han C, Shi J, Chen Y, et al. Increased flare of acne caused by long-time mask wearing during COVID-19 pandemic among general population. Dermatol Ther 2020;33(4):3–5.

32. Trepanowski N, Larson AR, Evers-Meltzer R. Occupational dermatoses among front-line health care workers during the COVID-19 pandemic: a cross-sectional survey. J Am Acad Dermatol 2021;84:223–5.

33. Zuo Y, Hua W, Luo Y, et al. Skin reactions of N95 masks and medial masks among health-care personnel: a self-report questionnaire survey in China. Contact Dermatitis 2020;83(2):145–7.

34. Foo CCI, Goon ATJ, Leow YH, et al. Adverse skin reactions to personal protective equipment against severe acute respiratory syndrome - a descriptive study in Singapore. Contact Dermatitis 2006;55(5): 291–4.

35. Toyoda M, Morohashi M. Pathogenesis of acne. Med Electron Microsc 2001;34(1):29–40.

36. Tan KT, Greaves MW. N95 acne. Int J Dermatol 2004;43(7):522–3.

37. Wayne BB, Pelletier AL. Rosacea: a common, yet commonly overlooked, condition. Am Fam Physician 2002;66(3):435–40.

38. Lin P, Zhu S, Huang Y, et al. Adverse skin reactions among healthcare workers during the coronavirus disease 2019 outbreak: a survey in Wuhan and its surrounding regions. Br J Dermatol 2020;183(1): 190–2.

39. Mawhirt SL, Frankel D, Diaz AM. Cutaneous manifestations in adult patients with COVID-19 and dermatologic conditions related to the COVID-19 pandemic in health care workers. Curr Allergy Asthma Rep 2020;20(12):75.

40. Warshaw EM, Schlarbaum JP, Silverberg JI, et al. Safety equipment: when protection becomes a problem. Contact Dermatitis 2019;81(2):130–2.

41. Donovan J, Kudla I, Holness DL, et al. Skin reactions following use of N95 facial masks. J Child Neurol 2006;21(3):261–73.

42. Yan Y, Chen H, Chen L, et al. Consensus of Chinese experts on protection of skin and mucous membrane barrier for health-care workers fighting against coronavirus disease 2019. Dermatol Ther 2020;33(4):1–7.

43. Zhang B, Zhai R, Ma L. 2019 Novel coronavirus disease epidemic: skin protection for healthcare workers must not be ignored. J Eur Acad Dermatol Venereol 2020;34(9):e434–5.

44. Bhoyrul B, Lecamwasam K, Wilkinson M, et al. A review of non-glove personal protective equipment-related occupational dermatoses reported to epiderm between 1993 and 2013. Contact Dermatitis 2019;80(4):217–21.

45. Donovan J, Skotnicki-Grant S. Allergic contact dermatitis from formaldehyde textile resins in surgical uniforms and nonwoven textile masks. Dermatitis 2007;18(1):40–4.

46. Bui ATN, Yu Z, Lee K, et al. A pilot study of the impact of facial skin protectants on qualitative fit testing of N95 masks. J Am Acad Dermatol 2021; 84(2):554–6.

47. Pacis M, Azor-Ocampo A, Burnett E, et al. Prophylactic dressings for maintaining skin integrity of healthcare workers when using N95 respirators while preventing contamination due to the novel coronavirus: a quality improvement project. J Wound Ostomy Continence Nurs 2020;47(6): 551–7.

48. LeBlanc K, Heerschap C, Butt B, et al. Prevention and management of person protective equipment skin injury: update 2020. NSWOCC. Available at: www.nswoc.ca/ppe. [Accessed 16 January 2021].

49. Cuddigan J, Black J, Deppisch M, et al. NPIAP position statements on preventing injury with N95 masks. Available at: https://npiap.com/page/COVID-19Resources. [Accessed 10 January 2021].

50. Alves, P, Moura A, Ferreira A, et al: PRPPE Guidelines | COVID 19. Journal of Tissue Healing and Regenration 2020. 1-8. Available at: https://serenagroupinc.com/covid-19/white-paper-prppe-guideline-covid-19/. Accessed January 13, 2021.

51. Desai SR, Kovarik C, Brod B, et al. COVID-19 and personal protective equipment: treatment and prevention of skin conditions related to the occupational use of personal protective equipment. J Am Acad Dermatol 2020;83(2):675–7.

52. Two AM, Wu W, Gallo RL, et al. Rosacea: part I. Introduction, categorization, histology, pathogenesis, and risk factors. J Am Acad Dermatol 2015; 72(5):749–58.

53. Zaenglein AL, Pathy AL, Schlosser BJ, et al. Guidelines of care for the management of acne vulgaris. J Am Acad Dermatol 2016;74(5):945–73.

54. Wilkin J, Dahl M, Detmar M, et al. Standard classification of rosacea: Report of the National Rosacea Society Expert Committee on the Classification and Staging of Rosacea. J Am Acad Dermatol 2002; 46(4):584–7.

55. Rusiecka-Ziółkowska J, Nokiel M, Fleischer M. Demodex - an old pathogen or a new one? Adv Clin Exp Med 2014;23(2):295–8.

56. List N Tool: COVID-19 disinfectants. Available at: https://www.epa.gov/pesticide-registration/list-n-disinfectants-coronavirus-covid-19. [Accessed 20 January 2021].

57. Goh CF, Ming LC, Wong LC. Dermatologic reactions to disinfectant use during the COVID-19 pandemic. Clin Dermatol 2020. Available at: https://www.sciencedirect.com/science/article/abs/pii/S0738081X20301796.

58. Rundle CW, Presley CL, Militello M, et al. Hand hygiene during COVID-19: recommendations from the American Contact Dermatitis Society. J Am Acad Dermatol 2020;83(6):1730–7.

59. Lampel HP, Powell HB. Occupational and hand dermatitis: a practical approach. Clin Rev Allergy Immunol 2019;56(1):60–71.

60. Kadivar S, Belsito DV. Occupational dermatitis in health care workers evaluated for suspected allergic contact dermatitis. Dermatitis 2015;26(4): 177–83.

61. Patrick DR, Findon G, Miller TE. Residual moisture determines the level of touch-contact-associated bacterial transfer following hand washing. Epidemiol Infect 1997;119(3):319–25.

62. Rundle CW, Bergman D, Goldenberg A, et al. Contact dermatitis considerations in atopic dermatitis. Clin Dermatol 2017;35(4):367–74.

63. Siddharta A, Pfaender S, Vielle NJ, et al. Virucidal activity of world health organization-recommended formulations against enveloped viruses, including zika, ebola, and emerging coronaviruses. J Infect Dis 2017;215(6):902–6.

64. Voller LM, Schlarbaum JP, Hylwa SA. Allergenic ingredients in health care hand sanitizers in the United States. Dermatitis 2021;32(3):151–9.

65. Rodriguez-Homs LG, Atwater AR. Allergens in medical hand skin cleansers. Dermatitis 2019;30(6):336–41.

66. Sanghvi AR. COVID-19: an overview for dermatologists. Int J Dermatol 2020;59(12):1437–49.

67. Kersh AE, Helms S, De La Feld S. Glove-related allergic contact dermatitis. Dermatitis 2018;29(1): 13–21.

68. Smylie AL, Gill N, Oosterhuis R, et al. Glove-induced allergic contact hand dermatitis: a quality improvement initiative. J Cutan Med Surg 2021; 25(2):216–7.

69. Long H, Zhao H, Chen A, et al. Protecting medical staff from skin injury/disease caused by personal protective equipment during epidemic period of COVID-19: experience from China. J Eur Acad Dermatol Venereol 2020;34(5):919–21.

70. Mauleón C, Mauleón P, Chavarría E, et al. Airborne contact dermatitis from n-alkyl dimethylbenzylammonium chloride and n-alkyl dimethylethyl-

benzylammonium chloride in a detergent. Contact Dermatitis 2006;55(5):311–2.

71. White JML, Goossens A. Occupational airborne allergic contact dermatitis to linalyl acetate in a disinfectant spray. Contact Dermatitis 2020;83(5): 412–3.

72. Lodén M. Role of topical emollients and moisturizers in the treatment of dry skin barrier disorders. Am J Clin Dermatol 2003;4(11):771–88.

Coronavirus Disease 2019 and Race in Dermatology

Seemal R. Desai, MD[a,b,*], Amy J. McMichael, MD[c], Rayva Khanna, BA[d]

KEYWORDS

- COVID-19 • Race • COVID-toes • Pernio • Chilblains • Racial disparities • Healthcare inequities
- Dermatologic literatures

KEY POINTS

- Coronavirus Disease 2019 (COVID-19) disproportionately affects Black and Hispanic/Latino populations.
- Racial disparities in health care and dermatology have further become evident through the COVID-19 pandemic.
- The lack of clinical images of COVID-19 cutaneous manifestations, along with other dermatologic diseases, in patients of color represents an unmet need in medical literature.

BACKGROUND

Structural and systemic racism has subsequent harmful effects on patients of color.[1–3] Spurred by racial injustices in the United States of America in the past year, racial inequities have finally come to the forefront of dialog within health care.[4,5] Particularly, there has been an increased focus on structural racism; the way in which societies foster discrimination through reinforcing inequitable systems and stereotypes.[1] The Coronavirus Disease 2019 (COVID-19) pandemic highlighted the importance of recognizing the role structural racism plays in amplifying and uncovering power imbalances that already exist among vulnerable racial and ethnic groups. For example, access to education, housing, and environmental stress all impact quality health care, comorbid medical conditions, ability to obtain personal protective equipment, and capability to quarantine in a safe space.[6] The synergistic effects of the pandemic in conjunction with the political, economic, and social inequalities in the United States have led to detrimental consequences for patients of color.[7]

Current literature documents the increased morbidity and mortality in Black and Hispanic/Latino populations as an outcome of the pandemic.

- Notably, Price-Haywood and colleagues documented that in a large cohort in Louisiana, a startling 70.6% of individuals who died from COVID-19 were Black, although Black patients comprised only 31% of the hospital system population.[8]
- Furthermore, in early April, Sachdeva and colleagues reported that in Chicago, Illinois, 51.5% of COVID-positive patients and 67.3% (n = 132) of those who died were Black.[9]
- The Centers for Disease Control and Prevention's statement regarding the racial disparities in COVID-19 and race similarly acknowledged a greater burden of disease for non-white individuals. They noted that among individuals youger than 50 years, a markedly higher percentage of patients who tested positive for COVID-19 were Hispanic

Patient consent: Patient consent not required.
[a] Innovative Dermatology, PA, 5425 West Spring Creek Parkway, Suite 265, Plano, TX 75024, USA; [b] Department of Dermatology, University of Texas Southwestern Medical Center, Dallas, TX, USA; [c] Wake Forest School of Medicine, Winston-Salem, NC, USA; [d] Georgetown University School of Medicine, Washington, D.C., USA
* Correspondence author.
E-mail address: seemald@yahoo.com

Dermatol Clin 39 (2021) 569–574
https://doi.org/10.1016/j.det.2021.05.003

or Latino. In addition, Black Americans had the highest percent test positive among their racial or ethnic groups.[10]

Therefore, COVID-19 has highlighted the innate imbalances that exist within the medical field.

The medical community has called on dermatologists to increase skin of color representation in the literature.[11] Currently, there is a paucity of images of cutaneous manifestations of COVID-19 for skin of color patients. Thus, dermatologists are encouraged to photograph and disseminate these images among the medical community.[12]

It is important to note that skin of color dermatology has long been championed by board-certified dermatologists as well as by organized dermatologic associations. The need for more attentiveness, education of the physician workforce, public awareness, and advocacy has historically been highlighted as key needs by experts in skin of color. For example, the Skin of Color Society, now the largest international organization dedicated to skin of color dermatology, was founded many years ago to specifically foster collaboration among dermatologists that are key opinion leaders in skin of color dermatology while simultaneously looking at ways to address the educational needs of dermatologists who may not specialize in skin of color. In addition, increasing diversity within the dermatology workforce, providing critical research opportunities to underrepresented minority physicians and medical students and fostering mentorship to advance skin of color dermatology are at the core of this specific organizations' mission.

The social injustices of recent times, in combination with glaring health inequities during the pandemic, have presented a historic opportunity for the skin of color discipline: to take these tragedies and use them as an opportunity for true and meaningful change. This article aims to summarize the cutaneous manifestations of COVID-19 in skin of color patients and recognize the gaps in dermatologic literature and need for further research.

RACIAL INEQUITIES IN DERMATOLOGY
Medical Education

Before addressing the cutaneous manifestations of COVID-19, it is important to discuss the racial/ethnic barriers that inherently exist in dermatology. Dermatology education regarding cutaneous manifestations in patients of color is limited by a lack of racial diversity in dermatology and dearth of educational material representing patients of color. Remarkably, a previous study noted that 47% of dermatologists felt that their training was

inadequate to diagnose disease in skin of color patients.[13] In order to elucidate why such health care disparities exist in diagnosing patients of color, Lester and colleagues analyzed the pages of common dermatology textbooks commonly used in resident education:[13]

- Of 5026 images reviewed, independent image reviewers categorized photos from two common textbooks. Upon analyzing these images, skin of color representation was estimated to be 22% to 32% in textbooks.
- However, for images of sexually transmitted infections (STIs), the proportion of skin of color varied from 47% to 58%, compared with 28% for images of infections that were not STIs.
- Therefore, the depiction of skin of color images in common educational literature remains unequal and may reflect implicit bias.[4]

An updated analysis by Adelekun and colleagues showed that dermatology textbooks contained a mere 4%-18% of images of patients with dark skin.[14] Lack of imagery of common dermatologic conditions across a wide variety of skin types can lead to adverse outcomes for patients due to delayed diagnosis and treatment in these populations. A study of patients with Lyme Disease noted that patients of color had a later date of presentation.[15] In part, delayed diagnosis and treatment of Lyme disease in patients with darker skin tones may be due to the different presentation of the "characteristic" erythema migrans rash.[11] It is important to recognize the dangers of labeling the cutaneous manifestations as "typical" or "classic" based on the clinical presentation of a certain condition in a white population. Specifically, the effect of pigmentation on erythema should be considered when diagnosing even common dermatologic conditions such as acne and psoriasis.[16] Overall, lack of skin of color patient representation in dermatologic imagery not only affects the knowledge of the trainee population but also narrows the scope of the field.

Patient Attitudes and Beliefs

Patient attitudes regarding dermatology may vary based on racial or ethnic background. Importantly, although skin of color patients are often categorized into Fitzpatrick skin phototypes IV to VI, it is important to note that ethnicity and race are not synonymous. For example, some individuals who identify as Hispanic/Latino may be patients with Fitzpatrick phototype I. Furthermore, skin cancer can still occur in darker phenotypes and often leads to poor outcomes in these populations because of lack of early detection and treatment.[17]

Buster and colleagues administered a survey to categorize patient attitudes and behaviors regarding skin cancer.[17,18] They found that Black individuals had different viewpoints than white patients regarding lifestyle influence on skin cancer and the utility of skin examinations and that Black and Hispanic/Latino individuals were less likely to believe they could change their own risk of skin cancer with personal interventions.

Previous literature has noted there is a low rate of dermatology outpatient visits for Asian Americans as well despite Asian Americans representing the fastest growing minority group in the United States. Lingala and colleagues reported that skin cancer has a delayed detection in Asian Americans[19]: Notably, of 506 patients, 48% of respondents reported having their skin checked by a dermatologist, and only 60% of the participants performed a self-skin examination.

In combatting skin-care myths and beliefs, studies have shown that educational interventions can help improve photoprotection practices. Kundu and colleagues performed a study in which patients of color were educated on how to find atypical moles with cutaneous self-examinations. Through the interventions, monthly skin checks improved across the study sample, thus emphasizing the importance of patient education in decreasing adverse outcomes in skin of color populations.[17]

Currently, in the COVID-19 pandemic in conjunction with pre-existing systemic racism, we are witnessing an increase in the medical mistrust by Black populations—specifically in regard to receiving COVID-19 vaccinations.[20–22] In a study of HIV-positive Black Americans, 97% endorsed at least one general COVID-19 mistrust belief.[21] This generalized distrust regarding COVID-19 management could likely transcend to Black patients' care-seeking behavior in context of COVID manifestations of the skin.

Imbalances Within Dermatology

Health care disparities and structural racism are widespread in medicine, with causes ranging from barriers to access to care, mistrust between the patient and physician, and implicit bias inherent in medicine. The groups that tend to be most impacted by these inequities are racial minorities and people of lower socioeconomic status.[23] Within dermatology specifically, there is a lack of diversity among practicing dermatologists. Although 12% of Americans are Black, Black dermatologists make up 3% of dermatologists,

making dermatology one of the least medically diverse specialties.[4] Residents and practicing dermatologists have called for academic institutions to promote mentorship and selection of Black students to increase racial representation throughout the field.[4,5] This lack of racial representation can lead to adverse outcomes in patients of color. Distrust of the medical system is one of the issues of concern, potentially resulting in part from race discordance between patients and providers, as patients with providers of a different race are more likely to be uncomfortable with treatment plans because of the fear of their symptoms not being taken seriously by their physicians.[16,24]

Furthermore, it is important to consider the financial burden of outpatient dermatologic visits. Studies have shown that Black patients are more likely to report a cost as an obstacle in obtaining dermatologic care, with a greater percentage of Black patients receiving insurance from government payers (Medicare and Medicaid).[25,26] Creadore and colleagues recently reported patients with Medicaid had less success getting appointments and longer appointment wait times than those with Medicare or Blue Cross/Blue Shield. With the increased reliance of telemedicine in dermatology due to the pandemic, there may be isolation of individuals without access to a computer.[27] There is some evidence that the Fee For Service reimbursement policies in US dermatology practice may promote procedures for a subset of the population and exacerbate disparities for ethnic minorities.[26] Therefore, if a patient's dermatologic condition is not causing active functional impairment, they may be less likely to seek care.

IMAGES OF SKIN OF COLOR IN COVID-19
Lack of COVID-19 Images of Skin of Color Patients

The importance of increased racial representation in dermatologic education has been widely discussed in the literature. There are clear discrepancies in the current dermatologic literature with a shortage of imagery from skin of color patients in dermatologic journals textbooks.[11] Owing to the strongly visual nature of dermatologic medicine, this decreased representation in the dermatologic literature can impact patient care by hindering potential differential diagnoses.

Specifically, in the COVID-19 pandemic, there is a demand for dermatology images of skin of color patients with COVID-19 dermatologic manifestations due to the concern that if COVID patients and care providers do not personally visualize an array of images in different skin tones, they may not recognize COVID manifestations in darker skin tones.

Owing to the racial disparities in COVID-19 infections, all clinical manifestations of COVID-19 should be documented and recognized to provide timely quality care. A recent literature review by Lester and colleagues noted that 92% of the 130 images included in their review of COVID-19 cutaneous manifestations included Fitzpatrick Phototypes I-III.[12] Only 6% of patients were classified with Fitzpatrick phototype IV skin, and 0% of the images were from patients with Fitzpatrick phototype V or VI skin.[12] In order to combat this lack of information, dermatologists should document all cutaneous COVID-19 manifestations in skin of color patients and widely distribute these findings.

COVID-19 Dermato-Epidemiology Across Different Countries and Populations

Systemic manifestations of COVID-19 documented in the literature include rashes containing macules and papules, urticarial, vesicular, and vaso-occlusive lesions, maculopapular rash, petechiae/purpura, livedoid/necrotic lesions, chilblain-like lesions (COVID toes), erythema multiforme-like lesions, and aphthous ulcers.[28] A meta-analysis by Tan and colleagues described the skin manifestations of COVID-19 worldwide.[29] At present, given the lack of population-level data or large cohort studies with a known denominator, we do not yet know if reported differences between different populations represent a true genetic difference in response to severe acute respiratory syndrome coronavirus 2 (SARS-CoV-2), or merely demonstrates trends in access to care and/or reporting in different countries.

For example, we do not yet know if the reporting of COVID-19-associated vaso-occlusive disease, such as fixed livedo racemosa or retiform purpura, in the United States (6.4%) and Spain (5.2%) is higher than that in India, where preliminary reports of a prospective cohort study put the prevalence at 1.4%.[29] Similarly, other vascular cutaneous manifestations, such as chilblain-like lesions, vasculitis, and vasculopathic ulcers, were rarely reported among Indian patients.[30] If not just due to reporting bias,[31,32] some pathophysiologic mechanisms that have been proposed are that increased levels of lipoprotein A in some populations could predispose patients to cardiovascular and peripheral arterial diseases or that Factor V Leiden in white populations compared with Asian populations could explain the differences in thromboembolic events.[29]

In addition, studies have noted a relative dearth of COVID toes in Hispanic and Black populations.[33] Daneshjou and colleagues published a series of 6 case reports (1 positive for COVID) to increase skin of color representation for dermatologic images.[31] However, additional literature notes that COVID-toes manifestations are uncommon in pigmented skin.[32] It is not yet clear if this paucity of COVID toes in skin of color is due to underrecognition by patients and providers of this phenomenon in darker skin, less access to health care, or truly less incidence of pernio/chilblains/COVID toes in some populations, or a multifactorial combination of all of these.

The underrepresentation of minority communities in dermatologic literature, difficulty in identifying cutaneous lesions in these individuals, and increased adverse outcomes in Black and Hispanic/Latino populations demands further investigation into potential biases in recognizing and reporting skin manifestations of COVID-19, including COVID-toes, in patients of color. Poor access coupled with nonrecognition of erythema by clinicians in patients with darker skin tones likely contribute. This further complicates clinical diagnosis of other cutaneous manifestations of COVID-19 infection, including morbilliform, urticarial, exanthematous, and even eczematous features. However, we additionally wonder about genetic polymorphisms accounting for varying immunologic responses to SARS-CoV-2 in different populations. Increased data and images are strongly encouraged to increase the sample size and power of future studies. Dermatologists should continue to document and distribute all cutaneous manifestations of COVID and report cases, including pernio-like lesions, in COVID-19-positive patients across a wide variety of skin types.

Recognizing, discussing, and developing ways to reduce health disparities should be a priority for the entire house of medicine, and studying COVID-19 under this lens allows a better understanding of current shortcomings and future calls to action. Dermatologic disease in patients of color has been an exceedingly important issue that has not gone unrecognized or unaddressed. In fact, the COVID-19 pandemic has brought so much attention to health disparities that goals and aspiration in the field have taken on even more importance for our specialty. The lack of images of cutaneous COVID-19 manifestations is just one example of a tangible paradigm that can be ameliorated to help dermatologists and other clinicians alike. However, the ultimate goal of eliminating health disparities in at-risk populations in medicine is a longitudinal journey that requires introspection, recognition, research, and resolve. Dermatology continues to do its part in creating a solution and advancing skin of color dermatology via multiple paradigms as a key part of helping this important cause.

CLINICS CARE POINTS

> Clinicians should be aware of health disparities that exist in skin of color populations. In addition, cutaneous manifestations of COVID-19 may be more difficult to detect in patients of color due to the clinical appearance of erythema, lack of clinical experience in detecting dermatologic disease in skin of color, and due to potential biases in diagnosis.

CONFLICT OF INTEREST

Dr. Desai is a member of the American Academy of Dermatology Ad Hoc Task Force on COVID-19. The other authors have no conflicts of interest to declare.

REFERENCES

1. Egede LE, Walker RJ. Structural Racism, Social Risk Factors, and Covid-19 — A Dangerous Convergence for Black Americans. N Engl J Med 2020. https://doi.org/10.1056/nejmp2023616.
2. Bailey ZD, Feldman JM, Bassett MT. How Structural Racism Works — Racist Policies as a Root Cause of U.S. Racial Health Inequities. N Engl J Med 2021; 384(8):768–73.
3. Paradies Y, Ben J, Denson N, et al. Racism as a Determinant of Health: A Systematic Review and Meta-Analysis. PLoS One 2015;10(9):e0138511.
4. Smith RJ, Oliver BU. Advocating for Black Lives—A Call to Dermatologists to Dismantle Institutionalized Racism and Address Racial Health Inequities. JAMA Dermatol 2021;157(2):155–6.
5. Lester JC, Taylor SC. Resisting Racism in Dermatology: A Call to Action. JAMA Dermatol 2021. https://doi.org/10.1001/jamadermatol.2020.5029.
6. Devakumar D, Shannon G, Bhopal SS, et al. Racism and discrimination in COVID-19 responses. Lancet 2020. https://doi.org/10.1016/S0140-6736(20)30792-3.
7. Gravlee CC. Systemic racism, chronic health inequities, and COVID-19: A syndemic in the making? Am J Human Biol 2020. https://doi.org/10.1002/ajhb.23482.
8. Price-Haywood EG, Burton J, Fort D, et al. Hospitalization and Mortality among Black Patients and White Patients with Covid-19. N Engl J Med 2020. https://doi.org/10.1056/nejmsa2011686.
9. Shah M, Sachdeva M, Dodiuk-Gad RP. COVID-19 and racial disparities. J Am Acad Dermatol 2020. https://doi.org/10.1016/j.jaad.2020.04.046.
10. COVID-19 Racial and Ethnic Health Disparities. Centers for Disease Control and Prevention.
11. Nolen L. How Medical Education Is Missing the Bull's-eye. N Engl J Med 2020. https://doi.org/10.1056/nejmp1915891.
12. Lester JC, Jia JL, Zhang L, et al. Absence of images of skin of colour in publications of COVID-19 skin manifestations. Br J Dermatol 2020. https://doi.org/10.1111/bjd.19258.
13. Lester JC, Taylor SC, Chren MM. Under-representation of skin of colour in dermatology images: not just an educational issue. Br J Dermatol 2019. https://doi.org/10.1111/bjd.17608.
14. Adelekun A, Onyekaba G, Lipoff JB. Skin color in dermatology textbooks: An updated evaluation and analysis. J Am Acad Dermatol 2021. https://doi.org/10.1016/j.jaad.2020.04.084.
15. Fix AD, Peña CA, Strickland GT. Racial Differences in Reported Lyme Disease Incidence. Am J Epidemiol 2000;152(8):756–9.
16. Jothishankar B, Stein SL. Impact of skin color and ethnicity. Clin Dermatol 2019. https://doi.org/10.1016/j.clindermatol.2019.07.009.
17. Agbai ON, Buster K, Sanchez M, et al. Skin cancer and photoprotection in people of color: A review and recommendations for physicians and the public. J Am Acad Dermatol 2014. https://doi.org/10.1016/j.jaad.2013.11.038.
18. Buster KJ, You Z, Fouad M, et al. Skin cancer risk perceptions: A comparison across ethnicity, age, education, gender, and income. J Am Acad Dermatol 2012. https://doi.org/10.1016/j.jaad.2011.05.021.
19. Lingala B, Li S, Wysong A, et al. Low rate of dermatology outpatient visits in Asian-Americans: an initial survey study for associated patient-related factors. BMC Dermatol 2014;14:13.
20. Fisher KA, Bloomstone SJ, Walder J, et al. Attitudes Toward a Potential SARS-CoV-2 Vaccine: A Survey of U.S. Adults. Ann Intern Med 2020;173(12):964–73.
21. Bogart LM, Ojikutu BO, Tyagi K, et al. COVID-19 Related Medical Mistrust, Health Impacts, and Potential Vaccine Hesitancy Among Black Americans Living With HIV. J Acquir Immune Defic Syndr 2021;86(2):200–7.
22. Momplaisir F, Haynes N, Nkwihoreze H, et al. Understanding Drivers of COVID-19 Vaccine Hesitancy Among Blacks. Clin Infect Dis 2021. https://doi.org/10.1093/cid/ciab102. ciab102.
23. Lopez L III, Hart LH III, Katz MH. Racial and Ethnic Health Disparities Related to COVID-19. JAMA 2021;325(8):719–20.
24. Benkert R, Peters RM, Clark R, et al. Effects of perceived racism, cultural mistrust and trust in

providers on satisfaction with care. J Natl Med Assoc 2006;98(9):1532–40.

25. Friedman LC, Bruce S, Weinberg AD, et al. Early detection of skin cancer: Racial/ethnic differences in behaviors and attitudes. J Cancer Educ 1994; 9(2):105–10.

26. Wang LL, Adelekun A, Taylor SC, et al. Fee-for-service and structural forces may drive racial disparities in US dermatology. Br J Dermatol 2020. https://doi.org/10.1111/bjd.19217.

27. Kind T, Huang ZJ, Farr D, et al. Internet and Computer Access and Use for Health Information in an Underserved Community. Ambul Pediatr 2005;5(2): 117–21.

28. Freeman EE, McMahon DE, Lipoff JB, et al. The spectrum of COVID-19–associated dermatologic manifestations: An international registry of 716 patients from 31 countries. J Am Acad Dermatol 2020. https://doi.org/10.1016/j.jaad.2020.06.1016.

29. Tan SW, Tam YC, Oh CC. Skin manifestations of COVID-19: A worldwide review. JAAD Int 2021;2: 119–33.

30. Pangti R, Gupta S, Nischal N, et al. Recognizable vascular skin manifestations of SARS-CoV-2 (COVID-19) infection are uncommon in patients with darker skin phototypes. Clin Exp Dermatol 2021. https://doi.org/10.1111/ced.14421.

31. Daneshjou R, Rana J, Dickman M, et al. Pernio-like eruption associated with COVID-19 in skin of color. JAAD Case Rep 2020. https://doi.org/10.1016/j.jdcr.2020.07.009.

32. Cline A, Berk-Krauss J, Keyes Jacobs A, et al. The underrepresentation of "COVID toes" in skin of color: An example of racial bias or evidence of a tenuous disease association? J Am Acad Dermatol 2021. https://doi.org/10.1016/j.jaad.2020.11.003.

33. Deutsch A, Blasiak R, Keyes A, et al. COVID toes: Phenomenon or epiphenomenon? J Am Acad Dermatol 2020;83(5):e347–8.

Dermatology COVID-19 Registries
Updates and Future Directions

Esther E. Freeman, MD, PhD[a,b],*, Grace C. Chamberlin, BA[b],
Devon E. McMahon, MD[a], George J. Hruza, MD, MBA[c],
Dmitri Wall, MB BCh BAO[d,e,f], Nekma Meah, MD, FACD[g,h],
Rodney Sinclair, MBBS, MD, FACD[i], Esther A. Balogh, MD[j],
Steven R. Feldman, MD, PhD[j], Michelle A. Lowes, MBBS, PhD[k],
Angelo V. Marzano, MD[l,m], Haley B. Naik, MD, MHSc[n],
Leslie Castelo-Soccio, MD, PhD[o], Irene Lara-Corrales, MD, MSc[p],
Kelly M. Cordoro, MD[n], Satveer K. Mahil, MD, PhD[q],
Christopher E.M. Griffiths, MD[r], Catherine H. Smith, MD[q],
Alan D. Irvine, MD, DSc[s], Phyllis I. Spuls, MD, PhD[t], Carsten Flohr, MD, PhD[u],
Lars E. French, MD[v,w]

KEYWORDS

- COVID-19 • SARS-CoV-2 • Dermatology • Global health • Registry • Psoriasis
- Hidradenitis suppurativa • Atopic dermatitis

Continued

[a] Department of Dermatology, Massachusetts General Hospital, Harvard Medical School, 55 Fruit St, Boston, MA 02114, USA; [b] Medical Practice Evaluation Center, Mongan Institute, Massachusetts General Hospital, Boston, MA, USA; [c] Department of Dermatology, Saint Louis University School of Medicine, Saint Louis, MO, USA; [d] Hair Restoration Blackrock, Dublin, Ireland; [e] National and International Skin Registry Solutions (NISR), Charles Institute of Dermatology, Dublin, Ireland; [f] School of Medicine, University College Dublin, Dublin, Ireland; [g] St Helens & Knowsley NHS Trust, Marshalls Cross Road, St. Helens WA9 3DA, UK; [h] Manchester University, Faculty of Biology, Medicine and Health, Oxford Road, Manchester, UK; [i] Sinclair Dermatology, East Melbourne, Victoria 3002, Australia; [j] Center for Dermatology Research, Department of Dermatology, Wake Forest School of Medicine, Winston Salem, NC, USA; [k] The Rockefeller University, New York, NY, USA; [l] Dermatology Unit, Fondazione IRCCS Ca' Granda Ospedale Maggiore Policlinico, Milan, Italy; [m] Department of Pathophysiology and Transplantation, Università degli Studi di Milano, Milan, Italy; [n] Department of Dermatology, University of California, San Francisco, CA, USA; [o] Section of Pediatric Dermatology, Children's Hospital of Philadelphia, Philadelphia, PA, USA; [p] Section of Pediatric Dermatology, Hospital for Sick Children, Toronto, Canada; [q] St John's Institute of Dermatology, King's College London and Guy's & St Thomas' NHS Foundation Trust, London, UK; [r] Dermatology Centre, Salford Royal Hospital, NIHR Manchester Biomedical Research Centre, University of Manchester, Manchester, UK; [s] Clinical Medicine, Trinity College Dublin, Dublin, Ireland; [t] Department of Dermatology, Public Health and Epidemiology; Immunity and Infections, Amsterdam University Medical Centers, Location Academic Medical Center, Amsterdam, the Netherlands; [u] Unit for Population-Based Dermatology Research, St John's Institute of Dermatology, King's College London and Guy's & St Thomas' NHS Foundation Trust, London, UK; [v] Department of Dermatology, University Hospital, Munich University of Ludwig Maximilian, Munich, Germany; [w] Dr. Philip Frost Department of Dermatology and Cutaneous Surgery, University of Miami Miller School of Medicine, Miami, Florida, USA
* Corresponding author. Massachusetts General Hospital, 55 Fruit Street, Boston, MA 02114.
E-mail address: efreeman@mgh.harvard.edu

Dermatol Clin 39 (2021) 575–585
https://doi.org/10.1016/j.det.2021.05.013
0733-8635/21/© 2021 Elsevier Inc. All rights reserved.

derm.theclinics.com

Continued

KEY POINTS

- Dermatology registries created during the COVID-19 pandemic have collected more than 8000 cases since they opened for case reporting in March and April of 2020.
- Information from these registries has informed scientific knowledge and medical practice on topics ranging from the spectrum of possible skin manifestations of COVID-19 to the safety of continued systemic treatments for dermatologic conditions in severe acute respiratory syndrome coronavirus 2 (SARS-CoV-2)–positive and suspected positive patients.
- Collaboration between registries—within and outside dermatology—has been critical to this rapid knowledge production and should set a precedent for future data collection harmonization.
- A majority of cases entered in these registries are white patients from North America and Europe, indicating the work still to be done on ensuring that registries and conclusions drawn from them are representative of the affected populations.

INTRODUCTION

The world has now been dealing with the unprecedented effects of the COVID-19 pandemic for more than a year, with a global case count that has surpassed 135 million as of April 2021.[1] Accurate reporting of cases, symptoms, and treatment of the causative virus, severe acute respiratory syndrome coronavirus 2 (SARS-CoV-2), has been critical to the development of knowledge and subsequent public health response. Registries have played an important role in collecting real-world evidence during the pandemic. Due to their rapid, harmonized, international response, the 7 dermatology groups included in this update have been managing and analyzing registry data for almost as long as the pandemic has been spreading. Launched during March and April of 2020, these registries—focused on the relationship between COVID-19 and dermatology—have now cumulatively collected more than 8000 case reports sourced from all over the world (**Table 1**). This article serves as an update[2] on their objectives, findings, and future goals in the ever-evolving COVID-19 landscape.

AMERICAN ACADEMY OF DERMATOLOGY (AAD)/INTERNATIONAL LEAGUE OF DERMATOLOGICAL SOCIETIES (ILDS) COVID-19 DERMATOLOGY REGISTRY

After initial reports from Italy and China of COVID-19 associated dermatologic manifestations, leaders from the American Academy of Dermatology (AAD) and the International League of Dermatological Societies (ILDS) founded a registry on April 9, 2020 in order to understand and better form hypotheses about this interplay between the skin and COVID-19.[3] Understanding that frontline health care workers needed reliable information, AAD and ILDS leadership worked rapidly to bring the registry from the idea generation phase to the collection of first patient data in just 8 days.[4] In an effort to capture as much data as possible, entries are crowdsourced internationally from any physician or other health care provider seeing patients with COVID-19 and possible related skin symptoms or patients who have preexisting dermatologic conditions that may be affected by COVID-19.

The AAD/ILDS COVID-19 Dermatology Registry has 1875 entries from 52 countries as of March 2021. Registry data have demonstrated the wide spectrum of dermatologic manifestations of COVID-19, ranging from pernio/chilblains in relatively mild COVID-19 to retiform purpura in ill, hospitalized patients.[5,6] The most common dermatologic morphologies in 716 patients, in the subset of COVID-19 laboratory-confirmed cases, included morbilliform (22%), pernio-like (18%), urticarial (16%), macular erythema (13%), vesicular (11%), papulosquamous (9.9%), and retiform purpura (6.4%) morphologies.[5] Other registry publications have focused on the importance of the time of testing in relation to the onset of dermatologic symptoms: polymerase chain reaction (PCR) test results earlier in the disease course were more likely to be positive, even when date of onset was defined by cutaneous manifestations rather than systemic symptoms.[7]

The registry also demonstrated that skin symptoms are experienced by long-haulers, those who experience COVID-19 symptoms for weeks or months after initial infection.[8] Pernio, or COVID toes, in particular, may last for many months,

Table 1
The status of 7 international COVID-19 dermatology registries, as of March 2021

Registry	Provider-Facing?	Patient-Facing?	Date First Case Was Entered	Cases in Registry	Open for New Entries?	Web Site
AAD/ILDS	✓		April 9, 2020	1875	✓	www.aad.org/covidregistry
SECURE-Alopecia	✓		April 8, 2020	229	✓	www.securealopecia.covidderm.org
SECURE-AD	✓	✓	April 1, 2020	261(provider) 639 (patient)	✓	www.covidderm.org
PsoProtect	✓		March 27, 2020	996	✓	www.psoprotect.org
PsoProtectMe		✓	May 4, 2020	3660	✓	https://psoprotectme.org/
SECURE-Psoriasis	✓		April 1, 2020	33	✓	www.covidpso.org
HS COVID	✓	✓	April 30, 2020	46 (provider) 184 (patient)	✓	https://hscovid.ucsf.edu/
PeDRA	✓		April 12, 2020	467	✓	www.pedsderm.net

raising the question about persistent inflammation in these patients.[9] In addition to these findings, data from the registry have been used to inform public health policy. In multiple states, COVID toes are now part of their testing criteria and have served to highlight the importance of dermatologic data for characterizing the different phenotypes of COVID-19.

A majority (75%) of registry entries were of new-onset dermatologic manifestations in the setting of COVID-19. The registry still collected, however, approximately 5% of total cases on outcomes of patients with dermatologic conditions on immunosuppressive medications and was able to collaborate with PsoProtect and Surveillance Epidemiology of Coronavirus Under ResearchExclusion–Atopic Dermatitis (SECURE-AD) to share these cases. Additionally, there were multiple cases of post–COVID-19 telogen effluvium (TE), which the AAD/ILDS registry has worked with SECURE-Alopecia to document.

Given the importance of data sharing and allowing other investigators to explore important COVID-19 dermatology questions, the AAD/ILDS registry has established a data request process whereby investigators can apply for access to registry data.[10] Additionally, the AAD/ILDS registry has added a new module on COVID-19 cutaneous vaccine reactions to characterize reactions to COVID-19 vaccines[11]; 526 vaccine reactions already have been reported. The aim of this characterization is to understand the types of reactions that can present and to provide data that may prove reassuring to patients and health care providers regarding the ability to receive a second dose (in vaccines that require 2 doses) for patients with cutaneous reactions to the first dose.

SECURE-ALOPECIA

Emerging evidence regarding the potential of multiple therapies utilized in patients with alopecia (including hydroxychloroquine, antiandrogens, and JAK inhibitors, such as baricitinib) to alter COVID-19 outcomes prompted a core team from Ireland, the United Kingdom, and Australia to launch Surveillance Epidemiology of Coronavirus Under Research Exclusion-Alopecia (SECURE-Alopecia). After engaging an internationally recognized network of hair experts to define a data set harmonized with SECURE-AD (described later), the registry was launched on April 8, 2020 to record data of COVID-19–positive patients with scarring and nonscarring alopecia, both on treatment and off treatment.[12–14] The primary objective was to uncover the underlying determinants of outcomes of COVID-19–positive patients with any form of alopecia and to assess the impact of COVID-19 on alopecia—such as the development of TE.

As of March 5, 2021, there were 229 cases from 14 countries in the SECURE-Alopecia registry. Although initial data have been presented at a meeting of the American Hair Research Society and numerous educational meetings, a formal analysis has not yet been published because the diversity of the data has necessitated greater recruitment. The international steering committee has led to 2 publications regarding alopecia therapeutics during the COVID-19 era and the development of patient registries during a pandemic.[15,16]

The pressure on health services to prioritize acute and emergency care during the pandemic understandably has reduced the capacity for clinicians to follow patients with alopecia. As the pandemic has progressed and services have become more accessible, the number of cases entered in SECURE-Alopecia has increased. The delayed emergence of TE also has contributed to greater reporting of cases with time. TE is a nonscarring alopecia that results in diffuse alopecia.[17] Immediate anagen release—when large numbers of anagen follicles are triggered to prematurely enter catagen and then telogen[18]—classically is associated with high fever and certain medications and the timing mirrors the mean time from SARS-CoV-2 diagnosis in a study of 195 patients who developed acute TE.[19] Although proinflammatory cytokines or medication were proposed as potential triggers, 10% of patients experienced subclinical disease.[19] A more immediate, presumed dystrophic anagen effluvium has been reported in a single case report, although further evidence is required to validate this.[20,21] It is expected that SECURE-Alopecia will contribute to a better understanding of this component of long COVID.

SECURE-Alopecia is based on a data set developed by SECURE–Inflammatory Bowel Disease (IBD), an international database used to track cases of COVID-19 in patients with IBD. SECURE-Alopecia is matched with SECURE-AD and also is aligned closely with PsoProtect, the AAD/ILDS registry, and other inflammatory disease registries in order to enable comparative analyses. SECURE-Alopecia is engaged in ongoing discussions with these and other registries to ensure collaboration as data collection progresses. Collaboration with other registries also is of considerable interest to the steering committee, particularly with respect to cases where immunomodulatory therapies have been utilized.

In view of the delayed reporting of cases of alopecia and the emerging cases of TE and anagen effluvium that are being described, SECURE-Alopecia intends to continue to recruit cases for the foreseeable future and also aim to extend its data set to analyze the impact of vaccination on alopecia.

SECURE-AD

The SECURE-AD registry went live on April 1, 2020, as an international collaboration of dermatologists, epidemiologists, and patient experts. The primary objective is to uncover the underlying determinants of outcomes of COVID-19 in patients with AD who are treated with systemic immunomodulating medications and to examine whether outcomes are influenced by age, sex, ethnicity, or comorbidities. A secondary aim is to determine the impact of COVID-19 on the disease course and severity of AD.

SECURE-AD has both patient-facing and physician-facing registries. To date, more than 900 patients from 22 countries have been enrolled in the 2 data entry platforms (261 in the physician registry and 639 in the patient registry). In the physician registry, a majority of patients (49.8%) had mild disease at baseline (moderate, 19.0%; severe, 6.8%; remission, 20.5%; and unknown, 3.9%). Only 18.0% of patients experienced an AD flare during their COVID-19 episode. Among the 163 patients on systemic immunomodulatory medication, most were treated with dupilumab (74%), whereas 9% of patients received a conventional immunosuppressive drug during their COVID-19 episode (methotrexate, cyclosporin, mycophenolate mofetil, azathioprine, or corticosteroids). The remainder were only on topical therapy for their AD. 33 patients attended a hospital emergency department (ED) and 7 patients were hospitalized, 4 of whom required ventilation. In examining comorbidities, 2 of the ventilated patients had a body mass index (BMI) over 30 kg/m2. None of the hospitalized patients died.

Data from the registry showed that COVID-19 symptom duration and resolution were not influenced by type of systemic medication (dupilumab vs conventional immunosuppressive treatments), although there was a trend toward a higher number of ED visits in the latter group. Overall, the risk of COVID-19 and its complications appears low in AD patients treated with systemic medications.

SECURE-AD has been collaborating with the SECURE-IBD, PsoProtect, SECURE-Alopecia, and AAD/ILDS registries and comparative analyses between these different data sets are planned for the future. SECURE-AD intends to continue to recruit cases for the foreseeable future and also aim to extend its data set to analyze the impact of vaccination on AD.

THE PsoProtect

The PsoProtect registry launched globally on March 27, 2020 as a platform for clinicians to report their patients with psoriasis and confirmed or suspected COVID-19. The PsoProtect registry sought to characterize the course of COVID-19 in people with psoriasis and identify factors associated with adverse outcomes. It was established as a collaborative research effort involving an international team of clinicians, epidemiologists, health data researchers Oxford, and patient representatives, and the registry's data fields are aligned with other immune-mediated inflammatory disease (IMID) COVID-19 registries (including SECURE-AD, SECURE-IBD, and Global Rheumatology Alliance [GRA]). PsoProtect*Me*, a separate patient-facing registry with aligned questions available in 10 languages, launched globally on May 4, 2020. PsoProtect*Me* aims to characterize the experiences and behaviors of those with psoriasis (whether or not they have had COVID-19) during the pandemic.

Analysis of the first 374 patients reported by clinicians to PsoProtect with confirmed or suspected COVID-19 and psoriasis was published in the *Journal of Allergy and Clinical Immunology*[22]; 71% of patients reported to PsoProtect were receiving a biologic, 18% were receiving a nonbiologic, and 10% were not receiving any systemic treatment of their psoriasis; 93% of reported patients fully recovered from COVID-19, 21% were hospitalized, and 9 patients (2%) died. There were no significant differences found between classes of biologics, but biologic use was associated with a lower risk of COVID-19–related hospitalization compared with nonbiologic systemic therapies. The PsoProtect investigators highlight the need for further investigation into this on account of potential selection biases (eg, most patients reported to PsoProtect were receiving biologics) and unmeasured confounding (eg, potential differences in risk mitigating behaviors between treatment groups).

An analysis of self-reported data from 2869 people with psoriasis reporting to PsoProtect*Me* subsequently was published in the *British Journal of Dermatology*.[23] Data from PsoProtect*Me* were pooled with self-reported data from 851 people with rheumatic diseases reporting to the aligned registry CORE-UK. Shielding, or stringent risk-mitigating behavior, during the pandemic was associated with use of targeted therapies compared with standard systemic agents or no treatment. This difference in behavior between treatment groups may contribute to the reported lower risk of adverse COVID-19 outcomes associated with use of targeted biologic treatment. Shielding also was associated with established risk factors for severe COVID-19 (male sex, obesity, and comorbidity burden) and a positive anxiety or depression screen.

Data from the PsoProtect registry has thus uncovered key demographic and clinical factors associated with severe COVID-19 outcomes in psoriasis, which have helped to inform clinical care during the pandemic. Reassuringly, these data suggested that most people with psoriasis receiving drugs that affect the immune system fully recovered from COVID-19. PsoProtect has informed clinical guidance statements from the International Psoriasis Council[24] and the National Psoriasis Foundation[25] and has engaged with patient organizations, such as the Psoriasis Association[26] and the International Federation of Psoriasis Associations.[27] Findings from PsoProtect*Me* on risk-mitigating behavior across treatment groups also have informed evidence-based communication with patients and have the potential to inform updated public health guidelines on shielding as the pandemic continues.

PsoProtect continues to collaborate with AAD/ILDS and SECURE-Psoriasis in order to optimize international case capture. There also is an ongoing collaboration between PsoProtect, SECURE-IBD, and GRA, which seeks to identify factors associated with severe COVID-19 outcomes across IMIDs and across systemic treatments.

SECURE-PSORIASIS

Surveillance Epidemiology of Coronavirus Under Research Exclusion-Psoriasis (SECURE-Psoriasis) is the other registry focused specifically on psoriasis in this group of contributors. It was launched on April 1, 2020, by a team from Wake Forest School of Medicine in North Carolina as an international, deidentified, provider-facing registry for psoriasis patients with concomitant confirmed COVID-19 infection. This registry was produced in partnership with SECURE-IBD[28] and was designed to better define the impact of COVID-19 on patients with psoriasis.

The SECURE-Psoriasis registry has recorded more than 30 reported cases in recent months, both from the United States and internationally. The registry has shared its data with several other COVID-19 registries for patients with dermatologic conditions, including PsoProtect, resulting in multiple internationally collaborative articles, such as the review of 374 psoriasis patients with confirmed COVID-19 (described previously).[22] Another shared publication discusses the importance of collaborative development of interoperable patient registries.[16]

The data gathered through SECURE-Psoriasis and other registries for psoriasis patients diagnosed with COVID-19 have helped inform the question of how patients on biologic therapy for chronic inflammatory conditions, such as psoriasis, fare during a global pandemic. SECURE-Psoriasis data also have helped to answer the question of which patient characteristics are associated with better and worse COVID-19 outcomes. Additionally, the registry has gathered data on COVID-19's possible effect on psoriasis symptoms.

As recently as December 2020, SECURE-Psoriasis shared a new collection of case data with PsoProtect in order to maximize collaboration between US and international registry efforts. Continued collaboration with other international registries is planned in the future in order to examine the question of biologics' effect on COVID-19 outcomes more comprehensively and in a larger patient population.

The main objective of the SECURE-Psoriasis registry continues to be the maximization of data sharing and collaboration with other registries for psoriasis patients diagnosed with COVID-19 in order to better understand the effects of a pandemic environment on patients with chronic inflammatory conditions.

GLOBAL HIDRADENITIS SUPPURATIVA COVID-19 REGISTRY

The Global Hidradenitis Suppurativa COVID-19 (HS COVID) Registry was established in order to identify predictors of COVID-19 outcomes and improve the care of patients with HS.[29] This international pediatric and adult registry was launched by a team of investigators and patient partners from the United States, Canada, United Kingdom, Australia, Italy, and Denmark in collaboration with the United States, Canadian, and Asia-Pacific hidradenitis suppurativa foundations; Hope for HS; and Hidradenitis Suppurativa Warriors. At registry inception, data collection instruments were harmonized with SECURE-Alopecia, PsoProtect, SECURE-AD, and AAD/ILDS to enable comparisons of outcomes with other patient populations, including those with inflammatory diseases. The registry went live on April 5, 2020.

Data from HS COVID have shown that biologics are not associated with greater COVID-19 severity or greater need for COVID-19 treatment. In patient-reported cases, after adjusting for age, sex, and comorbidities, hidradenitis suppurativa (HS) patients taking biologics did not have greater odds of in-hospital treatment compared with those not taking biologics (odds ratio [OR] 0.5; 95% CI [0.1, 2.4]; $P = .4$). HS patients taking biologics did not have significantly greater odds of requiring oxygen support compared with those not taking biologics (OR 0.52; 95% CI [0.2, 1.8]; $P = .5$). No differences in hospitalization, oxygen requirement, or complications were observed for those who continued versus discontinued biologics at the time of COVID-19 diagnosis ($P>.5$ for all).

In health care provider–reported cases, COVID-19 severity ranged from asymptomatic to moderate (11.1% asymptomatic, 77.8% mild, and 11.1% moderate). No difference in virus severity was observed between patients taking biologics and not taking biologics ($P = .3$). Shortness of breath and acute respiratory distress syndrome were reported infrequently (4 of 27 cases; 13.3%). There was no difference in COVID-19 severity between those who continued and those who discontinued biologics ($P = .3$). No instances of death, strokes, myocardial infarctions, heart failure, or sepsis were reported by patients or providers.

These initial findings have guided use of biologic therapies in patients with HS, and informed knowledge of the safety of tumor necrosis factor, interleukin (IL)-1, IL-17, and IL-12/23 inhibitors in the overall setting of COVID-19. By confirming the continued use of disease-altering therapies throughout the pandemic, these findings potentially have aided in reducing urgent care and emergency room health care utilization by HS patients with disease flares. Overall, initial findings from patient-reported and provider-reported cases indicate that COVID-19 severity in HS patients was mild to moderate, with no difference in COVID-19 severity between those taking and not taking biologics nor between those who continued versus discontinued biologic treatment.

The team plans to examine HS outcomes in comparison with other inflammatory skin disease outcomes. As an extension of this work, HS COVID is considering collecting data on the vaccination preferences and experiences of people living with HS. These data will inform HS management for this and future pandemics and public health crises.

PeDRA REGISTRY

With a goal of creating a pediatric-specific international registry for acral skin changes, the Pediatric Dermatology COVID-19 Response Task Force—a collaborative effort by members of the Society for Pediatric Dermatology (SPD) and Pediatric Dermatology Research Alliance (PeDRA), further supported by the British Society for Paediatric Dermatology—established the PeDRA registry on April 12, 2020.

To date, 467 patients have been entered into the pediatric (2 months to 18 years) acral change registry. A majority (60%) of patients entered were white men with an average age of 13 years (±3.6 y). A minority of patients had been tested for SARS-Cov-2 and only 1.6% of those tested had a positive PCR or antibody test. Generally, COVID-19–positive children had minimal other symptoms, no hospitalizations, and no mortality. Ten children who presented in the spring had recurrence of acral changes in the late fall and early winter without other symptoms. This work was presented at the PeDRA October 2020 meeting.[30]

The PeDRA registry has been instrumental in understanding the short-term and long-term sequelae of acral pernio. Reassuringly, pediatric patients presenting with acral pernio-like changes have an excellent prognosis. Rare patients with systemic signs or symptoms did not have significant complications or lasting systemic sequelae, but a subset have had persistent or recurrent acral changes weeks to months after initial presentation. Acral pernio in otherwise healthy pediatric patients does not need to be comprehensively evaluated with skin biopsy and laboratory work because it is not suggestive of the severe ischemic coagulopathies observed in critically ill COVID-positive adults. In certain clinical contexts, COVID-19 testing by PCR or serology may be appropriate.

In the future, the registry aims to track all entries for updated clinical data about course and prognosis and evaluate cases comprehensively in order to assist in the ongoing work of determining the precise nature of the relationship between COVID-19 and acral pernio in otherwise healthy children.

DISCUSSION: WHERE DO WE GO FROM HERE?

There certainly are limitations to the conclusions that can be drawn from registry data. For example, an important limitation of these registries is their lack of information on the total population at risk for any event of interest, be it dermatologic manifestations of COVID-19 or outcomes, such as death or hospitalization. Thus, the data cannot be used to calculate the incidence or prevalence of any complications of COVID-19 in the population at large. Additionally, the fact that most registries are available only in English—despite being open for global submissions—introduces a reporting bias, which further curtails generalizability, exemplified by the fact that many of the cases entered in these registries are white patients from North America and Europe. For example, although the AAD/ILDS registry has entries from 52 countries on all continents other than Antarctica, 87.8% of those cases are from the United States, and 79.9% of the patients are white

(9.4% Asian, 8.1% Hispanic/Latino, and 2.7% black). Other registries follow a similar racial breakdown, with 78.1% of SECURE-AD, 77.8% of SECURE-Psoriasis, 72% of PeDRA, 68% of HS COVID, and 64% of SECURE-Alopecia cases being white patients. Geographically, 87% and 56%, respectively, of SECURE-Psoriasis and HS COVID cases are from North America, and 70% of PEDRA cases are from the United States. This homogeneity has implications for the ability of registries to contribute generalizable scientific knowledge, especially for a pandemic that has touched all continents and disproportionately afflicted communities of color. In the end, conclusions drawn from these registries are only as good as the data entered. There still is work to be done in ensuring equitable representation of the global dermatologic patient community.

That said, registry data have been instrumental in enhancing scientific knowledge during the pandemic. By providing a platform where physicians and, in some cases, patients can enter their observations, a registry can crowdsource disparate findings from around the world, facilitating the recognition of recurrent patterns. Registry data led to the understanding of the spectrum of cutaneous manifestations of the virus: pernio-like lesions are associated with mild COVID-19 whereas retiform purpura is seen only in severe COVID-19 patients requiring intensive care.[5] Other hypotheses generated from this real-world evidence have influenced the advancement of scientific knowledge about the virus, its various manifestations, and patient care, as in the cases of recognizing COVID toes as a symptom of the

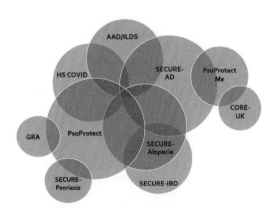

Fig. 1. Every group collaborated with at least 1 other in developing their registry or analyzing data. Overlap between circles represents collaboration between registries; circle size corresponds to number of collaborations, with PsoProtect and SECURE-AD each having 6 and SECURE-Psoriasis having 1.

Table 2
The registries have a shared objective of understanding the interplay between COVID-19 and skin conditions

Registry	Objective
AAD/ILDS	To capture observations from health care providers worldwide in order to understand dermatologic manifestations of COVID-19 and form hypotheses about the virus
SECURE-Alopecia	To capture observations from health care providers worldwide in order to understand the impact of alopecias and their therapies on COVID-19 and whether the virus induces alopecia
SECURE-AD	To uncover the underlying determinants of the outcomes of COVID-19 in patients with AD who are treated with systemic immunomodulating medication, and—through the patient survey—to better understand how COVID-19 affects AD patients and improve their care
PsoProtect	To characterize the course of COVID-19 in people with psoriasis and the factors associated with adverse outcomes through a physician-reported registry
PsoProtectMe	To characterize the behaviors and experiences of people with psoriasis during the COVID-19 pandemic, regardless of COVID-19 infection, through a patient-reported registry
SECURE-Psoriasis	To collect cases of psoriasis patients diagnosed with COVID-19 and examine the disease course and clinical outcomes in psoriasis patients, and to evaluate patient factors that may lead to better or worse COVID-19 outcomes
HS COVID	To identify predictors of COVID-19 outcomes and improve the care of patients with HS
PeDRA	To collect cases of acral pernio-like changes identified in pediatric patients through a registry for health care providers in order to capture and document this newly observed phenomenon and determine its relationship to COVID-19 by symptoms, exposure, and formal testing

virus or providing reassuring data on use of biologics and immunosuppressive medications during the pandemic.[22] Furthermore, the synthesized data generated by these registries have been made widely accessible to professionals and the public through peer-reviewed publications and informative online platforms,[31,32] thus providing important guidance concerning COVID-19 disease symptoms in the general population and in patients with chronic skin diseases.

The immense amount of collaboration (**Fig. 1**) between registries—both within dermatology and with external registries documenting nondermatological conditions—was instrumental to this production of knowledge and should set a precedent for the harmonization of data collection in the international dermatology community moving forward. When the need for evidence-based answers is high and the availability of time and resources is low, collaboration can enhance the ability of researchers and medical professionals to provide quality information and care. Due to democratized access and less stringent inclusion criteria (compared with clinical trials and studies), registries can better reflect real-world evidence, especially when it comes to rare diseases or long-term complications and outcomes.[2,16]

All the registries included in this article intend to remain open for further case reporting. As the global vaccine rollout continues, at least 5 registries—AAD/ILDS, SECURE-Alopecia, SECURE-AD, PsoProtect, and HS COVID—are collating information on patients' COVID-19 vaccine complications and experiences into their work. The biggest and most critical shared goal is the continued collaboration between registries as they work toward their shared objectives (**Table 2**) of understanding COVID-19 in the context of dermatologic diseases and better serving patients worldwide.

DISCLOSURE

Dr L.E. French is president of the ILDS. Dr E.E. Freeman is principal investigator of the AAD/ILDS COVID-19 Dermatology Registry. The ILDS provides financial support for the AAD/ILDS registry.

Dr E.E. Freeman is an author for UpToDate. Drs S.R. Feldman, C.E.M. Griffiths, S.K. Mahil, H.B. Naik, and C.H. Smith have received funding or support from and Drs L.E. French, A.D. Irvine, and P.I. Spuls have been consultants for AbbVie; Dr M.A. Lowes has served on the advisory board for AbbVie. Drs S.R. Feldman, L.E. French, C.E.M. Griffiths, S.K. Mahil, R. Sinclair, and C.H. Smith have received funding or support from Novartis. Drs S.R. Feldman, C.E.M. Griffiths, R. Sinclair, C.H. Smith, and D. Wall have received funding from Pfizer. Drs S.R. Feldman, S.K. Mahil, and C.H. Smith have received funding from and Drs A.D. Irvine and P.I. Spuls have been consultants for Sanofi. Drs S.R. Feldman, C.E.M. Griffiths, A.D. Irvine, S.K. Mahil, R. Sinclair, and D. Wall have received funding or honoraria from Eli Lily; Drs S.R. Feldman, L.E. French, C.E.M. Griffiths, S.K. Mahil, R. Sinclair, and D. Wall have received funding or honoraria from Janssen. Drs S.R. Feldman and C.E. M. Griffiths have received funding or support from BMS, Almirall, Amgen, Galderma, LEO Pharma, Stiefel GSK, and Sun Pharmaceuticals. Drs C.E.M. Griffiths and S.K. Mahil have received funding or support from Celgene and UCB Pharma. Dr C.E.M. Griffiths has received honoraria and/or research grants from MSD and Sandoz. Dr S.R. Feldman received research, speaking and/or consulting support from Alvotech, Boehringer Ingelheim, Mylan, Ortho Dermatology, Samsung, Menlo, Helsinn, Arena, Forte, Merck, Regeneron, Novan, Qurient, National Biological Corporation, Caremark, Advance Medical, Suncare Research, Informa, UpToDate, and National Psoriasis Foundation. Dr S.R. Feldman is founder and majority owner of www.DrScore.com and is founder and part owner of Causa Research, a company dedicated to enhancing patients' adherence to treatment. Dr L.E. French received speaking and/or consulting support from Galderma, Amgen, Leo Pharma, Biotest, and Pincell Srl. Dr H.B. Naik has received consulting fees from 23andme, Abbvie, and DAVA Oncology and advisory board fees from Boehringer Ingelheim and is an investigator for Pfizer. She also is an associate editor for *JAMA Dermatology*. Dr M.A. Lowes has served on the advisory boards for Abbvie, InflaRx, Janssen, and Viela Bio, and consulted for Almirall, BSN medical, Incyte, Janssen, Kymera, and XBiotech. Dr C.H. Smith is an investigator on Medical Research Council and Horizon 2020–funded consortia with industry partners (see psort.org.uk and biomap-imi.eu). Drs H.B. Naik (board member) and M.A. Lowes (vice president) are unpaid members of the US Hidradenitis Suppurativa Foundation. Drs L. Castelo-Soccio, K.M. Cordoro and I. Lara-Corrales are part of the PeDRA COVID-19 Response Task Force, a collaboration between the SPD and the PeDRA. Dr C. Flohr is President of the British Society for Paediatric Dermatology and Chief Investigator of the UK-Irish Atopic Eczema Systemic Therapy Register (A-STAR) (ISRCTN11210918). Dr C. Flohr and the patient-facing part of the SECURE-AD registry are supported by the National Institute for Health Research Biomedical Research Centre at Guy's and St Thomas' NHS Foundation Trust, London, UK. Dr A.D. Irvine is the unpaid Chairman of National and International Skin Registry Solutions (NISR) Ltd, a not-for-profit charity dedicated to developing registries for patients with skin disease. NISR supports the Secure-AD registry. Dr A.D. Irvine is a co–principal investigator on the A-STAR and has been a consultant or speaker for Regeneron and LEO Pharma outside of the scope of the current work. Dr P.I. Spuls has received departmental independent research grants from a few pharmaceutical companies for the TREAT NL registry, is involved in performing clinical trials with many pharmaceutical industries that manufacture drugs used for the treatment of conditions like psoriasis and atopic dermatitis, for which financial compensation is paid to the department/hospital, and is chief investigator of a systemic and phototherapy atopic eczema registry (TREAT NL) for adults and children and one of the main investigators of the SECURE-AD registry. Drs D. Wall and R. Sinclair colead and are members of the steering committee, along with Dr N. Meah, of the SECURE-Alopecia registry. Drs R. Sinclair, D. Wall, and N. Meah are leading the development of the Global Registry of Alopecia Areata Disease Severity and Treatment Safety. Dr D. Wall is an employee of the charity NISR. Dr R. Sinclair also reports serving as a consultant or paid speaker for or participating in clinical trials sponsored by LEO Pharma, Amgen, Merck & Co, Celgene Corporation, Coherus BioSciences, Regeneron Pharmaceuticals, MedImmune, GlaxoSmithKline, Cutanea, Samson Clinical, Boehringer Ingelheim, Merck Sharpe & Dohme, Oncobiologics, F. Hoffman–La Roche, and Bayer AG and serves as the current president of the Australasian Hair and Wool Research Society. G.C. Chamberlin and D.E. McMahon and Drs E.A. Balogh and A.V. Marzano have no conflicts of interest to declare.

REFERENCES

1. WHO Coronavirus (COVID-19) Dashboard. Available at: https://covid19.who.int. Accessed April 7, 2021.

2. Freeman EE, McMahon DE, Hruza GJ, et al. International collaboration and rapid harmonization across dermatologic COVID-19 registries. J Am Acad Dermatol 2020;83(3):e261–6.

3. Freeman EE, McMahon DE, Fitzgerald ME, et al. The American Academy of Dermatology COVID-19 registry: Crowdsourcing dermatology in the age of COVID-19. J Am Acad Dermatol 2020;83(2):509–10.

4. AAD Registry for Skin Manifestations of COVID-19: Q&A With Dr Freeman. The Dermatologist. Available at: https://www.the-dermatologist.com/article/aad-registry-skin-manifestations-covid-19-qa-dr-freeman. Accessed February 25, 2021.

5. Freeman EE, McMahon DE, Lipoff JB, et al. The spectrum of COVID-19–associated dermatologic manifestations: An international registry of 716 patients from 31 countries. J Am Acad Dermatol 2020;83(4):1118–29.

6. Freeman EE, McMahon DE, Lipoff JB, et al. Pernio-like skin lesions associated with COVID-19: A case series of 318 patients from 8 countries. JAAD 2020;83(2):486–92.

7. Freeman EE, McMahon DE, Hruza GJ, et al. Timing of PCR and antibody testing in patients with COVID-19 associated dermatologic manifestations. J Am Acad Dermatol 2020;0(0). https://doi.org/10.1016/j.jaad.2020.09.007.

8. McMahon DE, Gallman AE, Hruza GJ, et al. Long COVID in the skin: a registry analysis of COVID-19 dermatological duration. Lancet Infect Dis 2021; 21(3):313–4.

9. Freeman EE, McMahon DE, Lipoff JB, et al. Cold and COVID: Recurrent Pernio during the COVID-19 Pandemic. Br J Dermatol 2021;bjd.19894. https://doi.org/10.1111/bjd.19894.

10. Freeman EE, McMahon DE. COVID-19 Dermatology Registry Data Request Application. Available at: https://redcap.partners.org/redcap/surveys/index.php?s=HC7R44JJLT. Accessed February 25, 2021.

11. McMahon DE, Amerson E, Rosenbach M, et al. Cutaneous reactions reported after Moderna and Pfizer COVID-19 vaccination: A registry-based study of 414 cases. J Am Acad Dermatol 2021. https://doi.org/10.1016/j.jaad.2021.03.092.

12. Meah N, Wall D, York K, et al. The Alopecia Areata Consensus of Experts (ACE) Study: Results of an International Expert Opinion on Treatments for Alopecia Areata. J Am Acad Dermatol 2020. https://doi.org/10.1016/j.jaad.2020.03.004.

13. Meah N, Wall D, York K, et al. The Alopecia Areata Consensus of Experts (ACE) Study PART II: Results of an International Expert Opinion on Diagnosis and Laboratory Evaluation for Alopecia Areata. J Am Acad Dermatol 2020;83(1):123–30.

14. Wall D, Meah N, York K, et al. A Global eDelphi Exercise to Identify Core Domains and Domain Items for the Development of a Global Registry of Alopecia Areata Disease Severity and Treatment Safety (GRASS). JAMA Dermatol 2021. https://doi.org/10.1001/jamadermatol.2020.5839.

15. Fagan CN, Meah N, York K, et al. Shedding light on therapeutics in alopecia and their relevance to COVID-19. Clin Dermatol 2020;114(June):e00146.

16. Wall D, Alhusayen R, Arents B. Learning from disease registries during a pandemic: moving towards an international federation of patient registries. Clin Dermatol 2021.

17. Cranwell WC, Sinclair R. Telogen effluvium. In: Alopecia. St. Louis, Missouri: Elsevier; 2019. p. 83–93.

18. Headington JT. Telogen effluvium: new concepts and review. Arch Dermatol 1993;129(3):356.

19. Moreno-Arrones OM, Lobato-Berezo A, Gomez-Zubiaur A, et al. SARS-CoV-2-induced telogen effluvium: a multicentric study. J Eur Acad Dermatol Venereol 2021;35(3). https://doi.org/10.1111/jdv.17045.

20. Trüeb RM, Dutra Rezende H, Gavazzoni Dias MFR. What can the hair tell us about COVID-19? Exp Dermatol 2021;30(2):288–90.

21. Shanshal M. COVID-19 related anagen effluvium. J Dermatol Treat 2020;1–2. https://doi.org/10.1080/09546634.2020.1792400.

22. Mahil SK, Dand N, Mason KJ, et al. Factors associated with adverse COVID-19 outcomes in patients with psoriasis—insights from a global registry–based study. J Allergy Clin Immunol 2021;147(1):60–71.

23. Mahil SK, Yates M, Langan SM, et al. Risk mitigating behaviours in people with inflammatory skin and joint disease during the COVID-19 pandemic differ by treatment type: a cross-sectional patient survey. Br J Dermatol 2020;bjd.19755.

24. IPC - IPC Statement on COVID-19 and Psoriasis. IPC. Available at: https://www.psoriasiscouncil.org/blog/COVID-19-Statement.htm. Accessed February 11, 2021.

25. Gelfand JM, Armstrong AW, Bell S, et al. National psoriasis foundation COVID-19 task force guidance for management of psoriatic disease during the pandemic: Version 1. J Am Acad Dermatol 2020; 83(6):1704–16.

26. PsoProtect & PsoProtectMe - April 2021 Update. Psoriasis Association. Available at: https://www.psoriasis-association.org.uk/news/psoprotect-psoprotectme-april-2021-update. Accessed April 7, 2021.

27. COVID-19. International Federation of Psoriasis Associations. Available at: https://ifpa-pso.com/covid-19/. Accessed April 7, 2021.

28. SECURE-IBD Database. SECURE-IBD Database. Available at: https://covidibd.org/. Accessed February 11, 2021.

29. Naik HB, Alhusayen R, Frew J, et al. Global Hidradenitis Suppurativa COVID-19 Registry: a registry to inform data-driven management practices. Br J Dermatol 2020;183(4):780–1.

30. Castelo-Soccio L, Lara-Corrales I, Paller AS. Acral Changes in pediatric patients during COVID 19 pandemic: Registry report from the COVID 19 response task force of the Society for Pediatric Dermatology (SPD) and the Pediatric Dermatology Research Alliance (PeDRA). Pediatr Dermatol 2021;00:1–7.

31. Resource Centre. ILDS. Available at: https://ilds.org/resource-centre/. Accessed April 5, 2021.

32. Coronavirus Resource Center. Available at: https://www.aad.org/member/practice/coronavirus. Accessed April 5, 2021.

Coronavirus Disease 2019 and Dermatology Practice Changes

Angeli Eloise Torres, MD[a,b,*], David M. Ozog, MD[b],
George J. Hruza, MD, MBA[c]

KEYWORDS

- COVID-19 • Dermatology practice • Guidelines • New normal • Pandemic • Phototherapy
- Procedural dermatology • Teledermatology

KEY POINTS

- Dermatology practice adjustments during the COVID-19 pandemic have involved measures to facilitate physical distancing and curtail viral transmission.
- Telemedicine utilization has increased tremendously and has continued to account for a significant proportion of overall visits even as clinics began to reopen.
- Face-to-face consultations are unlikely to be replaced entirely by teledermatology, particularly for conditions that require closer inspection/palpation, microscopy, or biopsy.
- During the early phases of the COVID-19 pandemic and associated lockdowns, dermatology procedures declined dramatically and were limited mostly to nonelective surgeries, whereas cosmetic procedures became exceedingly rare.
- The decision to resume phototherapy should be made based on the weight of its perceived benefit versus the potential risks to both the patient and staff. Until widespread vaccination has been rolled out, patients may opt to forego phototherapy sessions and risk disease flares over fears of contracting COVID-19.

INTRODUCTION

The coronavirus disease 2019 (COVID-19) pandemic has substantially impacted medical practice worldwide. At its peak, lockdown measures were implemented in an effort to curb viral spread and reallocate resources and manpower toward the pandemic response. This situation entailed the closure of ambulatory sites that are deemed nonessential, which included dermatology outpatient clinics. As clinics began to reopen, dermatologists were faced with the challenge of navigating clinical practice while adhering to enhanced safety protocols (ie, physical distancing, mask wearing, frequent hand washing), and teledermatology, often referred to as the "new normal." In this article, we describe how the COVID-19 pandemic has restructured the practice of dermatology and provide a summary of expert guidelines on the safe conduct of dermatology consultations, procedures, and phototherapy in the midst of this global health crisis.

The Rise of Teledermatology

During the height of the COVID-19 pandemic, many workers switched to working remotely to minimize in-person encounters and limit viral transmission. The medical field was no exception, as face-to-face patient encounters have been

a Department of Dermatology, Makati Medical Center, Makati City, Philippines; b Department of Dermatology, Henry Ford Health System, 3031 W Grand Blvd, Detroit, MI 48202, USA; c Department of Dermatology, Saint Louis University, 1 N Grand Blvd, St. Louis, MO 63103, USA
* Corresponding author. Department of Dermatology, Makati Medical Center, 2 Amorsolo St., Legaspi Village, Makati City 1229, Philippines
E-mail address: angelieloise@gmail.com

Dermatol Clin 39 (2021) 587–597
https://doi.org/10.1016/j.det.2021.05.004

minimized to reduce the need for personal protective equipment (PPE) in short supply, whereas telemedicine was maximized. Telemedicine is defined as "the use of electronic information and communications technologies to provide and support health care when distance separates the participants."[1] This definition encompasses radio dispatching of emergency personnel, robotic surgery, and telephone and/or video consults.[1] Being a highly visual field, dermatology is a field well suited to maximize telemedicine. The term "teledermatology" has been used to describe the use of telemedicine to evaluate skin lesions, review laboratory findings, and diagnose and treat patients remotely.[2]

First developed during the 1960s, the practice of teledermatology has increased exponentially in recent years.[2] Teledermatology has proved to be vital during the peak of COVID-19 restrictions and, even as clinics have reopened, teledermatology continued to account for a significant proportion of overall dermatology visits.[3] A recent analysis of trends in teledermatology use found that from May 2020 to June 2020, teledermatology consults for common dermatoses (ie, acne, rosacea, psoriasis, atopic dermatitis, and eczema) increased, whereas consults for skin malignancies decreased.[3] This finding indicates that despite the availability of in-person consultation as an option, both patients and physicians felt comfortable addressing benign skin conditions via teledermatology.[3] It is therefore reasonable to expect the long-term integration of telemedicine into dermatology practice, which necessitates the development of guidelines for optimal delivery of this service (**Box 1**).

Teledermatology aims to improve access and accessibility to care, increase efficiency, and reduce cost[2,4]; however, it also has limitations. These limitations include technical difficulties (ie, poor Internet connection), privacy concerns, patient challenges with technology, access to technology, and lack of insurance coverage.[5,6] In addition, there is potential for misdiagnosis due to incomplete history taking, poor photograph/video quality, and inability to perform physical examination (eg, lesion palpation) and diagnostic procedures.[6] One review reports that more than half of teledermatology consultations require a subsequent in-person visit.[2] Hence, clinicians must assess the appropriateness of teledermatology on a case-to-case basis.[7]

In-Person Consultation

Trends in average weekly patient visits during the initial phase of the pandemic (mid-February to mid-April) showed an 81% decline (from 149.7 to 28.2), with an uptick observed in mid-May (96.5 patients seen per week), commensurate with the gradual easing of lockdown restrictions in the United States[8]; this means that from February to May 2020, a potential 10.2 million patient visits were missed, which equates to an estimated decrease in revenue of $2.3 billion.[8] In addition, a global Web-based survey of 733 dermatologists revealed that in-person consultation decreased by 54% following the onset of the pandemic, whereas teledermatology use increased 3-fold.[9] More than two-thirds of survey respondents expect continued use of teledermatology in the future, further emphasizing its role in dermatology practice beyond the pandemic.[9]

Nonetheless, despite its increasing acceptability among both patients and practitioners alike, it is unlikely for teledermatology to entirely replace traditional face-to-face consultation. One study found that when presented with the same patient, there was a high degree of concordance (72%) between the diagnosis made by a dermatologist through teleconsultation and another dermatologist through face-to-face visit.[10] However, it was also noted that 20% of the patients were deemed unfit for teleconsultation. These patients included those with conditions that cannot be sufficiently diagnosed without closer inspection and palpation, dermoscopy, fungal or viral microscopy, and biopsy.[10] Hence, dermatology practice during the "new normal" involves determining whether a patient is suitable for teledermatology or in-person consultation.

Dermatology practices generally fall under the low-risk category for COVID-19 exposure.[11] However, according to a study by Gerami and Liszewski,[12] a dermatologist is likely to encounter 1 active COVID-19 case per week in the outpatient clinic, given an average of 165 new COVID-19 cases a day in a population of 100,000. Hence, during the pandemic, it is still prudent to have administrative and engineering measures in place to ensure the safety of both patients and staff. The American Academy of Dermatology recommended steps for running dermatology practice during the COVID-19 pandemic, first shared on their Web site in December 2020 (**Box 2**).[11]

Most interim guidelines, when COVID-19 community spread was high, recommended seeing only urgent and essential cases, decreasing opening days and/or hours, reducing the number of staff per shift, and limiting the number of patients seen per day. Intervals in between appointments were lengthened, whereas the actual patient encounter was limited to as little time as possible

---

Box 1
American Telemedicine Association clinical practice guidelines for teledermatology

Informed consent and data privacy

- Secure a verbal or written informed consent from the patient before the start of the telemedicine encounter.

Physical environment

- Both patient and health care provider should stay in a room or environment that ensures visual and auditory privacy.
- Before commencing with the consult, both parties should identify all persons present in the room and verify that all can be clearly seen and heard.
- Seating and lighting should be conducive for a professional interaction between the patient and provider. There should be minimal background light from windows or other sources.
- Cameras should be placed at eye level on a stable platform to minimize unnecessary movement and allow clear visualization for both parties.

Patient evaluation and examination

- The provider should obtain all data necessary to arrive at a diagnosis, differential diagnosis, appropriate workup, and treatment plan.
- Although a full-body skin examination is feasible through video consult or photographs, it may not show all skin lesions and surfaces with sufficient detail. Such examination may help to obtain multiple images from several angles and enhance lighting.
- For examination of hair-bearing skin, the patient may be required to physically displace or even remove hair. Special lighting may be helpful.
- Examination and diagnosis of pigmented lesions may be challenging and require a high index of suspicion.
- For examination of mucosal lesions and orifices (including genitalia), special attention should be given to adequate lighting and exposure.
- Note that certain lighting and background conditions may alter the color of skin lesions when captured in a photograph or video.

Follow-up and care coordination

- Coordinate care with the patient's usual physician (if applicable).
- Make referrals as indicated.
- Communicate encounter notes to the referring physician and/or the patient.
- Formulate a follow-up plan and communicate it to the patient and/or referring physician.

Documentation

- Document each patient encounter in a secure HIPAA-compliant form and location.
- At a minimum, documentation should include a summary of findings, diagnosis and/or differential diagnosis, and management/treatment plan.
- Recording of video consults is optional and should be done only with patient consent.

Data from McKoy K, Antoniotti NM, Armstrong A, et al. Practice Guidelines for Teledermatology. Telemed J E Health. 2016;22(12):981–90.

(10–15 minutes). With appointment slots limited, triaging of patients for scheduling of in-person consultation became a necessity. Guidelines for prioritizing limited in-person appointments during the height of the pandemic suggested that precedence should be given to the following[13]:

- Health care workers with skin diseases that interfere with their delivery of service.
- Patients with severe skin diseases that are potentially life-threatening, functionally debilitating, or cause significant impairment to quality of life.

Box 2
Steps for running dermatology practice during the coronavirus disease 2019 pandemic

Step 1: Be aware of the COVID-19 prevalence in the community.

- Areas with higher prevalence will likely require more stringent infection control measures.

Step 2: Clean and disinfect your practice in accordance with WHO standards.

- Use 70% ethyl alcohol, 0.5% sodium hypochlorite, or any disinfectant product that meets standard criteria for use against SARS-CoV-2.
- In the examination room, clean commonly touched surfaces (eg, tabletop, examination bed/table, door handle/knob, light switch) in between patients.
- Clean all other common areas (eg, bathroom, reception, waiting area) at the end of each day.

Step 3: Reorganize your practice to minimize patient contact and increase sterilization.

- Provide signs and/or floor markings to direct patient traffic and maintain appropriate physical distancing.

Step 4: Maintain proper PPE for staff.

- Ensure adequate PPE for all staff members.
- Mask and eye protection should be worn during patient encounters, and patients should be wearing masks.
- Consider measures to conserve PPE as needed (ie, decontamination and reusing of masks).

Step 5: Schedule all patients, including virtual consultations.

- Prioritize urgent cases.
- Consider transitioning nonurgent cases and follow-ups to telemedicine.

Step 6: Organize your staff.

- Limit the number of staff members per room to facilitate physical distancing.
- Screen staff daily.
- Staff members who are experiencing COVID-19 symptoms should refrain from reporting to work and be referred to employee health services.

Step 7: Screen patients.

- Unless a companion or caregiver is needed (eg, minors or elderly in need of assistance), patients should come to the appointment alone.
- As much as possible, patients should come on their allotted schedule to minimize patient traffic and time spent in the waiting areas.
- All patients should be screened for COVID-19 (temperature and symptom check) before entering the clinic.
- Treat all patients as potentially infectious even if they pass screening.

Step 8: Communicate with your patients.

- Update your patients regarding practice adjustments and the possibility of any future changes as the pandemic situation evolves.

SARS-CoV-2, severe acute respiratory syndrome coronavirus 2; WHO, World Health Organization.

Data from American Academy of Dermatology. Running Dermatology Practices During COVID-19. 2020. Available at: https://assets.ctfassets.net/1ny4yoiyrqia/1VQd8nAZqLCiLe7fGNlXrQ/230fd02e0b8d908b84905e57765 ff57f/Running_Practices_During_Covid-19_12.03.20.pdf. Accessed February 12, 2021.

- Diagnostic procedures for confirmatory purposes, especially when the differential diagnosis includes high-risk conditions (eg, melanoma, severe infection, mycosis fungoides, autoimmune blistering diseases).
- Patients with skin disease resulting in significant functional and/or emotional impairment who have no access to or cannot effectively use telemedicine.
- Patients with similar prognoses should be selected randomly as to who gets a particular appointment.

In addition, COVID-19 screening (temperature and symptom check) and wearing of masks became a routine, and in most cases even a prerequisite for a patient or staff member to be allowed entry into the clinic. It is recommended that staff members who are suspected to have COVID-19, either through positive screening or exposure to an infected individual, be sent home and follow the Centers for Disease Control and Prevention (CDC) guidelines for returning to work following a COVID-19 exposure (Fig. 1).[14] Overall, these adjustments were made

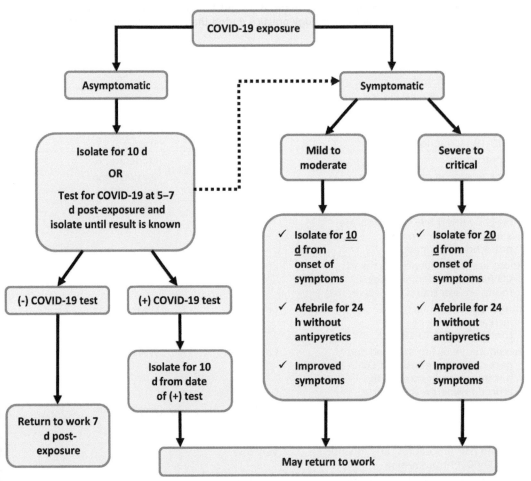

Fig. 1. Summary of CDC return to work criteria for health care staff who have been exposed to COVID-19. Exposure through close contact is defined by the CDC as being within 6 ft of an infected individual for at least 15 minutes without PPE. A previously asymptomatic staff member who starts to develop symptoms during 10-day isolation or while waiting for COVID-19 test results (dotted arrow) should follow the algorithm for symptomatic health care workers. Per CDC, fully vaccinated individuals (ie, ≥ 2 weeks and < 3 months from receiving requisite vaccine doses) or who have recovered from COVID-19 infection less than 3 months earlier do not have to quarantine after a meaningful COVID-19 exposure as long as they remain asymptomatic. Data from Centers for Disease Control and Prevention (CDC). Return to work criteria for healthcare personnel with SARS-CoV-2 infection (interim guidance). 2021. Available at: https://www.cdc.gov/coronavirus/2019-ncov/hcp/return-to-work.html?CDC_AA_refVal=https%3A%2F%2Fwww.cdc.gov%2Fcoronavirus%2F2019-ncov%2Fhealthcare-facilities%2Fhcp-return-work.html. Accessed February 27, 2021.

to facilitate physical distancing and curtail viral transmission.

Procedural Dermatology

Based on a global Web-based survey, only 25% of dermatologists performed procedures during the height of the pandemic.[9] Of these, biopsies and Mohs micrographic surgeries (MMSs) were the most commonly performed, whereas cosmetic procedures became exceedingly rare,[9] which comes as no surprise, because most interim guidelines in 2020 recommended deferring elective cosmetic and surgical procedures to reduce the risk of COVID-19 transmission and preserve PPE. The International League of Dermatologic Societies defines elective dermatologic procedures as those performed on skin lesions that pose no imminent danger to the patient if not surgically removed within 3 months[15]; these include acne surgery, chemical peels, laser hair removal, and injectables (botulinum toxin and cosmetic filler

Table 1
American Society of Dermatologic Surgery Association and American Society for Laser Medicine and Surgery guidelines for cosmetic dermatology practice during the coronavirus disease 2019 pandemic

Recommendation	Level of Evidence	Strength of Recommendation
Use of masks by patients, physicians and staff	Moderate	Strong
Physician and staff masking for procedures near the nose and mouth	Moderate	Strong
Handwashing	Moderate	Strong
COVID-19 vaccination	Moderate	Strong
Eye protection	Moderate	Moderate
Use of air suction or HEPA filters	Moderate	Weak/Option
Use of upper-room UVGI	Moderate	Weak/Option
During prolonged skin procedures, properly fitted N95 respirators are a more effective form of protection than masks	Low	Weak/Option
Room size can influence the risk of COVID-19 infection (ie, larger rooms are associated with lower risk)	Low	Weak/Option
Longer patient contact time increases the risk of contracting COVID-19	Low	Weak/Option
Procedures involving the head and neck carry greater risk of COVID-19 transmission compared with procedures below the clavicle	Low	Weak/Option
Forced air cooling increases the risk of COVID-19 transmission vs contact cooling during laser procedures	Very low	Weak/Option
Skin and hair procedures carry low risk of COVID-19 transmission	Very low	None
No documented risk of contracting COVID-19 from blood during procedures	Very low	None
No evidence that ablative laser procedures or liposuction increase the risk of COVID-19 infection	Very low	None

Abbreviations: ASDSA, American Society of Dermatologic Surgery Association; ASLMS, American Society for Laser Medicine and Surgery; HEPA, high-efficiency particulate air; UVGI, ultraviolet-C germicidal irradiation.

Data from Narla S, Alam M, Ozog D, et al. American Society of Dermatologic Surgery Association (ASDSA) and American Society for Laser Medicine & Surgery (ASLMS) Guidance for Cosmetic Dermatology Practices During COVID-19. 2021. Available at: https://www.aslms.org/docs/default-source/for-professionals/resources/asdsa-and-aslms-final-cosmetic-reopening-guidance-june2020.pdf?sfvrsn=c879e53b_2. Accessed February 12, 2021.

injections). Conversely, lesions such as melanoma, atypical melanocytic lesions, or abscess drainage may necessitate prompt management with surgery or other procedures, which should be done during the pandemic under strict infection prevention and control measures (see **Box 2**).

With regard to MMS, a United Kingdom-based nationwide survey revealed that almost half of surgeons performing MMS completely ceased services during the height of the pandemic, whereas 36% and 15% had reduced and normal operations, respectively.[16] To minimize patient visits, those who continued to perform MMS showed an increased preference toward the use of absorbable sutures for wound closure, as well as telecommunications (telephone/video) for follow-up visits compared with before COVID-19.[16] On the other hand, post-Mohs reconstructions performed by other specialties were significantly decreased

(74%) together with face-to-face consultations (91% decrease).[16]

In early 2021, the American Society for Dermatologic Surgery together with the American Society for Laser Medicine and Surgery, Inc, released guidelines for the safe practice of cosmetic dermatology during COVID-19 (**Table 1**).[17] The document detailed and graded ancillary evidence on various infection prevention and control measures (eg, mask/respirator use, eye protection, and handwashing), as well as the risk of viral transmission associated with certain dermatologic procedures.[17]

Phototherapy

The COVID-19 pandemic significantly impacted the use of chronic dermatologic treatments, including phototherapy. Many phototherapy

---

Box 3
Recommendations for phototherapy during the coronavirus disease 2019 pandemic

General recommendations

- All patients should be scheduled.
- Schedule appointments not more than every 30 min to limit the number of patients treated per day, and allow adequate time for disinfection in between patients.
- Have all patients screened for COVID-19 symptoms before entering the phototherapy unit. Patients with symptoms may be refused treatment and referred to the appropriate COVID-19 referral unit.
- Patients should ideally come alone for their phototherapy appointment. If a companion is necessary (ie, patient is a minor, an elderly who requires assistance, or disabled), only 1 is allowed.
- All patients should wear a face mask, except during total-body phototherapy treatment.
- All staff and patient companions (if any) should wear a face mask.
- All patients, patient companions, and staff must practice strict hand hygiene at all times. These should include, but are not limited to, the following instances: before entering the phototherapy unit, before and after treatment (for patients), before and after the patient encounter (for staff), after touching high-touch surfaces, before exiting the phototherapy unit.
- Maintain physical distancing at all times.

Recommendations for phototherapy treatment

- Provide all patients with individual goggles to be stored in individualized bags inside the phototherapy unit. Goggles should be disinfected according to manufacturer's instructions before storage.
- Provide a bag for storage of the patient's clothes upon disrobing. Discard the bag at the end of treatment.
- Avoid turning on the fan in the phototherapy unit. Treatments may be fractionated if needed to avoid excessive heat build-up inside the unit.
- Staff should disinfect all high-touch areas and surfaces after each patient.

Data from Lim HW, Feldman SR, Van Voorhees AS, Gelfand JM. Recommendations for phototherapy during the COVID-19 pandemic. J Am Acad Dermatol. 2020;83(1):287–88 and Laconico-Tumalad LL, Sabido PWM, Sison-de Jesus C. Philippine Dermatological Society Photodermatology Subspecialty Core Group Post-Quarantine Guidelines for Phototherapy Centers. 2020. Available at: https://pds.org.ph/pds_new/wp-content/uploads/2020/06/PDS-Photodermatology-Post-ECQ-Guidelines-for-Phototherapy-FINAL.pdf. Accessed January 29, 2021.

centers worldwide were closed during the height of the pandemic, whereas the few that remained open experienced a decline in patient census. In one of the biggest health systems in Israel, the number of patients coming in for phototherapy decreased by more than 50% since March 2020.[18] This decrease was found to be primarily driven by patients declining treatment continuation because of fear of contracting the virus; the interruption in care posed the risk of a skin disease flare.[18] Photoimmunosuppression may also be of particular concern amid the pandemic, because it is one of the mechanisms by which phototherapy controls skin disease. However, based on clinical experience with human immunodeficiency virus-positive patients, phototherapy is a safe and reasonable option during this time.[19]

The risk of severe acute respiratory syndrome coronavirus 2 (SARS-CoV-2) transmission in phototherapy units is currently unknown.[20] Although safety protocols observed in other hospital units are largely applicable, there are certain elements unique to phototherapy that require special attention. First, phototherapy involves having a patient come to the clinic multiple times a week, which potentially increases exposure to both the patient and staff. Second, localized treatments (ie, excimer laser or light) entail close contact between the patient and the staff for a prolonged period, and treatment of the face and periorificial areas where patients need to be unmasked puts the staff at even higher risk. Third, full-body treatments, although generally preferred during the pandemic, are typically administered in enclosed booths where patients stand in close proximity to phototherapy equipment surfaces made of plastic or steel.[21] This proximity can potentially facilitate viral transmission because SARS-CoV-2 has been found to survive for up to 9 days on these surfaces,[21] even though evidence of COVID-19 transmission through inanimate objects is limited. In addition, phototherapy booths normally have fans that are turned on during treatment to prevent overheating, which is potentially aerosolizing and could facilitate viral spread.[22]

Therefore, the decision to resume phototherapy should be made based on the weight of its perceived benefit versus the potential risks to both patient and staff. Most guidelines recommend prioritizing patients with severe skin disease, those who are more likely to respond to phototherapy, and in cases wherein other options besides phototherapy are limited or unavailable.[20] Home phototherapy is also a reasonable option and may even be preferable during this time; however, it may not be feasible for all patients.

If in-office phototherapy is deemed necessary, efforts must be taken to conduct operations as safely as possible. **Box 3** lists expert recommendations for operating phototherapy clinics during the COVID-19 pandemic.[22,23]

SUMMARY

	Before COVID	New Normal
Dermatology consultation	• Appointments for face-to-face consultation far outnumbered telemedicine visits • Clinics follow normal office hours • Patients can schedule in-person appointments regardless of the reason for consult • Screening, physical distancing, and wearing of face masks are generally not required • Appointments have short intervals and double bookings are acceptable • Patients are allowed to bring companions	• Increased utilization of telemedicine • Limited in-person appointments • Decreased clinic opening days and/or hours • Prioritization of urgent and essential cases for face-to-face visit • Screening of patients for COVID-19 before clinic entry • Physical distancing • Wearing of face masks • Increased time interval between appointments for disinfection • Patients are advised to come alone whenever possible
Dermatology procedures	• Elective procedures are acceptable • Postoperative patients have sutures removed in-office • In-person postoperative visits are the norm	• Elective procedures are deferred to reduce viral transmission risk • Use of absorbable sutures to eliminate additional visit for removal • Virtual postoperative visits are more frequent
Phototherapy	• Patients share a common set of goggles • Fans are turned on during treatment to avoid overheating • Multiple patients can be treated at once (ie, one patient in UV-B and one in UV-A)	• Patients are given individual goggles • Turning on of the fan is avoided to minimize potential aerosolization • Only one patient at a time is

(continued on next page)

(continued)

	Before COVID	New Normal
	• No restrictions on treating localized lesions on the face and periorificial areas	allowed with no <30-min intervals between patients • Localized treatment to the face and periorificial areas is avoided as much as possible

Future Perspectives

As of February 2021, a total of 72.8 million doses of COVID-19 vaccine have been administered in the United States, most which were first given to health care workers (HCWs).[24] In Israel, which was the first country to vaccinate most of their population, fully vaccinated HCWs (2 doses of the Pfizer BioNT vaccine) comprised only 2% of those who contracted COVID-19; this compared favorably to partially vaccinated (1 dose received) and unvaccinated HCWs who comprised 46% and 52% of infections, respectively.[25] Hence, with HCWs almost universally vaccinated, it is reasonable to expect that some easing of restrictions may take place. Per CDC guidance as of March 2021, individuals who are at least 2 weeks and less than 3 months from receiving the requisite doses of vaccine, or who have recovered from COVID-19 infection less than 3 months earlier, do not have to quarantine after a meaningful COVID-19 exposure as long as they remain asymptomatic.[26,27] However, given its unpredictable nature, COVID-19 resurgence is a possibility and may warrant reinstatement of administrative and engineering measures detailed herein. Experts advise that even after receiving 2 doses of COVID-19 vaccine, individuals must still wear masks and practice physical distancing until more information becomes available.[28]

CLINICS CARE POINTS

- COVID-19 is a rapidly evolving situation with expert recommendations changing at an almost daily basis, therefore, dermatologists must update themselves periodically and make necessary adjustments in accordance with local, state, and federal guidelines and

mandates. The points summarized herein represent expert recommendation at the height of the pandemic.

- The appropriateness of teledermatology must be assessed on a case to case basis. Many patients and dermatologists feel comfortable using teledermatology to address common dermatoses; however, lesions which require closer examination (i.e. suspected malignancy) may warrant a face-to-face visit.
- Triaging of patients for scheduling in-person visits may be necessary. COVID-19 screening, wearing of masks, and physical distancing should still be practiced.
- Elective procedures should be deferred in order to reduce the risk of COVID-19 transmission and preserve personal protective equipment, while necessary procedures should be done under strict infection control and prevention measures.
- Many patients are reluctant to resume phototherapy for fear of contracting COVID-19. Home phototherapy, if feasible, is a reasonable option. Otherwise, in-office therapy should be resumed based on the perceived benefit versus potential risks, and should be conducted with safety protocols in place.
- Despite health care workers almost universally vaccinated, COVID-19 resurgence is still a possibility. Experts recommend that fully-vaccinated individuals continue to wear masks and practice physical distancing until more information becomes available.
- As the pandemic winds down, many of these recommendations/precautions can be safely relaxed.

DISCLOSURES

Dr Torres has no relevant disclosures. Dr Ozog is an investigator for Biofrontera. Dr Hruza has no financial disclosures. He is Chair of the American Academy of Dermatology COVID-19 Ad-Hoc Task Force.

REFERENCES

1. Field MJ. Telemedicine: a guide to assessing telecommunications in health care. Washington, DC: National Academies Press (US); 1996.
2. Romero G, Garrido JA, Garcia-Arpa M. [Telemedicine and teledermatology (I): concepts and applications]. Actas Dermosifiliogr 2008;99(7):506–22.
3. Su MY, Smith GP, Das S. Trends in teledermatology use during clinic reopening after COVID-19 closures. J Am Acad Dermatol 2021;84(4):213–4.

4. Landow SM, Mateus A, Korgavkar K, et al. Teledermatology: key factors associated with reducing face-to-face dermatology visits. J Am Acad Dermatol 2014;71(3):570–6.

5. Gupta R, Ibraheim MK, Doan HQ. Teledermatology in the wake of COVID-19: Advantages and challenges to continued care in a time of disarray. J Am Acad Dermatol 2020;83(1):168–9.

6. Ng JN, Cembrano KAG, Wanitphakdeedecha R, et al. The aftermath of COVID-19 in dermatology practice: What's next? J Cosmet Dermatol 2020; 19(8):1826–7.

7. McKoy K, Antoniotti NM, Armstrong A, et al. Practice guidelines for teledermatology. Telemed J E Health 2016;22(12):981–90.

8. Litchman GH, Marson JW, Rigel DS. The continuing impact of COVID-19 on dermatology practice: Office workflow, economics, and future implications. J Am Acad Dermatol 2021;84(2):576–9.

9. Bhargava S, McKeever C, Kroumpouzos G. Impact of covid-19 pandemic on dermatology practices: results of a web-based, global survey. Int J Womens Dermatol 2021;7(2):217–23.

10. Nordal EJ, Moseng D, Kvammen B, et al. A comparative study of teleconsultations versus face-to-face consultations. J Telemed Telecare 2001;7(5):257–65.

11. American Academy of Dermatology. Running Dermatology Practices During COVID-19. 2020. Available at: https://assets.ctfassets.net/1ny4yoiyrqia/1VQd8nAZq LCiLe7fGNIXrQ/230fd02e0b8d908b84905e57765f f57f/Running_Practices_During_Covid-19_12.03.20. pdf. Accessed February 12, 2021.

12. Gerami P, Liszewski W. Risk assessment of outpatient dermatology practice in the setting of the COVID-19 pandemic. J Am Acad Dermatol 2020; 83(5):1538–9.

13. Stoff BK, Blalock TW, Swerlick RA, et al. Guiding principles for prioritization of limited in-person dermatology appointments during the COVID-19 pandemic. J Am Acad Dermatol 2020;83(4): 1228–30.

14. Centers for Disease Control and Prevention (CDC). Return to Work Criteria for Healthcare Personnel with SARS-CoV-2 Infection (Interim Guidance). 2021. Available at: https://www.cdc.gov/coronavirus/2019-ncov/hcp/return-to-work.html?CDC_AA_refVal=https %3A%2F%2Fwww.cdc.gov%2Fcoronavirus%2F2019-ncov%2Fhealthcare-facilities%2Fhcp-return-work.html. Accessed February 27, 2021.

15. International League of Dermatological Societies. Guidance on the practice of dermatosurgery and cosmetic procedures during the COVID-19 (SARS-CoV-2, Coronavirus) pandemic (updated June 2020). 2020. Available at: https://ilds.org/wp-content/uploads/2020/06/ILDS-Guidance-on-the-practice-of-dermatosurgery-and-cosmetic-procedures-COVID-19-Update-June-2020.pdf. Accessed February 12, 2021.

16. Nicholson P, Ali FR, Mallipeddi R. Impact of COVID-19 on Mohs micrographic surgery: UK-wide survey and recommendations for practice. Clin Exp Dermatol 2020;45(7):901–2.

17. Narla S, Alam M, Ozog D, et al. American Society of Dermatologic Surgery Association (ASDSA) and American Society for Laser Medicine & Surgery (ASLMS) Guidance for Cosmetic Dermatology Practices During COVID-19. 2021. Available at: https://www.aslms.org/docs/default-source/for-professionals/resources/asdsa-and-aslms-final-cosmetic-reopening-guidance-june2020.pdf?sfvrsn=c879e53b_2. Accessed February 12, 2021.

18. Fisher S, Ziv M. COVID-19 effect on phototherapy treatment utilization in dermatology. J Dermatol Treat 2020;1–3.

19. Torres AE, Lyons AB, Hamzavi IH, et al. Role of phototherapy in the era of biologics. J Am Acad Dermatol 2021;84(2):479–85.

20. Aguilera P, Gilaberte Y, Perez-Ferriols A, et al. Management of phototherapy units during the COVID-19 pandemic: Recommendations of the AEDV's Spanish Photobiology Group. Actas Dermosifiliogr 2021; 112(1):73–5.

21. Tursen U, Tursen B, Lotti T. Ultraviolet and COVID-19 pandemic. J Cosmet Dermatol 2020;19(9):2162–4.

22. Lim HW, Feldman SR, Van Voorhees AS, et al. Recommendations for phototherapy during the COVID-19 pandemic. J Am Acad Dermatol 2020;83(1): 287–8.

23. Laconico-Tumalad LL, Sabido PWM, Sison-de Jesus C. Philippine Dermatological Society Photodermatology Subspecialty Core Group Post-Quarantine Guidelines for Phototherapy Centers. 2020. Available at: https://pds.org.ph/pds_new/wp-content/uploads/2020/06/PDS-Photodermatology-Post-ECQ-Guidelines-for-Phototherapy-FINAL.pdf. Accessed January 29, 2021.

24. Centers for Disease Control and Prevention (CDC). COVID-19 Vaccinations in the United States. 2021. Available at: https://covid.cdc.gov/covid-data-tracker/#vaccinations. Accessed February 27, 2021.

25. Amit S, Regev-Yochay G, Afek A, et al. Early rate reductions of SARS-CoV-2 infection and COVID-19 in BNT162b2 vaccine recipients. Lancet 2021; 397(10277):875–7.

26. Centers for Disease Control and Prevention (CDC). When to Quarantine. 2021. Available at:

https://www.cdc.gov/coronavirus/2019-ncov/if-you-are-sick/quarantine.html. Accessed February 28, 2021.

27. Centers for Disease Control and Prevention (CDC). Interim Clinical Considerations for Use of mRNA COVID-19 Vaccines Currently Authorized in the United States. 2021. Available at: https://www.cdc. gov/vaccines/covid-19/info-by-product/clinical-considerations.html. Accessed February 28, 2021.

28. Centers for Disease Control and Prevention (CDC). Frequently Asked Questions about COVID-19 Vaccination. 2021. Available at: https://www.cdc. gov/coronavirus/2019-ncov/vaccines/faq.html. Accessed February 27, 2021.

The Impact of COVID-19 on Teledermatology: A Review

Cassandra B. Yeboah, BS, MBS[a], Nailah Harvey, BS[a], Rohan Krishnan[b], Jules B. Lipoff, MD[b,c,*]

KEYWORDS

- Teledermatology • COVID-19 • Telemedicine • Telehealth • Store-and-forward teledermatology
- Live-interactive teledermatology • Digital divide

KEY POINTS

- Before the coronavirus disease 2019 pandemic, teledermatology was limited by lack of insurance reimbursement for telemedicine visits, concern about liabilities, and licensing restrictions.
- Coronavirus disease 2019 prompted regulatory and policy changes; health systems created and adapted protocols to continue care, save personal protective equipment, and decrease unnecessary exposures.
- Teledermatology has been conducive to the constraints imposed by coronavirus disease 2019, but telemedicine may worsen care access for patients without adequate digital connections.
- Expansion of telemedicine reimbursements favored synchronous video visits rather than store-and-forward teledermatology.
- Policy changes established during the coronavirus disease 2019 pandemic, although likely temporary, have set new precedents that will have long-term impacts on teledermatology use.

INTRODUCTION

Coronavirus disease 2019 (COVID-19) has changed the way that medicine is practiced throughout the world. In March of 2020, the World Health Organization declared COVID-19 a pandemic and created guidelines in an effort to mitigate the spread of the virus. Among these guidelines were recommendations to socially distance, quarantine, and suspend all nonurgent in-person medical visits.[1] As the information known about COVID-19 has evolved, so have the safety guidelines. The unprecedented situation has forced health care providers across all fields of practice to critically look at how to maintain continuity of services in the changing landscape,

and dermatology is no exception. Certainly, dermatology has always been well-suited for telemedicine owing to its reliance on visual examinations. Changes imposed by these recommendations will remain for the foreseeable future; thus, many dermatologists have adopted telemedicine to adhere to social distancing while remaining engaged with their patient populations. Indeed, telemedicine seems especially well-suited for maintaining care during a pandemic.

This accelerated implementation and use of teledermatology during COVID-19 has met with successes and challenges. This review explores, first, how telemedicine was used in dermatology before

Funding sources: None.
Conflicts of Interest: Dr. Lipoff is the outgoing chair of the American Academy of Dermatology's Teledermatology Task Force and a member of the Ad Hoc COVID-19 Task Force. He has served as a paid consultant on telemedicine for Havas Life Medicom and as telemedicine advisor for AcneAway, a direct-to-consumer teledermatology start-up.
[a] Philadelphia College of Osteopathic Medicine, 4170 City Avenue, Philadelphia, PA 19131, USA;
[b] Department of Dermatology, Perelman School of Medicine, University of Pennsylvania, 4170 City Avenue, Philadelphia, PA 19131, USA; [c] Leonard Davis Institute of Health Economics, University of Pennsylvania, Philadelphia, PA, USA
* Corresponding author. Penn Medicine University City, 3737 Market Street, Suite 1100, Philadelphia, PA 19104.
E-mail address: jules.lipoff@pennmedicine.upenn.edu

Dermatol Clin 39 (2021) 599–608
https://doi.org/10.1016/j.det.2021.05.007

the pandemic, evaluates the regulatory adaptions made in response to the pandemic and the effectiveness of the rapid implementation of teledermatology, and, finally, considers how teledermatology may have expanded for the long term as a result of COVID-19. In addition, we examine lessons learned, how teledermatology's reliance on digital technologies might paradoxically exacerbate health care disparities, and consider the future outlook.

TELEDERMATOLOGY BEFORE CORONAVIRUS DISEASE 2019

With approximately 1 in 3 people in the United States suffering from skin diseases,[2] new and innovative methods of increasing patient outreach are essential to adequately meet the needs of the patient population. In the decades before the COVID-19 pandemic, the incorporation of teledermatology into practices' offerings was inconsistent and sparse. Limiting factors to implementation included a lack of adequate reimbursement, concerns about liability, and licensing restrictions.[3]

In the United States, teledermatology was first described in the literature as an adequate avenue for care in 1994, when it was used to deliver care in rural Oregon.[4] The use of teledermatology increased through the 2010s, but remained limited.[3,5] A 2018 review article found that only 40 nongovernment sanctioned teledermatology programs were active in the United States in 2016, with a median yearly volume of 263 consultations.[3] Although the number of teledermatology programs available was limited, consultations did show an upward trend. In 2011, the total estimated teledermatology consultations conducted by these nongovernment programs was 6500, and by 2016, the number increased to 20,000.[5] Globally, teledermatology has proven a useful tool, especially given significant variability in patient access to local dermatologists for in-person visits. In the United States, the average dermatologist to population ratio is 1:30,000, whereas in Central and South America the ratio is 1:76,000 in nonrural areas and 1:1.66 million in rural areas.[6] A trend of physician maldistribution is found throughout the world, with high-income countries and regions generally richly abundant with dermatologists, whereas middle- and low-income countries and regions lack such access. This general lack of access to specialists echoes the bigger problem of health care equity. Teledermatology has been implemented in myriad government-sanctioned health systems, commercial telemedicine services, and nonprofit and charitable organizations.[7] In countries with government-established health systems, teledermatology is primarily used to triage patients.[6] Similarly, the KSYOS Telemedical Center in the Netherlands, a commercial company, has had more than 2000 general practitioners refer more than 25,000 patients for their teledermatology service, decreasing in-person referrals by 65% to 70%.[7] Nonprofit and charitable programs, such as the Institute of Tropical Medicine in Antwerp, Belgium, the Swinfen Charitable Trust, and the African Teledermatology Project, have provided local health professionals in underserved countries with educational resources, training, and decision making support to ensure that the needs of these communities are met.[7]

Before COVID-19, teledermatology research had closely examined its efficacy for diagnosis and treatment. Evidence generally found teledermatology to be reasonably equivalent in diagnosis and management compared with traditional in-person visits.[3,8] Despite this success, adoption remained slow before the pandemic. An academic dermatology clinician may see perhaps 100 patients per week, on average, and by comparison, in 2018 the average program conducted an estimated 283 virtual visits for the entire year, thus indicating significant barriers to implementation.[3] Still, teledermatology programs have succeeded in diverse practice systems: capitated, charitable, and government.[3] A systematic review published in 2010 identified structural barriers to teledermatology implementation in the Department of Veteran Affairs, notably a lack of understanding of organization revenue models and how they might be affected by adaptive changes in workload and compensation.[8] For teledermatology to succeed, the review argued that targeted efforts must address both compensation and workload, with operating budgets possibly reallocated to support changes.[8] However, the predominant fee-for-service health care model in the United States had not adapted the changes necessary for teledermatology to succeed, especially given lack of adequate reimbursement before the COVID-19 pandemic to incentivize use.[3]

TELEMEDICINE REGULATORY CHANGES IN RESPONSE TO THE CORONAVIRUS DISEASE 2019 PANDEMIC

Before the COVID-19 pandemic, many states had parity laws through Medicare, Medicaid, and private insurance companies that allowed for telemedicine reimbursements, but the level of reimbursement varied by state and payer.[9] In fact, Medicare only paid for telemedicine if the patient lived in a rural area and when they left their home to go to a designated clinic, hospital, or medical center for the telemedicine service.[10] By 2019, the American Telemedicine Association had found that 40 states increased their coverage parameters to accommodate the increased use of telemedicine.[11] Sixteen states had limited reimbursement to only synchronous telemedicine (real-time video or telephone visits).

Despite the slow progress over the previous decade, with COVID-19, these telemedicine regulatory and policy restrictions evaporated essentially overnight, with the Centers for Medicaid and Medicare Services (CMS) enacting bold changes.[10] In all states, laws were relaxed that required that telemedicine physicians had to have preexisting in-person relationships with patients before any prescription could be written for patients after virtual visits.[9] Some states have even relaxed or eliminated interstate licensure limits, which barred physicians from providing care to patients who lived outside of their jurisdictions, thus providing patients with increased options for care.[12] For example, New Jersey provided a temporary waiver of telemedicine rules to allow for out of state licensed physicians to continue, and perhaps expand, patient care.[13]

Another pre-pandemic law, the Health Insurance Portability and Accountability Act (HIPAA), requires teledermatology visits to meet certain personal health information confidentiality standards (eg, encryption), but with COVID-19 policy relaxations, the necessity of HIPAA compliance was decreased. Specifically, the CMS waived the enforcement of HIPAA health privacy violations against providers acting in good faith.[12,14,15] Many platforms for telemedicine visits had previously opted out of these agreements, which left the liability for security and privacy breaches solely on the physician.[14] CMS's waiver of HIPAA enforcement during the public health emergency thus allowed telemedicine, for the moment at least, to be conducted over non–HIPAA-compliant platforms.[15] Other regulatory changes brought on during the COVID-19 pandemic included an increased consideration of good faith defenses in relation to HIPAA violations,[12] meaning that leniency would be applied to telemedicine-related HIPAA violations that were made nonmaliciously. Collectively, these regulatory changes led to the increased adoption of telehealth owing to necessity to continue care, expanded financial remuneration, and decreased risk of financial loss, allowance for the use of nonencrypted platforms to conduct patient visits, and the ability to reach patients without geographic restrictions (**Table 1**).

IMPLEMENTATION OF TELEDERMATOLOGY DURING THE CORONAVIRUS DISEASE 2019 PANDEMIC

The COVID-19 pandemic has led to innovations in teledermatology that will most certainly set new precedents in how it is practiced for years to come. Not only has teledermatology served as a patch to help patients in a difficult time, but these disruptive changes pushed telemedicine into the forefront of conversations for reshaping best practices for dermatology care overall as well.

As an intended effect of regulatory changes implemented during the pandemic, patients were given increasingly diverse options for telemedicine care. These new telemedicine options have been met with satisfaction by both patients and dermatologists. Pre-pandemic studies had revealed equivocal patient satisfaction ratings with teledermatology relative to traditional in-person evaluations, finding no significant differences in satisfaction between patients using solely teledermatology and patients receiving in-person care.[16,17] During the pandemic, dermatology patients reported positive satisfaction using teledermatology; for example, an observational study conducted in Italy found that 93% of surveyed patients were satisfied with these virtual visits during the pandemic.[18] An observational study of dermatology patients in Cairo, Egypt, found a 91% overall satisfaction and likelihood for future teledermatology use, with 94% remarking on its usefulness, 87% describing its allowance for quality interaction, 88% noting its ease of use, and 87% expressing its reliability.[19] For US dermatologists practicing during the pandemic, a study of 184 practices found that 89% used teledermatology, and 71% intended to use teledermatology in the future.[20] In a survey of members conducted by the American Academy of Dermatology, 14.1% of dermatologists had used teledermatology before COVID-19, compared with 96.9% since the pandemic began.[21]

Teletriage in dermatology practices may also increase practice efficiency by decreasing wait times and allowing for patient inquiries to be stratified according to their acuity.[22] During the pandemic, physicians leveraged remote patient monitoring models to collect patient data and triage visits according to importance and severity.[23] One study evaluating the effectiveness of dermatoscopic photos for the diagnosis of skin lesion found that this method increased the urgency score for malignant neoplasms, prioritizing them for in-person visits and thus increasing efficiency for both patients and physicians.[24]

Table 1
Regulatory changes in teledermatology in response to COVID-19

	Regulations before COVID-19	Regulation Changes Made During COVID-19
Reimbursements	Reimbursement schedules varied by state and payer	Expansion to accommodate increased use of teledermatology, namely, video visits
Interstate licensure limits	Physicians were limited to providing services to patients within their jurisdictions	Physicians were able to provide services to patients outside of their jurisdictions
HIPAA regulations	Services could only be conducted on encrypted platforms	Relaxed limits allowed services to be performed over nonencrypted platforms

Moreover, an analysis of teledermatology triage implementation at Zuckerberg San Francisco General Hospital determined that the remote system saved $140 per newly referred patient compared with conventional care systems.[25]

EXPANSION OF TELEDERMATOLOGY DURING THE CORONAVIRUS DISEASE 2019 PANDEMIC

During the pandemic, teledermatology has proven capable of successfully managing diagnosis, triage, and subsequent checkups for many visits, with in-person appointments still being offered to patients with more pressing concerns or visits unable to be conducted remotely (namely, skin checks and procedures).[26] Skin conditions proving especially well-suited to telemedicine have included chronic inflammatory conditions such as acne and psoriasis.[27] At the George Washington Medical Faculty Associates' Dermatology department, a study of 168 patients found the most popular reasons for telehealth appointments to be new rash (12%), eczema (10%), and psoriasis (9%).[28] A study of 153 U.S. dermatology practices operating during the pandemic found that 87% of practices offered teledermatology as an option to patients.[29] Across 12 dermatology clinics affiliated with Massachusetts General Hospital, virtual visits increased from 0 in April 2019 to 1564 in April 2020, and in-person visits for April 2020 represented less than 1% of the in-person visit volume from the year prior.[30] Before March 11, 2020, when the World Health Organization officially declared COVID-19 a pandemic, skin conditions were not listed among the most common telehealth diagnoses in the United States. However, by April 2020, skin conditions were ranked the fifth most common telehealth diagnosis in the United States.[31] Similarly, on July 21, 2020, 13 of the top 50 ranked medical applications in the US Apple App Store were useable for telemedicine, an increase of mean of 210.92 ranked positions compared with January 1, 2020.[32]

PROGRAM-SPECIFIC APPROACHES TO TELEDERMATOLOGY

Both private and academic practices used teledermatology only sporadically before COVID-19, and relied mostly on in-person visits as their standard care. In fact, in October of 2019, a J.D. Power consumer report found that about 10% of health care workers in the United States provided any telehealth services.[33] During COVID-19, a global web-based survey of 733 dermatologists found that use of teledermatology increased to 75% of all visits compared with a previous 26% of visits before the pandemic.[34] Such rapid and widespread adaptation opened opportunities for varied implementation. In this section, we analyze some of the ways that specific programs implemented teledermatology differently during the COVID-19 pandemic to consider different strategies to adapt, refine, and perfect teledermatology.

At the start of the pandemic, most planned, nonurgent in-person medical procedures were halted to prioritize the treatment of patients with COVID-19 and decrease transmission of the disease. In dermatology, most visits were considered non-urgent, and some American dermatologists worried their practices might be "vectors for the transmission of COVID-19."[35] Dermatology practices thus turned to video and store-and-forward (SAF) visits, and hybrid models using both, to adapt to the constraints on in-person visits. Across 12 dermatology clinics affiliated with Massachusetts General Hospital, most visits were scheduled live telephone calls where providers conversed with patients while viewing photographs uploaded in advance; asynchronous telemedicine visits comprised a minority (1 in 5) of all visits during April 2020. The potential advantages of asynchronous visits were the convenience of providers and patients operating on their own schedules.[36] Similarly, the Department of Dermatology at Yale School of Medicine concluded that a hybrid between SAF and video proved most effective, using

SAF before scheduled video calls to expedite visits.[27] Similarly, a survey of American Academy of Dermatology member dermatologists found that 72% (406 of 564) perceived the hybrid combination of video visits with stored photographs had the greatest accuracy.[21]

The need for a sudden change in the delivery of care forced new operationalization, especially for those with limited prior telemedicine experience. At Yale, for example, there were no teledermatology services available before COVID-19, so they created their own teledermatology training and office-based teledermatology practice algorithm.[27] Yale developed training videos for staff, departmental algorithms for patient visits, and call scripts for providers. Using a hybrid method, all new patients uploaded videos and images of lesions to their electronic medical records, and could speak directly to a provider. In total, the department's number of telemedicine visits increased from 225 during their first week after implementation to almost 500 during their third week.[27]

Similarly, the Ohio State University Division of Dermatology developed a SAF inpatient algorithm combined with subsequent chart review to assess teledermatology consult appropriateness using physician judgment.[37] If not deemed appropriate, follow-up questions stratified COVID-19 status and/or other respiratory illnesses to triage in-person consults. Other measures reduced physician and patient COVID-19 risk; by minimizing the number of people in rooms, they decreased any potential spread of respiratory droplets, as well as preserved more personal protective equipment.[37]

The SAF method has the largest body of evidence for both triaging and maintaining established care with a patient.[25,38] With COVID-19, SAF proved especially helpful with patients with stable chronic diseases and/or longer term medications (eg, patients doing well and simply needing refills).[19] SAF was also useful in recognizing certain common diagnoses, including acne, dermatitis, psoriasis, rashes, and rosacea. In contrast, as a limitation, pigmented lesions could be triaged but often not definitively diagnosed, requiring in-person visits.[37,39] Similarly, the vast majority of American Academy of Dermatology members surveyed felt that total body skin examination required in-person visits; in contrast, conditions such as acne did not require an in-person evaluation.[21] Indeed, total body skin examinations were a major limitation of teledermatology visits of all kinds, requiring an in-person evaluation. The need to triage skin checks may have led the specialty to reconsider the appropriateness, for individuals and all patients, default recommendations for yearly skin checks and other regular appointments.

THE IMPACT OF TELEMEDICINE FOR CORONAVIRUS DISEASE 2019 ON RESIDENT EDUCATION

The pandemic and its subsequent guidelines caused academic dermatology programs to reevaluate resident involvement and education.[40] Any significant changes to resident education that lasted more than 4 weeks had to be reported to the Executive Director of the Accreditation Council for Graduate Medical Education, because it would affect board certification eligibility. Thus, a focus on adjusting resident education through teledermatology allowed for residents and fellows to maintain the quality of their education.[40] Not unlike the standard of studying unknown photographs with kodachromes practicing teledermatology with both the asynchronous and synchronous methods allowed residents to triage diagnosis, conduct examinations, discuss assessments and plans, and present information to patients.[37,41] Programs also instituted virtual grand rounds featuring teledermatology to aid in resident education,[40,41] thus expanding telemedicine's reach in new ways.

The impact of the COVID-19 pandemic was not limited to current dermatology residents. Major adjustments to the residency application process were suggested in a dermatology program director consensus statement, which was released ahead of the application cycle. These changes included limiting the number and availability of away rotations, encouraging virtual rotations where applicable, and planning for remote interviews.[41]

LESSONS LEARNED DURING THE CORONAVIRUS DISEASE 2019 PANDEMIC

Early in the COVID-19 pandemic, some felt that dermatology practices could serve as vectors for COVID-19 transmission and recommended that all nonessential visits be canceled for the safety of patients and staff.[35] Many dermatology practices heeded this warning by converting to telemedicine for patient care. This pivot to teledermatology directly helped to mitigate the spread of COVID-19 by decreasing the risk of exposure of patients and staff.[18] Evidence shows that, within the inpatient setting, the use of teledermatology, when compared with in-person dermatology visits, saved personal protective equipment and decreased unnecessary exposure to patients and health care professionals.[37] One study also found that newly implemented COVID-19 teledermatology algorithms allowed for the most effective triaging and preparation for in the event that it may necessitate an in-person visit, increasing the efficiency of practices.[22]

Teledermatology's efficacy may vary in different populations. The elderly, for instance, may require assistance using digital devices.[42] A lack of education into the proper use of technology can limit the efficacy of teledermatology. We must also consider the emerging American population whose first language is not English. Even without the constraints of a pandemic, language barriers can be a social determinant of health impeding the delivery of optimal care. Thus, we must anticipate and proactively address how a lack of English fluency may affect proficiency and the ability to partake in teledermatology.[42]

Despite these challenges, these new approaches during the pandemic to teledermatology implementation serve as proof of concept with the intention to revise and adapt. For instance, additional services could provide caregivers for the elderly and translators for non-English speakers to improve adaptation.

Patient Data Security

When the CMS relaxed HIPAA regulations for telemedicine, the intention was to expand access to care.[15] Still, we must remain vigilant about quality standards to prevent security breaches. Many platforms being used for telemedicine appointments were developed primarily for insecure chats and are not encrypted or have security standards inadequate to protect patient information. These include FaceTime, Facebook Messenger, Google Hangouts, Zoom, and Skype.[43] The major benefits of these platforms include their low barrier for entry and ease of use for most patients and providers. Encryption standards vary; guidance must be provided to avoid any compromise of patient information. An uptick in cyber attacks on health care networks during COVID-19 certainly warrants additional scrutiny. Many hospitals have been targeted in ransomware attacks, in which patient data have been captured and withheld in exchange for money.[44]

Teledermatology and the Digital Divide

Telemedicine may overcome the barriers of distance and time, but it may also paradoxically worsen access for some people in unanticipated ways. Essentially, the most well-resourced patients may be overrepresented among telemedicine visits given their access and literacy, whereas other populations (resource limited) may have greater more difficulty adapting to this new system.[45] Barriers to health equity exist across many sectors including education, planning, housing, labor, and health. Unfortunately, this well-described digital divide may be an important contributing factor in disparities. Access to a reliable, high-quality Internet connection and a smart device correlates with income. In fact, in 2019, 26% of Americans in households earning less than $30,000 per year were solely reliant on smartphones for their Internet access.[44] That same year, it was also reported that 37% of adults in rural areas in the United States lacked broadband Internet and 31% lacked access to a computer. In addition, 25% of adults in urban areas lacked access to broadband Internet and 27% lacked access to a computer.[46]

Although both rural and urban populations may have limited Internet access, many specific populations may be especially at risk when care depends on this access, namely, Medicare patients, minorities, and patients whose first language is not English. Measures taken by agencies such as the CMS had their intended impact by allowing physicians to expand telemedicine access; for instance, Medicare patients are able to complete visits from the comfort and safety of their homes. However, it is important to note that 26% of Medicare patients lack home digital access.[47] Additionally, Medicare patients older than 85 years of age, those with a high school education or less, patients experiencing homelessness, Black and Hispanic patients, and patients with disabilities all have decreased digital access.[48] During the COVID-19 pandemic, the number of Spanish-speaking patients seeking teledermatology services was decreased when compared with 2019.[49] In 2019, 1 study found that 9% of Spanish-speaking patients scheduled teledermatology appointments through an outpatient academic clinic compared with 2020, where only 5% scheduled appointments.[49] Dependence on digital frameworks may disproportionately affect these populations already experiencing health disparities; in a specific example, many of these patients do not have reliable email addresses, making it harder to create teledermatology portals for communication.[49]

Certainly, it remains important to consider how different telemedicine models could mitigate any possible exacerbation in disparities. A study from Sao Paulo, Brazil, focused on the use of teledermatology consultation by primary care providers in individuals older than 60 years of age and they found that 67% of patients were treated via teledermatology without in-person visits and subsequently sent back to primary care providers for continued care.[50,51] Another retrospective study, assessing primary care provider use of the American Academy of Dermatology's free Access-Derm program looked at the initiation of SAF tele-dermatology consults in a clinic serving uninsured patients.[52] In this study, 65% of patients did not require an in-person evaluation.[52] Additionally, they found an 82% discordance between primary care provider and teledermatologist preconsult management plans.[52] The use of teledermatology decreased the costs and wait time associated with in-person visits and inappropriate care.[52] These provider-to-provider teledermatology models can circumvent any limited patient access to broadband Internet. Even as demand may push the market toward more direct-to-consumer or direct-to-patient models, direct partnerships between primary care providers and dermatologists may prove valuable in many ways—for example, as a learning outlet for primary care providers who frequently participate in referrals,[51] with 1 study demonstrating how primary care providers learned to manage dermatologic concerns from the repeated use of such a system.[53]

Moving forward, many other barriers can be anticipated and addressed to ensure care continues with telemedicine. For example, financial barriers that limit access can be decreased by offering waivers that cover devices and Internet access in underserved populations.[54] In addition to funding, training programs can promote technologic and health literacy for both patients and providers, done through the mail, or in person with a technology support team.[54] For patient populations with especially difficult circumstances (eg, those experiencing homelessness), telemedicine programs may need to work directly with other established centers, such as housing shelters, to ensure successful connections.[55]

Last, we must be especially mindful of cultural and language barriers in telemedicine implementation. Platforms should operate in multiple languages so that patients can easily navigate systems. To better direct focus toward local needs, governments and programs should work directly with local public health organizations that know and understand the people they wish to serve. These organizations' preexisting relationships may not only facilitate culturally competency and community buy-in, but may also help with implementation directly.

Addressing the digital divide to ensure telemedicine does not worsen disparities will require a concerted effort from physicians, regulatory bodies, and public health services to ensure access is not limited, and that Internet access does not become a new social determinant of health[52] (**Table 2**).

FUTURE OUTLOOK FOR TELEDERMATOLOGY

Before the COVID-19 pandemic, teledermatology was an already expanding field, albeit used sparingly compared with in-person visits. The option to use teledermatology had been stymied by limited insurance reimbursement for telemedicine visits,[9] concern about medicolegal liabilities,[9] and medical licensing restrictions.[3] Thus, without adequate support before the COVID-19 pandemic, most physicians opted out of using teledermatology.[14]

The COVID-19 pandemic prompted disruptive changes in the regulatory and policy landscapes, opening a new age of telemedicine growth and innovation. Dermatology practices and health systems created and adapted new protocols of care for both inpatient and outpatient settings.[26,27] Practices were able to save personal protective equipment and decrease unnecessary exposure of staff and patients to the coronavirus.[27,48] Residency programs were also able to institute teledermatology into resident education,[27] which further ameliorated the concern of exposure. Additionally, the implementation of teledermatology resulted in improved efficiency[37]; practices and health systems found that they were able to better prepare in advance for procedures and triage patients, thus saving both time and money while continuing follow-ups with established patients.[22] The increased use of teledermatology may open up spots to patients who require in-person visits and increase the efficiency of daily practice. Evidence

Table 2 Areas for improvement in the digital divide	
Area of Concern	Suggestions for Improvement
Financial assistance	Financial waivers could mitigate cost of devices and internet access
Interpretation services	Modeled after interpretation services used in patient, can increase quality of communication during the visit.
Community-based interventions	Community-based teledermatolgy programs can serve as an adjunct to assist with ease of use

also showed that teledermatology was an excellent option for common skin diagnoses and follow-up treatments; these common skin disorders include acne, rosacea, psoriasis, and eczema.[27,36]

Continuity of care has proven a primary concern during the pandemic, and teledermatology allows physicians to continue patient follow-up, especially for patients with chronic diseases and for patients on medium- to long-term treatment regimens.[22,51] Many of these patients are on immunomodulatory drugs, so teledermatology also conveys increased protection against COVID-19 for these patients. Moreover, teledermatology at its core allows physicians to care for patients at a distance, in situations where they may live far from a dermatologist or if they are quarantining.[51]

Teledermatology has been well-suited to the constraints of the COVID-19 pandemic, but limitations must be addressed. In addition to the medicolegal concerns, one rate-limiting step to teledermatology is access. Patient access to both secure Internet and the necessary technology for teledermatology visits limits many patients who lack digital access in their home or who lack the technological insight to participate in teledermatology.[46,51] Additionally, the expansion of telemedicine reimbursements frequently favored synchronous video visits and not SAF. Furthermore, evidence has shown that SAF is much more efficient in terms of response time for consultations, where a SAF dermatology consultation integration improved dermatology consultation time from 84 days to about 5 hours.[17] Reimbursement expansion was an important outcome to boost teledermatology, but the prioritization of synchronous visits over SAF could lead to the possible overuse of synchronous visits in situations where a SAF would be more appropriate for day-to-day efficiency.

Telemedicine policy changes will continue for at least the duration of the public health emergency. This uncertainty poses a potential threat to teledermatology advancement. However, there is a growing need for dermatology services, and during this pandemic teledermatology has proven to be efficient and effective. Therefore, as in-person care returns closer to prepandemic levels, we anticipate that teledermatology's use will remain significantly higher than before the pandemic and that it will continue to grow, especially for follow-up care and triaging visits. In the long term, the success of teledermatology will depend on federal and state policies and laws, as well as payers. Future policies must consider telemedicine expansion beyond geographic restrictions and further reimbursement increases and the use of SAF.

For sustained growth, government policymakers, physicians, insurance companies, and patient advocacy organizations must partner to create a system to fortify telemedicine with the many challenges of reimbursement, HIPAA compliance, and disparities in patient access to telemedicine.

CLINICS CARE POINTS

- Before the COVID-19 pandemic, the use of teledermatology was limited, presumably due to a lack of parity in reimbursement, liability concerns, and geographic licensing restrictions.

- The increased use of teledermatology during the pandemic was incentivized by the desire to maintain continuity of care, relaxation of regulatory restrictions which allowed for expanded financial reimbursement, and expanded options for communication methods used to conduct patient visits.

- The store and forward method has the most evidence-based support for superiority in both triaging patient inquiries and continuity of care with established patients. This method proved to be especially suitable for patients with chronic illness and was helpful in diagnosis of common diseases. More complex diagnoses still required in-person consultation.

- The expansion of teledermatology during the COVID-19 pandemic may have paradoxically increased access for some patients while leaving other vulnerable populations unaddressed.

- Measures taken during the pandemic have provided a framework that can be used to guide possible expansion of teledermatology use post-pandemic. Extra care should be taken in susceptible populations such as Medicare patients, those with a high school education or less, undomiciled patients, Black and Hispanic patients, and those with disabilities.

- A concerted effort must be taken by multiple stakeholders to thoroughly investigate and remedy the digital divide in order to avoid exacerbating pre-existing health care disparities and avoid creating new ones.

REFERENCES

1. Cucinotta D, Vanelli M. WHO declares COVID-19 a pandemic. Acta Biomed 2020;91(1):157–60.

2. Bickers DR, Lim HW, Margolis D, et al. The burden of skin diseases: 2004 a joint project of the American Academy of Dermatology Association and the Society for Investigative Dermatology. J Am Acad Dermatol 2006;55(3):490–500.

3. Lipoff J. "It's telemedicine or no medicine, whether doctors like it or not. Covid-19 ushers in age of telemedicine." *Barron's*. 2020. Available at: https://www.barrons.com/articles/telemedicine-on-the-rise-in-era-of-social-distancing-coronavirus-51589906377. Accessed January 30, 2021.

4. Perednia DA, Brown NA. Teledermatology: one application of telemedicine. Bull Med Libr Assoc 1995;83(1):42–7.

5. Yim KM, Florek AG, Oh DH, et al. Teledermatology in the United States: an update in a dynamic era. Telemed J E Health 2018;24(9):691–7.

6. Gaffney R, Rao B. Global teledermatology. Glob Dermatol 2015;2(5):209–14.

7. Desai B, McKoy K, Kovarik C. Overview of international teledermatology. Pan Afr Med J 2010;6:3.

8. Warshaw EM, Hillman YJ, Greer NL, et al. Teledermatology for diagnosis and management of skin conditions: a systematic review. J Am Acad Dermatol 2011;64(4):759–72.

9. Ogabechie O. The legal landscape of teledermatology. AJMC. 2017. Available at: https://www.ajmc.com/view/the-legal-landscape-of-teledermatology. Accessed January 5, 2021.

10. Centers for Medicare & Medicaid Services. Medicare telemedicine healthcare provider fact sheet: Medicare coverage and payment of virtual services. Available at: https://www.cms.gov/newsroom/fact-sheets/medicare-telemedicine-health-care-provider-fact-sheet?inf_contact_key1/438ca3f198618fc3aeb a4091611f5b055680f8914173f9191b1c0223e68310 bb1. Accessed January 30, 2021.

11. Wicklund E. ATA releases 2019 update of state-by-state telehealth report cards. mHealthIntelligence. Available at: https://mhealthintelligence.com/news/ata-releases-2019-update-of-state-by-state-telehealth-report-cards. Accessed January 5, 2021.

12. Puri P, Yiannias JA, Mangold AR, et al. The policy dimensions, regulatory landscape, and market characteristics of teledermatology in the United States. JAAD Int 2020;1(2):202–7.

13. COVID-19 waivers of licensing rules. Available at: https://www.njconsumeraffairs.gov/COVID19/Pages/C19-Waivers-of-Licensing-Rules.aspx. Accessed January 30, 2021.

14. Bhate C, Ho CH, Brodell RT. Time to revisit the Health Insurance Portability and Accountability Act (HIPAA)? Accelerated telehealth adoption during the COVID-19 pandemic. J Am Acad Dermatol 2020;83(4):e313–4.

15. Lipoff J. "Why loosening HIPAA requirements in response to the coronavirus was urgent and necessary." Slate. 2020. Available at: https://slate.com/technology/2020/03/hipaa-requirements-coronavirus-telemedicine.html. Accessed January 25, 2021.

16. Mounessa JS, Chapman S, Braunberger T, et al. A systematic review of satisfaction with teledermatology. J Telemed Telecare 2018;24(4):263–70.

17. Jariwala NN, Snider CK, Mehta SJ, et al. Prospective implementation of a consultative store-and-forward teledermatology model at a single urban academic health system with real cost data subanalysis. Telemed J E Health 2020. https://doi.org/10.1089/tmj.2020.0248.

18. Ruggiero A, Megna M, Annunziata MC, et al. Teledermatology for acne during COVID-19: high patients' satisfaction in spite of the emergency. J Eur Acad Dermatol Venereol 2020;34(11):e662–3.

19. Mostafa PIN, Hegazy AA. Dermatological consultations in the COVID-19 era: is teledermatology the key to social distancing? An Egyptian experience. J Dermatolog Treat 2020;1–6.

20. Sharma A, Jindal V, Singla P, et al. Will teledermatology be the silver lining during and after COVID-19? Dermatol Ther 2020;33(4):e13643.

21. Kennedy J, Arey S, Hopkins Z, et al. Dermatologist perceptions of teledermatology implementation and future use after COVID-19: demographics, barriers, and insights. JAMA Dermatol 2021;157(5):595–7.

22. Chansky PB, Simpson CL, Lipoff JB. Implementation of a dermatology teletriage system to improve access in an underserved clinic: a retrospective study. J Am Acad Dermatol 2017;77(5):975–7.

23. Bressler M, Siegel D, Markowitz O. Virtual dermatology: a COVID-19 update. Cutis 2020;105(4):163–4. E2.

24. McCrary MR, Rogers T, Yeung H, et al. Would dermoscopic photographs help triage teledermatology consults in the COVID-19 era? [abstract]. In: Proceedings of the AACR Virtual Meeting: COVID-19 and Cancer; 2020 Jul 20-22. Philadelphia (PA): AACR; Clin Cancer Res 2020;26(18_Suppl):Abstract nr PO-042.

25. Zakaria A, Miclau TA, Maurer T, et al. Cost minimization analysis of a teledermatology triage system in a managed care setting. JAMA Dermatol 2021;157(1):52–8.

26. Gupta R, Ibraheim MK, Doan HQ. Teledermatology in the wake of COVID-19: advantages and challenges to continued care in a time of disarray. J Am Acad Dermatol 2020;83(1):168–9.

27. Perkins S, Cohen JM, Nelson CA, et al. Teledermatology in the era of COVID-19: experience of an academic department of dermatology. J Am Acad Dermatol 2020;83(1):e43–4.

28. Yeroushalmi S, Millan SH, Nelson K, et al. Patient perceptions and satisfaction with teledermatology during the COVID-19 pandemic: a survey-based study. J Drugs Dermatol 2021;20(2):178–83.

29. Elsner P. Teledermatology in the times of COVID-19 - a systematic review. J Dtsch Dermatol Ges 2020; 18(8):841–5.

30. Su MY, Das S. Expansion of asynchronous teledermatology during the COVID-19 pandemic. J Am Acad Dermatol 2020;83(6):e471–2.

31. Monthly telehealth regional tracker: FAIR health. Monthly telehealth regional tracker. Available at: https://www.fairhealth.org/states-by-the-numbers/telehealth. Accessed January 30, 2021.

32. Pulsipher KJ, Presley CL, Rundle CW, et al. Teledermatology application use in the COVID-19 era. Dermatol Online J 2020;26(12). 13030/qt1fs0m0tp.

33. 2019 U.S. telehealth satisfaction study. J.D. Power. Available at: https://www.jdpower.com/business/press-releases/2019-us-telehealth-satisfaction-study. Accessed January 30, 2021.

34. Bhargava S, McKeever C, Kroumpouzos G. Impact of covid-19 pandemic on dermatology practices: results of a web-based, global survey. Int J Womens Dermatol 2020;7(2):217–23.

35. Kwatra SG, Sweren RJ, Grossberg AL. Dermatology practices as vectors for COVID-19 transmission: a call for immediate cessation of nonemergent dermatology visits. J Am Acad Dermatol 2020;82(5): e179–80.

36. Su MY, Smith GP, Das S. Trends in teledermatology use during clinic reopening after COVID-19 closures. J Am Acad Dermatol 2020;84(4):e213–4.

37. Rismiller K, Cartron AM, Trinidad JCL. Inpatient teledermatology during the COVID-19 pandemic. J Dermatolog Treat 2020;31(5):441–3.

38. Mufti A, Maliyar K, Sachdeva M, et al. Modifications to dermatology residency education during the COVID-19 pandemic. J Am Acad Dermatol 2020; 83(3):e235–6.

39. Farshchian M, Potts G, Kimyai-Asadi A, et al. Outpatient teledermatology implementation during the COVID-19 pandemic: challenges and lessons learned. J Drugs Dermatol 2020;19(6):683.

40. Oldenburg R, Marsch A. Optimizing teledermatology visits for dermatology resident education during the COVID-19 pandemic. J Am Acad Dermatol 2020;82(6):e229.

41. Rosman IS, Schadt CR, Samimi SS, et al. Approaching the dermatology residency application process during a pandemic. J Am Acad Dermatol 2020; 83(5):e351–2.

42. Simpson CL, Kovarik CL. Effectively engaging geriatric patients via teledermatology. J Am Acad Dermatol 2020;83(6):e417–8.

43. Calton B, Abedini N, Fratkin M. Telemedicine in the Time of Coronavirus. Journal of Pain and Symptom Management 2020;60(1). https://doi.org/10.1016/j.jpainsymman.2020.03.019.

44. Jalali MS, Landman A, Gordon WJ. Telemedicine, privacy, and information security in the age of COVID-19. J Am Med Inform Assoc 2021;28(3): 671–2.

45. Bakhtiar M, Elbuluk N, Lipoff JB. The digital divide: how COVID-19's telemedicine expansion could exacerbate disparities. J Am Acad Dermatol 2020; 83(5):e345–6.

46. Perrin A. Digital gap between rural and nonrural America persists. Pew Research Center. 2020. Available at: https://www.pewresearch.org/fact-tank/2019/05/31/digital-gap-between-rural-and-nonrural-america-persists/. Accessed March 24, 2021.

47. Anderson M, Kumar M. Digital divide persists even as lower-income Americans make gains in tech adoption. Pew Research Center. 2020. Available at: https://www.pewresearch.org/fact-tank/2019/05/07/digital-divide-persists-even-as-lower-income-americans-make-gains-in-tech-adoption/. Accessed January 23, 2021.

48. Roberts ET, Mehrotra A. Assessment of disparities in digital access among Medicare beneficiaries and implications for telemedicine. JAMA Intern Med 2020;180(10):1386–9.

49. Blundell AR, Kroshinsky D, Hawryluk EB, et al. Disparities in telemedicine access for Spanish-speaking patients during the COVID-19 crisis. Pediatr Dermatol 2021. https://doi.org/10.1111/pde.14489.

50. Bianchi M, Santos A, Cordioli E. Benefits of teledermatology for geriatric patients: population-based cross-sectional study. J Med Internet Res 2020; 22(4). e16700.

51. Maddukuri S, Patel J, Lipoff JB. Teledermatology addressing disparities in health care access: a review. Curr Dermatol Rep 2021;1–8. https://doi.org/10.1007/s13671-021-00329-2.

52. Holmes AN, Chansky PB, Simpson CL. Teledermatology consultation can optimize treatment of cutaneous disease by nondermatologists in under-resourced clinics. Telemed J E Health 2020;26(10): 1284–90.

53. Armstrong AW, Kwong MW, Chase EP, et al. Teledermatology operational considerations, challenges, and benefits: the referring providers' perspective. Telemed J E Health 2012;18(8):580–4.

54. Zhai Y. A call for addressing barriers to telemedicine: health disparities during the COVID-19 pandemic. Psychother Psychosom 2021;90(1):64–6.

55. Tierney AA, Kyalwazi MJ, Lockhart A. Tackling the digital divide by improving internet and telehealth access for low-income populations. Berkeley, CA: California Initiative for Health Equity & Action; 2020. Available at: https://healthequity.berkeley.edu/sites/default/files/tacklingthedigitaldivide.pdf. Accessed April 7, 2021.

Impact of COVID-19 on Dermatology Residency

Sara Samimi, MD[a],*, Juliana Choi, MD, PhD[a], Ilana S. Rosman, MD[b], Misha Rosenbach, MD[a]

KEYWORDS

- COVID-19 • Education • Wellness • Clinical experiences • Safety • Residency

KEY POINTS

- The pandemic declaration by the Accreditation Council for Graduate Medical Education (ACGME) redefined expectations of programs and approach to residency training.
- Graduate Medical Education (GME) programs shifted their didactics to virtual platforms, given in-person limitations.
- Clinical experiences were altered due to COVID-19-related clinical care, use of telemedicine, and changes in patient volumes.
- The pandemic brought a new focus and emphasis on trainee wellness and safety.
- The future of dermatology remains bright, but with new considerations in order to support our trainees during these evolving times.

INTRODUCTION

The COVID-19 pandemic challenged the world to navigate a new normal state. Residency and fellowship programs across the country faced many obstacles, including flexing trainees into new patient care roles, short staffing due to illness or quarantine, increased workloads, shifting responsibilities outside of work, and altered educational experiences. Many trainees were put in unfamiliar environments, including redeployment to provide care outside of their area of expertise.[1] For dermatology residents specifically, many felt uncomfortable being thrust into less familiar clinical roles.[2] Early in the pandemic, different parts of the country were discrepantly affected with surges in COVID-19 rates and strains on healthcare systems. In a survey from April 2020 by Li and colleagues, 18% of programs that responded had experienced reassignments to nondermatological healthcare activities,[2] as compared to 32% during the same time from Shaw and colleagues with a concentration of respondents in the Northeast, an early epicenter of the pandemic.[3] The majority redeployed served on inpatient wards (76%) with more than half volunteering (51.9%).

On March 13, 2020, the Accreditation Council for Graduate Medical Education (ACGME) cancelled all site visits, including accreditation visits and clinical learning environment reviews. The ACGME took unprecedented steps to adjust program requirements in response to the increased demands within local institutions to care for patients with COVID-19. On March 24, 2020, the ACGME issued a modified framework for how graduate medical education (GME) can effectively operate. Three stages were defined along a continuum: "business as usual," increased clinical demands, and pandemic emergency status[4] (**Table 1**). Graduate medical education committees (GMECs) across the country worked to define needs at their institutions and request modified status when necessary.[5] Notably, the extent and timing of pandemic-associated effects on healthcare systems, education, and local restrictions and laws varied by state, region, and setting (eg, urban vs rural), leading to disparate impacts on trainees across the country.

[a] University of Pennsylvania, 3400 Civic Center Boulevard, Philadelphia, PA 19104, USA; [b] Washington University, 660 South Euclid Avenue, CB 8118, Saint Louis, MO 63110, USA
* Corresponding author.
E-mail address: Sara.samimi@pennmedicine.upenn.edu

Dermatol Clin 39 (2021) 609–618
https://doi.org/10.1016/j.det.2021.05.002

Table 1
Modified framework for how graduate medical education (GME) can effectively operate

	Stage 1: "Business as Usual"	Stage 2: Increased Clinical Demands Guidance	Stage 3: Pandemic Emergency Status Guidance
Definition	No significant disruption of patient care and educational activities; planning underway for increased demands	Some residents/fellows need to shift to patient care duties; some educational activities are suspended	Most or all residents/ fellows need to shift to patient care; majority of educational activities are suspended
Requirements in effect	Governed by the common and specific program requirements	Governed by the common and specific program requirements and variances; see https:// acgme.org/Stage-2-Increased-Clinical-Demands-Guidance	Governed by 4 overriding requirements: work hour limit requirements, resources and training requirements, supervision requirements, fellows allowed to function in core specialty
Flexibility	ACGME activities suspended: site visits, self-study, ACGME surveys. Telemedicine requirements in effect	Stage 1 plus variances (see above) on the following: fellows working as attendings; residents/ fellows reassigned, fail to accrue required minimums, graduation; educational program changes; review committee evaluation of disruptions	Stages 1 and 2 plus specialty-specific requirements waived
ACGME notification			Sponsoring institutions can declare pandemic emergency status; contact institutional review committee executive director

Adapted from Accreditation Council for Graduate Medical Education. Three Stages of GME During the COVID-19 Pandemic. https://acgme.org/COVID-19/Three-Stages-of-GMEDuring-the-COVID-19-Pandemic.

The COVID-19 pandemic has impacted dermatology residency programs on an acute and chronic time scale. The acute effects were highlighted by abrupt changes to educational experiences to align with virtual learning, and altered clinical experiences—including changed rotations, implementation of teledermatology and virtual visits, and a reduction in patient volumes, in addition to potential redeployment outside of dermatology. The chronic effects include impact on mental health/wellness and their future careers. In this article, we attempt to tackle some of these effects through evidence in the literature as well as our own institutional experiences.

IMPACT ON EDUCATION

COVID-19 forced a complete paradigm shift in medical education, embracing new models of learning and exposing unforeseen educational opportunities in and out of dermatology.[6] As of April 2020, 90% of dermatology residents felt that their education was negatively impacted by COVID-19, though 92% still believed that remote learning was useful.[2] Notably, the perceived negative impact on education improved over time, with follow-up surveys as the pandemic progressed (surveyed May–July 2020) suggesting 59% of dermatology residents felt their didactics were negatively impacted.[7]

Learning Outside of Dermatology

Given demands across institutions to care for acutely ill patients, trainees have had to refocus on knowledge outside of their chosen disciplines.[6] In parallel, educational resources were developed to support the ability of trainees outside of medicine to flex into direct patient care roles.[8] At our institutions, the University of Pennsylvania (UPenn) and Washington University in St. Louis (WashU), electronic resources were created to facilitate learning for trainees redeployed outside of their specialty on how to care for patients on internal medicine floors and in the emergency department. At UPenn, an institution-specific COVID-19 learning homepage was created to collate carefully composed materials to support trainees flexing into new patient care roles. At WashU, a shared online folder was created to centrally house resources that residents could access. During this past year, trainees have not only had to continue in-depth learning in dermatology to facilitate certification exams, but have also had to be facile and up to date in caring for COVID-19 patients as an internist should the need arise.

Virtual Learning

Given the risk of presymptomatic spread of COVID-19, residency programs have adjusted their didactics to virtual platforms. A survey from May to July 2020 demonstrated that over 90% of dermatology residents reported having virtual didactics.[7] Of note, the majority of respondents were in the Northeast governed by stay-at-home orders. At our institutions (University of Pennsylvania [UPenn] and Washington University [WashU]), starting in March 2020, we adopted a virtual classroom. We adjusted other learning opportunities to be virtual when possible, including clinicopathologic conferences and our weekly live patient grand rounds, which shifted to clinical images rather than in-person patients. We encouraged those engaged in educating residents to use ancillary tools to augment participation, such as audience response systems and in-lecture quizzes and polls, to make sure residents were able to participate actively, even when physically separate.

Some learning experiences are more challenging in a virtual setting. These include dermatopathology and dermatologic surgery. We (at UPenn and WashU) shifted dermatopathology teaching, signout, and consensus conferences into experiences that could be streamed online. Slides were put on the scope and captured via an image viewer to allow for virtual live streaming. For procedural dermatology, UPenn also transiently shifted to virtual experiences with home kits with virtual oversight, where our procedural dermatology group would either review live, virtual sessions with the residents practicing surgical techniques, or the residents would record themselves for asynchronous review. Over time, as the pandemic case counts improved in the summer of 2020, we resumed in-person procedural sessions, but continued a virtual component. During in-person procedural sessions, including lasers, neurotoxin, and filler injections, we limited the number of on-site residents, but continued streaming the procedure sessions online for all residents to observe. Although there are challenges in clarity of images and lack of parallel hands-on experience, this allowed for a safer means of educating all residents on necessary procedures. All residents have had the opportunity to participate in hands-on sessions, but in smaller, socially distanced controlled groups of limited size.

The transition to virtual learning created unexpected challenges, including the need to carefully vet all images for any personal health identifiers (PHIs) and ensure that all platforms utilized for virtual education were HIPAA compliant and secure. Another unforeseen challenge of a push toward digital learning was a proliferation of online courses, educational videos, and conferences. Many of these were marketed directly to residents, some with unclear quality of educational content and obscured potential conflicts of interest. While having a multitude of resources has allowed for enhanced access to learning materials, we have witnessed information overload and digital fatigue in our own trainees.

Board Eligibility and Certification

Many residents expressed uncertainty at their ability to obtain the knowledge needed to pass their boards, and the potential impact time away from dermatology would have on their ability to graduate. The American Board of Dermatology (ABD) has strict criteria regarding training program structure and weeks away (vacation, maternity leave, illness). Notably, during the pandemic, some residents were exposed to SARS-CoV-2 and required to quarantine or isolate if infected. The ABD issued a statement on March 6th recognizing the very significant impact of COVID-19 on dermatology resident education.[9] They noted that time residents spent in mandated COVID-19 quarantine would be counted as clinical education if they could still work within their programs to have independent structured academic time.[9]

Additionally, for many residents graduating in July 2020, the pandemic limited their exposure to educational conferences, review courses, and in-person group studying. In March 2020, the American Academy of Dermatology (AAD) winter conference was cancelled.[10] This resulted in residents missing courses that are often viewed as high-yield content for board review, or opportunities for residents to round out their education with topics and content that is less well represented at their home institution. Some programs supported participation of their residents in virtual board reviews sponsored by other institutions and paid for resident access to question banks to bridge the gap. As a result, the boards became a rising source of anxiety and uncertainty. Initially there was uncertainty about whether the board exam would be held in person. Eventually, the date of the certification exam was adjusted from July to October, and transitioned to a completely virtual exam at testing sites across the country.

IMPACT ON CLINICAL EXPERIENCES
Redeployment of Dermatology Trainees

For some residents, the peak of the COVID-19 pandemic meant an abrupt shift to nondermatologic care in order to support the efforts of their respective health systems.[1] This shift translated to rotating through the intensive care unit (ICU), medicine floors, emergency departments (EDs), COVID-19 tents, or doing COVID-19 results management. However, as trainees have flexed in and out of their designated specialties, there has undoubtedly been a shift also in their dermatology-specific clinical experiences.

Changes in Volume and Procedural Experiences

At the start of the pandemic, dermatology practices had an abrupt, but necessary, decrease in their clinical volumes,[11] with up to a two-thirds drop in the number of outpatient visits.[7] While these shifts have been transient and dependent on case positivity rate, they continue to pose a challenge in ensuring adequate exposure to clinical experiences for trainees. At our institutions (UPenn and WashU), starting in March 2020, most visits were triaged to allow urgent, acute in-person visits, while other visits types were encouraged to be managed virtually, with the exception of necessary biopsies or procedures for malignancies that could not be delayed. Cosmetic procedures were subsequently put on hold in most places across the country. Procedural volume, as a result, notably decreased and/or stopped during that period. In combination with intermittent, state-by-state mediated suspension of elective procedures, trainees collectively have had altered, skewed, and/or reduced surgical experiences.[12] While volumes have now ramped back up, given the abrupt halt at the start of the pandemic, the cumulative experiences of some residents may be less. A lingering concern for these volume shifts is the ability to meet ACGME case log minimums, especially at smaller programs with lower prepandemic volumes and for less common procedures.

A reduction in procedural volume is especially important for new residents for whom hands-on practice and oversight is key for surgical safety. At our institution (UPenn), we distributed take-home surgical kits, had virtual oversight of common procedure types via live-streaming and recorded video observations, held in-person practice sessions in large open spaces with limited numbers of participants (divided groups), and prioritized hands-on experiences for first years (paired with senior "buddies") for low exposure risk surgical procedures. We (at UPenn and WashU) also secured COVID-19 testing for patients coming in for higher risk procedures to limit exposure risk, such as lengthy surgeries or cases on the head and neck, which may require patient mask removal.

Embracing Telemedicine

At the start of this global crisis, many dermatology programs and practices shifted to telemedicine to limit in-person exposures, conserve critical supplies of personal protective equipment (PPE), and reduce disease transmission according to guidelines issued by the Centers for Disease Control and Prevention (CDC) and the American Academy of Dermatology (AAD).[13] As a result, trainees have engaged in more telemedicine experiences through both synchronous and asynchronous care.[7] E-visits and e-consults using "store and forward" technology and live video virtual visits have increased dermatologic access during the pandemic for patients, while also enhancing educational exposure for trainees.[14] Trainees are able to delve into the clinical case, mirroring the flow of an in-person clinic, before presenting their differential and plan to the staff attending.[15,16] Trainees enter a virtual visit, obtain the history, and perform a clinical exam, whether it be by review of photographs submitted or video demonstration of the affected area(s). Then they are able to pause the visit to present their findings and assessment/plan to the attending. Subsequently, both the trainee and attending are able to enter back into the virtual visit to offer feedback to the patient and complete the visit.

Additionally, during the pandemic, numbers of persons under investigation (PUI), COVID-19-positive patients in the ED and admitted to the hospital have waxed and waned, leading to potential increased risk of exposure to hospital personnel. Inpatient dermatologists are a part of that at-risk group, and as a result, consideration of telemedicine to triage dermatologic care and increase access in the inpatient setting is also paramount.[17] Implementation of telemedicine in the inpatient setting also allows for conservation of critical PPE. Trinidad and colleagues highlight an algorithm to: prioritize the use of telemedicine consultation to minimize risk of COVID-19 exposure to patients and consulting dermatologists; identify high-risk patients; limit use of resources for low-risk patients; and provide a framework for outpatient dermatologists to use in the setting of an inpatient consult.[18] Algorithms like this are key to continue to champion both patient care and trainee safety in a pandemic setting.

SPOTLIGHT ON SAFETY

Now more than ever, the pandemic has put a spotlight on safety. Bringing attention to these issues remains integral to ensuring the safety of our trainees within dermatology and health systems as a whole.

Access to Personal Protective Equipment

In a survey by Stewart and colleagues, the majority of dermatology residents reported a hospital shortage of PPE, while only 74.5% felt that they had adequate PPE to perform their duties.[7] Similarly, when the dermatology program director listserv was surveyed, the responses were highly variable, ranging from no access to N95s to use of N95s with every dermatology patient. Even in those cases, most N95s were extensively reused. This highlights the need for institutions to continue to advocate for adequate PPE for trainees and suggests a national approach to this continued shortage is needed.

Dermatology residents are exposed to high-risk outpatient procedures, and PUIs and COVID-19-positive patients in the inpatient setting, but also potential high-risk exposures in the outpatient setting through procedures and evaluations around the nose and mouth for prolonged periods of time. Not only should there readily be access to

PPE (N95s, surgical masks, eye protection, powered air-purifying respirators), there should also be access to fit testing, and educational resources to ensure appropriate donning and doffing of protective gear. These resources should be available at all trainee practice sites.[19] Additionally, some institutions have developed guidelines for limiting exposure of trainees to COVID-19-positive patients in the inpatient setting to promote safety and to conserve PPE.[18]

Symptom Reporting and Testing

While transmission at the workplace is relatively low with universal masking, shared spaces—particularly during meals—can lead to risk of transmission at work. Programs have had to adapt existing spaces and rotations to ensure trainees have safe locations, preferably outdoors, or isolated singly, to eat and drink during the day. Community positivity rates have varied greatly over the course of the COVID-19 pandemic, and trainees remain at risk both at work, and outside of work. As such, residents should be encouraged to report their symptoms and to stay out of work with any concerning symptoms until further evaluation. Careful planning is required by programs to provide coverage for residents following an exposure, while they quarantine, or to isolate after a positive test. CDC guidelines have evolved during the course of the pandemic, and state or institutional guidance may vary, but trainees should be supported if they require time away after an exposure. Directly linked with that is access to and knowledge about institution-specific policies for COVID-19 testing and ensuring access for trainees to get testing done when appropriate.[19] How vaccine status may affect these policies remains unknown.

Access to the COVID-19 Vaccine

As of December 2020, the CDC updated their recommendations for access of healthcare personnel to the COVID-19 vaccine.[20] Based on recommendations by the Advisory Committee on Immunization Practices (ACIP), the CDC advised that healthcare professionals be offered the COVID-19 vaccine first. Trainees comprise a critical mass of personnel at risk. However, the methodology behind vaccine roll outs has differed by institution. In some cases, as at Stanford, a well-intended algorithm to identify those on the front lines only included seven out of 1300 trainees.[21] While this was ultimately remedied, it highlights the importance of institutions identifying those at risk to make sure there is appropriate access to the vaccine.

IMPACT ON WELLNESS

In recent years there has been increased awareness surrounding physician wellness. The ACGME has recognized its importance and subsequently placed greater emphasis on trainee wellness. This has been particularly important in dermatology, as our field has seen one of the largest increases in rates of burnout compared to other specialties.[22] COVID-19 has only accelerated the need to address wellness.

What Is Physician Wellness?

The answer is multifaceted and previously largely focused on negative mental aspects including burnout, depression, and emotional exhaustion. More recently there has been a shift in focus toward more positive aspects such as overall quality of life and work–life balance. In an attempt to synthesize the definition of physician wellness, Brady and colleagues conducted a systematic review of the literature.[23] They proposed defining physician wellness as "quality of life, which includes the absence of ill-being and the presence of positive physical, mental, social, and integrated well-being experienced in connection with activities and environments that allow physicians to develop their full potentials across personal and work-life domains."[23]

Stressors on Trainee Wellness

Wellness is different for each trainee. While dermatology trainees are not as commonly stressed, for example, by long overnight shifts and disrupted sleep, they have their own unique stressors, such as learning a new vocabulary, adjusting to seeing higher patient volumes in an outpatient setting, and needing to spend large amounts of nonclinic time to independently study less common diseases with dermatologic manifestations. COVID-19 has magnified these stressors. The decrease in outpatient clinic volumes including surgical procedures, the transition to telemedicine for outpatients as well as some inpatients, and redeployment to nondermatology services has led many trainees feeling as though their clinical training has been negatively impacted by COVID-19.[7] For incoming trainees there is the additional stress of adjusting to a new city and new job while being socially isolated. For upper level trainees there is heightened anxiety related to the uncertainties surrounding the board certification exam as well as obtaining fellowship positions and future employment.[24] For some there is also the added stress of starting a family and experiencing pregnancy during a pandemic or having childcare

issues due to school closures and possible COVID-19 exposures. And there have also been trainees who have needed to care for COVID-19-positive patients or family members, had sick family that they were unable to visit, or have even experienced loss of patients or loved ones from COVID-19. Some of these stressors have disproportionately fallen upon female trainees in the setting of a further dwindled support network during COVID-19.[25]

Furthermore, the pandemic has led to many restrictions across state lines, quarantine requirements, and institutional travel bans. As a result, many trainees have found themselves completely isolated and/or socially distanced from their typical support networks. In conjunction, many have experienced chronic anxiety around the uncertainty of the state of the world and where their expertise may be requested or required. Dermatology residents across the country, especially in certain hot spots, have had to transition onto medicine floors, intensive care units, and emergency rooms, putting them on the true frontlines of COVID-19 care. Additionally, for many, the social and celebratory aspects of residency were altered with reduced in-person gatherings, cancellation of graduation, and muted welcoming events for incoming first years. The discordance of what they expected their residency trajectory would be and their current reality further drives their anxiety and depression. As a result, mental health and wellness, more so than ever, need to be at the forefront of all residency programs, including dermatology.

Need for Action

At UPenn and WashU, preexisting institutional wellness initiatives have grown during COVID-19 to help combat some of the deleterious effects of this pandemic on wellness. Dedicated wellness websites are accessible to all trainees and include resources for self-care, family care, gratitude, as well as basic and life essentials including support for food, housing, and childcare. Additional institutional resources include free and confidential mental health counseling, virtual sessions to improve coping and resilience strategies, as well as group sessions on mindfulness and more. Furthermore, at the program level, we have been able to convert many wellness-related activities to virtual platforms or socially distanced events including an annual resident wellness retreat and monthly curated wellness activities (at UPenn). At WashU, we also formed "family groups," each comprised of a resident from each class and a faculty member to provide additional peer support and opportunities for social interactions outside of work.

In challenging times, clear and transparent communication from program leadership is critical to address trainee concerns, sustain relationships, and promote wellness. In the study by Li and colleagues, 22% of residents felt their program was not transparent in providing updates on COVID-19 impacts.[2] At UPenn and WashU, we implemented weekly virtual meetings with all trainees to ensure real-time information dissemination, validation of fears and concerns, and an open forum for discussion. Important faculty–trainee relationships have been further strengthened during this time by continued mentorship through digital platforms.

IMPACT ON CAREERS

The effects of COVID-19 on dermatology residents and their experiences have not only impacted their current state, but also their future career paths. With recommendations across health systems to remain grounded, away rotations, electives, and mentorship experiences were put on temporary hold. Many residents lost the opportunity to spend time with individuals who may have otherwise helped further shape their career or guide their decisions as to their areas of focus. Those who were awarded society mentorship grants opted to delay those experiences with the hopes that restrictions, and the pandemic itself, would not be long lasting.

Dermatology is a small world, allowing for connections forged across all academic and practice settings. These connections have been consistently strengthened by networking at various conferences, including the annual meeting of the AAD. While many meetings have been held virtually, residents are not able to get to know leaders in the field, potential mentors, and potential employers in the same way that an intimate conversation in person can bring.

While there is no shortage of qualified dermatology residents continuing to graduate from residency programs, hiring freezes at institutions and private practices are in place as a result of the financial strains imposed by the pandemic. This has likely shifted how residents have approached their job search, adjusted their expectations, and prioritized their career goals. The full impact of this is yet to be seen.

IMPACT ON RESIDENT RECRUITMENT AND SELECTION

The COVID-19 pandemic significantly disrupted undergraduate medical education (UME) with downstream effects on the UME-to-GME transition. Changes to clinical rotations, grading, and extracurricular activities impacted medical students as they navigated the application process amid the pandemic. Program directors responsible for addressing trainee and program needs were also tasked with reworking resident recruitment processes and counseling students concerned about their applications. With the pandemic entering its second year, it is clear there will be far-reaching consequences to resident recruitment and selection. Given prepandemic calls to address disparities in the application process, we have a unique opportunity to continue and expand upon COVID-19-related reforms beyond the current crisis.

Changes to Undergraduate Medical Education and the Application Process

Beginning in March 2020, medical schools implemented widespread changes including delayed and canceled rotations, shifts to virtual education, and expanded pass–fail grading. In-person away electives were cancelled, and there were delays or cancellations of United States Medical Licensing Exam (USMLE) Step administration. Pandemic-associated changes to institutional policies and faculty availability led to decreased opportunities for longitudinal service, advocacy, and research projects. These changes conceivably affected specialty choice, letters of recommendation, medical school rankings, and honor society elections, leading to significant impacts on the content and quality of individual applications, particularly in highly competitive specialties such as dermatology.

Continued travel restrictions and limitations to clinical and research activities directly affected the application process. To allow students to complete clinical rotations and acquire letters of recommendation, and to facilitate a comprehensive medical student performance evaluation (MSPE), the Association of American Medical Colleges (AAMC) delayed opening of the Electronic Residency Application Service by 5 weeks, to October 21, 2020. This delay significantly compressed the timeline for application review. Following a national call for virtual interviews, nearly all dermatology programs converted to a remote recruitment process.

Reforms Implemented During the Pandemic

Program directors from the Association of Professors of Dermatology (APD) released two statements to address applicants' concerns in spring 2020, which included recommendations for both applicants and programs.[26] Important recommendations for programs included: limiting in-person away rotations to applicants without a home dermatology program and creating virtual away experiences; performing holistic application review and considering COVID-19 related changes to individual applications; and conducting all-virtual interviews.[27] Applicants were encouraged to: continue with their application plans despite perceived weaknesses due to COVID-19; and to limit their number of applications and interviews to facilitate holistic review and equitable interview distribution.

While away rotations foster personal connections and facilitate letters of recommendation and research opportunities, financial costs, scheduling conflicts, and limited availability may lead to inequity in the process, hampering efforts to increase diversity in dermatology.[28,29] Programs introduced a variety of virtual options for this application cycle including electives, informational sessions, and participation in virtual didactics. Additionally, an initiative to increase transparency about dermatology residency programs led to guidelines for website information,[30] as well as an accessible Google doc with program-specific information about the application cycle.[31]

The COVID-19 pandemic inspired additional creative opportunities for virtual interaction between programs and applicants. Webinars hosted by national dermatology organizations addressed applicant concerns and offered recommendations on topics ranging from application content, pre- and postinterview communication, preference signaling, and interview etiquette.[32] Social media became both a powerful resource for mentorship and for outreach by dermatology programs, with many expanding their presence on popular platforms such as Twitter and Instagram.

The dual pandemics of COVID-19 and systemic racism unmasked the urgent need to address the lack of diversity in medicine. Holistic application review has been promoted as a means to increase diversity in medicine and shift emphasis away from standardized metrics toward qualities that have become even more critical during the current crisis, such as leadership, commitment to service, and resilience.[29,33,34] The compressed timeline for review challenged PDs to develop manageable but effective holistic review processes. Holistic review featured heavily at this year's Diversity Champions Workshop;[35] guidelines and best practices are currently being developed.

Match Outcomes

As of April 2021, limited data have been released from the National Resident Matching Program (NRMP). Early results suggest that overall match rates for dermatology decreased from prior years, given that the total number of PGY2 positions (478) was relatively stable in 2021 compared to 2020, yet there was an increase in applicants from 699 in 2020 to 734 in 2021.[36,37] Compared to 2020, the match rate for PGY2 dermatology positions decreased for US MD seniors from 78% to 74% and for DO applicants from 57% to 47%.[36,37] More granular data will be released by NRMP later this year and will allow for further analysis of match outcomes and application patterns during this cycle.

Future Directions in Resident Recruitment and Selection

The COVID-19 pandemic accelerated discussions about the resident application process, with increased calls for reform within dermatology and across all specialties.[38,39] Areas of particular interest include: preference signaling mechanisms, application and interview limits, virtual interviewing, increased transparency between programs and applicants, and an honest accounting of how we counsel dermatology hopefuls and weigh certain application parameters such as Step scores, research gap years, and publication numbers. Considerations to optimize the process are critical to address ongoing changes to UME and to create a more equitable and sustainable application process beyond the current crisis.

LOOKING TO THE FUTURE

We have yet to fully understand the long-term impact of COVID-19 on dermatology residency, but we know that we must remain transparent, adaptable, and engaged to ensure the best educational and clinical experiences for our trainees, and to secure a strong future for our specialty. The pandemic is not yet over, as is evidenced by surges in positivity rates across the country as of April 2020, but there is a light in the form of a vaccine. Questions remain regarding the duration of immunity, efficacy against various SARS-CoV-2 variants, and access to vaccines on a global level. That said, for an unknown period of time, as educators, we will need to continue to remain adaptable on shorter time scales given the continued unprecedented time we find ourselves in.

DISCLOSURE

The authors have no relevant commercial or financial conflicts of interest. M. Rosenbach is on the AAD's Ad Hoc COVID-19 task force and I.S. Rosman is the Chair of the APD Program Director

Section Steering Committee. This paper reflects the authors' views.

REFERENCES

1. Ammar A, Stock AD, Holland R, et al. Managing a specialty service during the COVID-19 qualitative study. J Gen Intern Med 2005;20(5):381–5.

2. Li Y, Galimberti F, Abrouk M, et al. US dermatology resident responses about the COVID19 pandemic: results from a nationwide survey. South Med J 2020;113(9):462–5.

3. Shaw K, Karagounis T, Yin L, et al. Exchanging dermatoscopes for stethescopes: has the COVID19 pandemic highlighted gaps in the US dermatology residency training. J Drugs Dermatol 2020;19(9):905–6.

4. Accreditation Council for Graduate Medical Education. Three stages of GME during the COVID-19 pandemic. Available at: https://acgme.org/COVID-19/Three-Stages-of-GMEDuring-the-COVID-19-Pandemic. Accessed April 9, 2021.

5. Accreditation Council for Graduate Medical Education. Stage 3: pandemic emergency status guidance. Available at: https://acgme.org/Stage-3-Pandemic-Emergency-Status-Guidance. Accessed April 9, 2021.

6. Botros M, Cooper A. The hidden curriculum of the COVID19 pandemic. J Grad Med Educ 2020; 12(5):550–2.

7. Stewart C, Lipner S. Experiences of resident dermatologists during the COVID19 pandemic: a cross sectional survey. Dermatol Ther 2020;34(1):e14574.

8. Steinbach TC, Albert TJ, Carmona HD, et al. Just-in-time tools for training non-critical care providers: troubleshooting problems in the ventilated patient. ATS Sch 2020;1(2). https://doi.org/10.34197/ats-scholar.2020-0038in.

9. American Board of Dermatology. Impact of COVID-19 on dermatology resident education. 2020. Available at: https://www.abderm.org/2978.aspx. Accessed April 9, 2021.

10. Hruza GJ. 2020 annual AAD meeting is canceled due to COVID-19 outbreak. American Academy of Dermatology website. Available at: https://www.aad.org/member/meetings/am2020/faqs/coronavirus. Accessed April 9, 2021.

11. Kwatra SG, Sweren RJ, Grossberg AL. Dermatology practices as vectors for COVID-19 transmission: a call for immediate cessation of nonemergent dermatology visits. J Am Acad Dermatol 2020;82(5):e179–80.

12. Aziz H, James T, Remulla D, et al. Effect of COVID19 on surgical training across the US: A national survey of general surgery residents. J Surg Educ 2020; 78(2):1–9.

13. American Academy of Dermatology Association Managing your practice through the COVID-19 outbreak. Available at: https://www.aad.org/member/practice/managing/coronavirus. Accessed April 9, 2021.

14. Mack S, Lilly E, Yu J, et al. Asynchronous teledermatology in medical education: lessons from the COVID19 pandemic. J Am Acad Dermatol 2020; 83(3):e267–8.

15. Oldenburg R, Marsch A. Optimizing teledermatology visits for dermatology resident education during the COVID-19 pandemic. J Am Acad Dermatol 2020;82(6):e229.

16. Hammond M, Sharma T, Cooper K, et al. Conducting inpatient dermatology consultations and maintaining resident education in the COVID19 telemedicine era. JAAD 2020;83(4):e317–8.

17. Wang RF, Trinidad J, Lawrence J. Improved patient access and outcomes with the integration of an eConsult program (teledermatology) within a large academic medical center. J Am Acad Dermatol 2020. https://doi.org/10.1016/j.jaad.2019.10.053.

18. Trinidad J, Kroshinsky D, Kaffenberger B, et al. Telemedicing for inpatient dermatology consultations in response to the COVID19 pandemic. J Am Acad Dermatol 2020;83(1):e69–71.

19. Anton M, Wright J, Braithwaite M, et al. Creating a COVID19 action plan for GME programs. J GME 2020;August:399–402.

20. Center for Disease Control. The Importance of COVID-19 Vaccination for Healthcare Personnel. The Importance of COVID-19 Vaccination for Healthcare Personnel | CDC. Available at: https://nam03. safelinks.protection.outlook.com/?url=https%3A% 2F%2Fwww.cdc.gov%2Fcoronavirus%2F2019-ncov %2Fvaccines%2Frecommendations%2Fhcp.html& data=04%7C01%7Cm.packiam%40elsevier.com% 7Ce86b759c4a7c418eb24308d9367477a1%7C927 4ee3f94254109a27f9fb15c10675d%7C0%7C0%7C 637600697210788130%7CUnknown%7CTWFpbG Zsb3d8eyJWIjoiMC4wLjAwMDAiLCJQIjoiV2luMzIiL CJBTiI6Ik1haWwiLCJXVCI6Mn0%3D%7C1000& sdata=IKEouy%2BimxtJFGDIOjoH7z3etPnPLEYZyL avfvC58fg%3D&reserved=0. Accessed June 23, 2021.

21. "Three lessons from Stanford's COVID-19 vaccine debacle". STAT. 3 lessons from Stanford's Covid-19 vaccine algorithm debacle (statnews.com). Available at: https://nam03.safelinks.protection.outlook. com/?url=https%3A%2F%2Fwww.statnews.com% 2F2020%2F12%2F21%2Fstanford-covid19-vaccine- algorithm%2F&data=04%7C01%7Cm.packiam% 40elsevier.com%7Ce86b759c4a7c418eb24308d9 367477a1%7C9274ee3f94254109a27f9fb15c10675 d%7C0%7C0%7C637600697210788130%7C Unknown%7CTWFpbGZsb3d8eyJWIjoiMC4wLjAw MDAiLCJQIjoiV2luMzIiLCJBTiI6Ik1haWwiLCJXVCI 6Mn0%3D%7C1000&sdata=CHzei3cyHR0UcWG zv0Fyj%2Bcw0jY9RLyH6k8I8Vbpb18%3D& reserved=0. Accessed June 23, 2021.

22. Stratman EJ, Anthony E, Stratman ZE, et al. The heightened focus on wellness in dermatology residency education. Clin Dermatol 2020;38(3):336–43.

23. Brady KJS, Trockel MT, Khan CT, et al. What do we mean by physician wellness? A systematic review of its definition and measurement. Acad Psychiatry 2018;42(1):94–108.

24. Adusumilli NC, Eleryan M, Tanner S, et al. Third-year dermatology resident anxiety in the era of COVID-19. J Am Acad Dermatol 2020;83(3):969–71.

25. Hickman A, Rosman I. Lean in or out: how to balance when the world turns upside down? Int J Womens Dermatol 2020;6(5):448–9.

26. Dermatology residency program director consensus statement and recommendations regarding the 2020-2021 application cycle. 2020. Available at: https://aamc-orange.global.ssl.fastly.net/production/media/filer_public/0f/7b/0f7b547e-65b5-4d93-8247-951206e7f726/updated_dermatology_program_director_statement_on_2020-21_application_cycle_.pdf. Accessed January 21, 2021.

27. Rosman IS, Schadt CR, Samimi SS, et al. Approaching the dermatology residency application process during a pandemic. J Am Acad Dermatol 2020;83(5):e351–2.

28. Phillips RC, Dhingra N, Uchida T, et al. The "away" dermatology elective for visiting medical students: educational opportunities and barriers. Dermatol Online J 2009;15(10):1.

29. Chen A, Shinkai K. Rethinking how we select dermatology applicants – turning the tide. JAMA Dermatol 2017;153(3):259–60.

30. Rosmarin D, Friedman AJ, Burkemper NM, et al. The association of professors of dermatology program directors task force and residency program transparency work group guidelines on residency program transparency. J Drugs Dermatol 2020;19(11):1117–8.

31. Dermatology program information for students; 2020-2021 application cycle. 2020. Available at: https://docs.google.com/spreadsheets/d/1iErSdHqAlPgH5is_MHN9F-qliqe-yknlsYZeR4FDDrY/edit#gid=1714351310. Accessed January 21, 2021.

32. Brumfiel CM, Jefferson IS, Wu AG, et al. A national webinar for dermatology applicants during the COVID-19 pandemic. J Am Acad Dermatol 2021;84(2):574–6.

33. Jones VA, Clark KA, Patel PM, et al. Considerations for dermatology residency applicants underrepresented in medicine amid the COVID-19 pandemic. J Am Acad Dermatol 2020;83(3):e247–8.

34. Kraisik D, O'Connor DM, Nathan NR. What matters most: why the COVID-19 pandemic should prompt us to revisit the dermatology resident selection process. J Am Acad Dermatol 2020;83(1):e55.

35. Diversity champion workshop focuses on inclusion to recruit minorities and care for underserved patients. 2020. Available at: https://www.aad.org/member/meetings/events/diversity-workshop/diversity-workshop-workforce-pipeline. Accessed January 22, 2021.

36. Results and data. 2020 main residency match. NRMP. 2020. Available at: https://mk0nrmp3oyqui6wqfm.kinstacdn.com/wp-content/uploads/2020/06/MM_Results_and-Data_2020-1.pdf. Accessed April 5, 2021.

37. Advance data tables. 2021 main residency match. NRMP. 2021. Available at: https://mk0nrmp3oyqui6wqfm.kinstacdn.com/wp-content/uploads/2021/03/Advance-Data-Tables-2021_Final.pdf. Accessed April 5, 2021.

38. Stewart CR, Chernoff KA, Wildman HF, et al. New insights into the dermatology residency application process amid the COVID-19 pandemic. Cutis 2020;106(1):35–6.

39. Hammoud MM, Standiford T, Carmody JB. Potential implications of COVID-19 for the 2020-2021 residency application cycle. JAMA 2020;324(1):29–30.

The Impact of the COVID-19 Pandemic on Global Health Dermatology

Claire Hannah, MD[a,b], Victoria Williams, MD[a,c],
Lucinda Claire Fuller, MA, FRCP(UK)[d,e], Amy Forrestel, MD[a],*

KEYWORDS

• COVID-19 • Global health • Dermatology • Pandemic • International

KEY POINTS

- The COVID-19 pandemic has affected patient care, research, education, and collaborations worldwide in dermatology.
- Many of the challenges that have arisen during the pandemic highlight inequalities and structural vulnerabilities that existed before COVID-19.
- Dermatologists around the world are working to adapt and innovate to overcome obstacles and to create more robust, sustainable systems that will benefit the field for years to come.

BACKGROUND

Skin disease is one of the most common human illnesses worldwide, affecting up to 70% of people.[1] Individuals living in resource-poor settings with limited access to health care face even higher rates of skin disease. Collectively, these diseases are a leading cause of morbidity across the globe and have been shown to result in more years lost because of disability than such diseases as diabetes mellitus, asthma, migraines, and chronic obstructive lung disease.[1] Additionally, skin conditions are among the most common reasons for presentation to a primary care setting and can serve as a valuable entry point into the health care system for individuals otherwise unlikely to seek care. The appropriate diagnosis and management of dermatologic disease can prevent physical disability, psychosocial distress, and even mortality.

Despite the significant global burden of skin disease, there is a critical shortage of dermatologists worldwide and the field is currently unable to meet demand for the care of these conditions, particularly in at-risk populations.[2,3] Global health dermatology is dedicated to addressing these health care discrepancies between and within countries to improve skin health for vulnerable populations worldwide. This growing community of dermatologists aims to reduce the global burden of skin disease through direct patient care and involvement with health policy organizations, research, and education of trainees domestically and abroad.[4,5]

In December 2019, the city of Wuhan in China identified a series of unexplained cases of pneumonia. This disease rapidly spread throughout China, followed shortly thereafter by an increasing number of cases in countries throughout the world. It is now known that this illness, designated COVID-19, is caused by a novel coronavirus, named SARS-CoV-2. At the time of this article, more than 150 million people have been infected with SARS-CoV-2 and more than 3 million have died. In addition to its direct impact on morbidity and mortality, the pandemic has also placed tremendous strain on health, economic,

[a] Department of Dermatology, Hospital of the University of Pennsylvania, 3600 Spruce Street, 2 Maloney, Philadelphia, PA 19104, USA; [b] Department of Internal Medicine, Hospital of the University of Pennsylvania, Philadelphia, PA, USA; [c] Merck & Co, Inc, Upper Gwynedd, PA, USA; [d] Chelsea and Westminster Hospital NHS Foundation Trust, London, UK; [e] International Foundation for Dermatology, London, UK
* Corresponding author. 3400 Civic Center Blvd, South Pavilion 7th Floor, Philadelphia, PA 19104.
E-mail address: amy.forrestel@pennmedicine.upenn.edu

Dermatol Clin 39 (2021) 619–625
https://doi.org/10.1016/j.det.2021.05.005
0733-8635/21/© 2021 Elsevier Inc. All rights reserved.

educational, and food systems, leading to a myriad of downstream consequences. Although the scope of the indirect effects of this pandemic cannot yet be fully grasped, it is already evident that vulnerable populations are suffering disproportionately because of such factors as poverty and socioeconomic disparities,[6,7] and that the care of patients with noncommunicable diseases has been markedly disrupted.[8] These effects have greatly impacted global health programs, collaborations, and projects.

In this article, we discuss some of the ways the COVID-19 pandemic has impacted global health dermatology. We surveyed more than 20 global health dermatologists via email and informal interviews, including dermatologists in the United States and Europe with various international collaborations, and dermatologists currently working in other regions of the world. In doing so, we gained insights into how COVID-19 has impacted patient care, control of neglected tropical diseases (NTDs), collaborations, education, and telemedicine across six continents, including programs in Botswana, China, Ethiopia, Fiji, Guatemala, Kenya, Mali, Nepal, Peru, Tajikistan, and Uganda.

IMPACT ON DIRECT PATIENT CARE

With most global health care resources focused on the COVID-19 crisis, routine care for chronic diseases has been markedly affected.[9] Nearly all dermatologists we interviewed reported either a significant reduction or complete cessation of outpatient dermatology services. For some, this period was limited to the peak of the pandemic, whereas others reported ongoing clinic closures. Although most places attempted to prioritize in-person visits for complex or serious skin conditions, this was not always possible for a variety of reasons. A dermatologist in South America noted that even their patients with pemphigus vulgaris, a potentially life-threatening disease, have been unable to receive face-to-face care. Although most private and academic dermatology practices are transitioning back toward full capacity, many nonprofit organizations that provide free or income-based health care to underserved populations remain closed. In the United States, dermatologists reported interruptions in face-to-face dermatology visits at free clinics. Even if patients are able to schedule in-person appointments, they face many barriers to successfully attending the visit, including public transportation closures and early mandatory curfews. These travel barriers have also prevented some dermatologists from participating in community outreach programs to rural and remote areas. In Botswana, one dermatologist noted that lockdown and travel restrictions disrupted an outreach clinic service, preventing visits to various rural sites for between 2 and 4 months. These community outreach programs provide vital care to patients who otherwise would not have access to dermatologic expertise in their area.

In addition to physical barriers, many patients are unwilling to be seen in person because of the risks of acquiring an infectious illness. The looming threat of contracting COVID-19 is a legitimate concern for patients and health care workers, particularly in low- and middle-income countries (LMIC) where access to clean water and severe shortages of expensive personal protective equipment limit basic hygiene practices.[10] Many interviewed dermatologists reported shortages or total absence of basic personal protective equipment across various countries. A dermatology clinic in East Africa did not have access to hand washing facilities, masks, or examination gloves in local hospitals for several months. Health care facilities in tropical climates have worked to maximize benefits from existing safety measures that have long been used to decrease transmission of diseases, such as tuberculosis. Examples include single-story facilities on large campuses with many outdoor spaces for patient waiting and triage, and open windows and doors to improve ventilation.

IMPACT ON NEGLECTED TROPICAL DISEASES

NTDs describe a group of mainly communicable diseases that affect individuals living in poverty, predominantly in LMIC.[11] Many NTDs involve the skin, either as the primary manifestation or as an associated clinical feature. Examples of skin NTDs include Buruli ulcer, cutaneous leishmaniasis, scabies, leprosy, deep mycoses, yaws, and lymphatic filariasis.[11] Although these diseases have historically been neglected in terms of funding, advocacy, research, and drug development, there has been growing public awareness of their considerable morbidity, social stigma, and economic effects. This has resulted in an enhanced global effort to prevent and eradicate them.[12] To efficiently and effectively target NTDs of the skin, global health dermatologists advocate for the use of integrated intervention strategies, which use a common pathway to simultaneously diagnose, treat, and prevent a group of two or more diseases.[11] The World Health Organization has recognized the benefits of integration around skin NTDs, and these strategies have been successfully used in a some settings.[13] However, the potential of this approach has not been fully realized and many countries are still in the early stages of developing and implementing integrated programs.

Dermatologists interviewed for this article expressed concern regarding the consequences of NTD program interruptions during the pandemic. COVID-19 has overwhelmed health systems worldwide, particularly in low-income countries that struggled to meet the demands of their population even before the pandemic. Research, funding, facilities, equipment, and personnel have been focused on preventing and treating the virus, which has diverted attention and resources from NTDs. In Ethiopia, community-based disease prevention and health promotion services have been stopped since the beginning of the pandemic.[14] At the national level, monitoring and supervision of key NTD programs were suspended. Mass drug administration programs were also affected, with planned community and school-based interventions for helminthiasis, trachoma, and onchocerciasis canceled because of COVID-19.[14] A colleague in Guatemala reported similar experiences, including suspension of government funding for the National Leprosy Program. Laudably, the program was able to continue its operations for 4 months without government financial support, and after multiple meetings and negotiations, a grant was secured.

The care of persons living with HIV has also been significantly impacted during the pandemic. There is a high degree of coinfection with HIV and NTDs, and certain NTDs may enhance the progression of HIV.[15] Given the close association between these diseases, disruptions in public health programs targeting HIV could affect the incidence and severity of NTDs, and vice versa. In many sub-Saharan African countries, government-supported HIV services were limited or closed during the pandemic, and access to antiretroviral therapy declined because of several factors, such as disruptions to the supply chain, personnel shortages, and patients' inability to or fear of traveling to central hospitals to pick up medications.[16] These same factors have likely contributed to a decline in HIV testing.[16,17] The long-standing implications of this period of decreased diagnosis, treatment, and prevention of NTDs, HIV, and other chronic diseases is unknown, but will likely be significant.

IMPACT ON COLLABORATIONS AND RELATIONSHIPS

Worldwide travel restrictions imposed since the beginning of the pandemic have resulted in the suspension of many in-person global health projects. The inability to be physically present with collaborators presented a variety of challenges to the global health community. Collaborations in the early stages of planning and implementation were perhaps most impacted by travel restrictions. To create sustainable, productive, mutually beneficial collaborations in another country, it is necessary to build relationships with local stakeholders and work together to identify priorities and set agendas. Face-to-face interactions and regular, in-person contact are invaluable for building the trust and respect needed to achieve these goals.

Some dermatologists were working to establish new collaborations on site when the pandemic began and were required to return home. Others were forced to cancel their first planned trips to a country. Although most attempted to continue building relationships remotely, many ultimately struggled to establish human connection and advance projects because of poor Internet connectivity, language barriers, and time zone differences. Additionally, most were simultaneously addressing pandemic-related challenges in their own clinical settings, which left limited time to dedicate to global health projects. For these reasons, tasks that would have been completed in a single face-to-face interaction have taken months to accomplish over email and telephone calls. Several of the interviewed physicians expressed concern and uncertainty about the chances of rebuilding relationships and restarting projects once global travel resumes.

In contrast, some well-established collaborations fared well during the pandemic. Several dermatologists voiced the perception that the global crisis fostered camaraderie between collaborators in different countries and resulted in increased dialogue to share information and resources. Others found that the pandemic exposed an underlying dependency on an in-person presence, resulting in stalled progress or complete dissolution of even long-standing projects. Although these setbacks were described as unexpected and disheartening, they ultimately allowed collaborators to identify weaknesses in project infrastructure that might have otherwise gone unrecognized. One colleague pointed out that an increasing number of US-based global health physicians are spending only weeks to months of the year physically present at a given project site, so the insights gained during the pandemic regarding productive virtual communication and project sustainability are helping to prepare for a future where this practice model is the norm.

IMPACT ON EDUCATION

Interviewees emphasized the pandemic's impact on education and mentorship. Because of international travel restrictions, there have been fewer clinical and research opportunities to foster trainee interest and expertise in global health dermatology. One of the biggest impacts has been the cancellation of international electives and exchanges, such as the American Academy of Dermatology Resident International Grant.[18] For more than 10 years, this grant has provided funding for multiple American and Canadian dermatology trainees to complete 4- to 6-week rotations in Botswana. In 2020, the program planned to expand to include three additional partner institutions from different regions of the world, and to support trainees from these institutions to rotate in the United States. These rotations have been on hold since the start of COVID-19. The US-based nonprofit organization PASHA,[19] which aims to increase access to skin care by strengthening health systems in Tajikistan and Nepal, was also required to cancel planned educational exchanges. One cancellation involved a recently received grant to send two dermatologists from Tajikistan to Nepal for an observational rotation to learn up-to-date evidence-based diagnostics, treatments, and alternative models of skin care delivery. Similarly, plans for a Tajik dermatologist to travel to the United States for a 1-year fellowship in dermatopathology were postponed because of COVID-19. PASHA instead had to focus its efforts on devising novel approaches to training; virtual case conferences were initiated and efforts to develop and fund remote pathology training are in progress.

These opportunities for cultural exchange, learning, and collaboration that occur during rotations often influence the course of participants' careers. It is uncertain when exchanges, such as these will resume, and when they do, there are multiple factors that may be altered long-term or permanently including trainee interest, funding availability, and institutional policies on hosting rotators. Additionally, many health systems in low-resource settings depend on the consistent presence of international rotators to assist with care delivery and to bring vital medical supplies. Many clinics are now short-staffed and unable to meet demands of patient care, which highlights long-standing concerns about the sustainability of global health projects that rely on foreign physicians, volunteers, or supplies.[20,21]

In addition to the cancellation of global health electives, there have been pandemic-induced setbacks in plans to establish dermatology training centers abroad. For example, in a long-standing collaborative project to create a Masters of Medicine in Dermatology program at Moi University School of Medicine in Kenya, the final approval process has been on hold because of the delays in the regulatory committee approval. The newly established Pacific Dermatology Training Center in Suva, Fiji has also faced multiple obstacles in the last year.[22] Starting in 2019, a Postgraduate Diploma of Dermatology program was initiated in partnership with Fiji National University to allow physicians from Fiji and surrounding Pacific island countries to specialize in dermatology, with a focus on skin conditions seen in the Pacific region. The curriculum was largely delivered by visiting dermatologists from Australia and New Zealand in collaboration with a local dermatology faculty member. At the start of the pandemic, just 1 year after opening, the program was temporarily suspended and trainees from other Pacific islands were requested to return home. The program pivoted to virtual teaching but has faced issues with poor Internet connectivity, large time differences between trainees and lecturers, and local government restrictions on educational activities for medical trainees.

The Regional Dermatology Training Center in Moshi, Tanzania was also required to send students back to their home countries. However, the Regional Dermatology Training Center, which has been graduating dermatovenerology officers for the past 30 years, was able to leverage well-established relationships and infrastructure to successfully transition to a virtual learning platform, maintain daily contact with collaborators, and deliver dermatology teaching throughout the initial surge of the pandemic. Through this platform, they were also able to deliver a virtual continuing medical education conference in January 2021, with 250 registered participants and 51 speakers from 12 different countries.

Adapting curricula to virtual formats was a common challenge identified by dermatologists around the world. One physician commented that becoming effective virtual teachers and learners has been a more difficult process than expected. Successful virtual education is contingent on teachers delivering engaging and interactive lessons, and students maintaining motivation and focus despite increased distractions and a more casual learning environment. Additionally, successful virtual teaching formats require equipment, software, and human resources. Project leaders have had to ensure that programs would have the computer literacy skills to ensure sustainability. Ultimately, the pandemic highlighted the potential for improving virtual education and research development between countries.

Lastly, the physical, psychological, and financial impacts of COVID-19 on educators and learners have been significant. Clinic closures, low patient volumes, and decreased educational activities were demoralizing for many of the interviewed physicians and trainees, and they struggled to reconcile their role during a global pandemic. Several dermatologists endorsed job insecurity and large pay reductions for several months during the peak of the pandemic. In some countries, the start of new residency cohorts was delayed by 5 months. Additionally, many of the physicians we interviewed lamented severe illness and death of beloved colleagues and teachers because of COVID-19.

IMPACT ON TELEMEDICINE

Telehealth refers to the delivery of health care by medical professionals using information and communication technologies, typically in situations where physical distance is a limiting factor. Because of its visual nature, dermatology is particularly well suited for telemedicine, and global health dermatologists have long been advocates for the use of telemedicine to increase access to quality skin care. In the United States, the full potential of telemedicine has not been realized and historically there has been little incentive to accelerate this process. Now, because of travel restrictions and stay-at-home mandates, there has been a tremendous rise in the use of telemedicine.[23,24] Health systems across the world have a renewed motivation to enhance their telehealth capacity and a surge of resources are being directed to improving technology and efficiency.[24] Additionally, public and private payer regulations surrounding reimbursement and telemedicine have significantly relaxed, further incentivizing the uptake of telemedicine in daily practice.[25]

Some global health dermatologists were able to use their prior experience in teledermatology to better adapt to the increased use of telehealth services in their country during the pandemic. However, those practicing in low-resource settings were often unable to transition to teledermatology because of a variety of factors, including poor Internet connectivity and inadequate information technology infrastructure.[26] Additionally, direct patient-to-provider telemedicine is often not feasible for patients in low-income settings because of costly cell phone data plans and weak home Internet connection. In areas lacking access to a local dermatologist, store-and-forward telemedicine platforms allow dermatologists in distant locations to serve as consultants. Store-and-forward systems rely on local health care providers to obtain digital pictures and pertinent medical history, then transmit the information electronically to consultants who assist with diagnosis and treatment.[27] During the pandemic, many of the dermatologists we interviewed reported a significant reduction in the volume of telemedicine consultations from primary care providers in developing countries, likely because of a combination of fewer patients seeking care and decreased availability of local providers to facilitate consultations. By serving as an intermediary between the patient and consultant, local primary care providers are critical for implementing effective and sustainable store-and-forward teledermatology systems. In the last year, many of these physicians were redeployed to other roles or required to stay at home, making it challenging for many teledermatology consulting systems to continue during the pandemic.

SUMMARY AND FUTURE DIRECTIONS

In this article, we discussed ways the COVID-19 pandemic has impacted patient care, NTD programs, professional collaborations, educational partnerships, and telemedicine delivery for global health dermatologists across the world. Many of the setbacks and hardships experienced by the global health community in the last year highlight long-standing global interdependencies and systems that perpetuate ethnic, economic, and social inequalities on local and global scales. The pandemic has brought discussions on global health colonialism to the forefront, a concept that acknowledges that the common power dynamic within collaborations of high-income countries pursuing their agendas to impose changes on LMICs reflects deeply engrained dynamics from former colonial relationships.[28] Most modern global health physicians recognize this approach is not effective, respectful, nor sustainable, and are working to identify tangible actions to increase equality and create mutually beneficial relationships.

Domestic health inequality has also been brought into sharp relief by the pandemic. In the United States, COVID-19 has caused disproportionately high morbidity and mortality in vulnerable and minority populations.[6,7] This has underscored and exacerbated the socio-politico-economic obstacles faced by these groups and increased levels of food, job, and housing insecurity. With the cancellation of international travel, many global health dermatologists valued the opportunity to explore health inequities present in their own communities and identify ways to deliver care to vulnerable populations.

Lastly, the participants in this study highlighted the potential benefits of improved telemedicine and virtual learning technology for supporting health care delivery, particularly in LMICs. The renewed focus on telemedicine has already resulted in creating more efficient, financially viable, and self-sustaining systems that will enhance the ability to provide quality patient care and education remotely.

These complex issues and their relationship to human health are at the core of global health work. Despite the many challenges, all global health dermatologists interviewed expressed hope that the COVID-19 pandemic will prompt critical reflection, discussion, and innovation that will lead to meaningful, lasting improvements to dermatology.

CLINICS CARE POINTS

- Based on interviews with dermatologists around the world, the COVID-19 pandemic has affected global health dermatology in many areas including patient care, education, research, and international collaborations.

- Generally, systems with fewer resources are suffering more severe negative impacts.

- Long-term effects of the pandemic on the field of global health dermatology, such as the effect of decreased services for neglected tropical diseases, remain to be seen.

- The pandemic highlighted existing structural inequalities within global dermatology and medicine and prompted ongoing discussion about systemic change.

ACKNOWLEDGMENTS

The authors thank Drs Elizabeth Bailey, Aileen Chang, Sarah Coates, Sigrid Collier, Huiting Dong, Wendemagegn Enbiale, Ousmane Faye, Alexia Knapp, Ali Lotfizadeh, Toby Maurer, Francisco Bravo Puccio, Garbiñe Riley, Rudolf Roth, Rustam Sultonov, Meciusela Tuicakau, and Karolyn Wanat for sharing their insights and experiences.

DISCLOSURE

None of the authors have commercial or financial conflicts of interest and there are no funding sources to report.

Funding: This research did not receive any specific grant from funding agencies in the public, commercial, or not-for-profit sectors.

Declarations of interest: none.

REFERENCES

1. Hay RJ, Johns NE, Williams HC, et al. The global burden of skin disease in 2010: an analysis of the prevalence and impact of skin conditions. J Invest Dermatol 2014;134(6):1527–34.

2. Fuller LC, Hay RJ. Global health dermatology: building community, gaining momentum. Br J Dermatol 2019;180(6):1279–80.

3. Mosam A, Todd G. Dermatology training in Africa: successes and challenges. Dermatol Clin 2021; 39(1):57–71.

4. Freeman EE. A seat at the big table: expanding the role of dermatology at the World Health Organization and beyond. J Invest Dermatol 2014;134(11): 2663–5.

5. McMahon DE, Oyesiku L, Amerson E, et al. Identifying gaps in global health dermatology: a survey of GLODERM members. Br J Dermatol 2021. https://doi.org/10.1111/bjd.19889.

6. Iacobucci G. Covid-19: increased risk among ethnic minorities is largely due to poverty and social disparities, review finds. BMJ 2020;371:m4099.

7. Shah GH, Shankar P, Schwind JS, et al. The detrimental impact of the COVID-19 crisis on health equity and social determinants of health. J Public Health Manag Pract 2020;26(4):317–9.

8. The Lancet: COVID-19: a new lens for noncommunicable diseases. Lancet 2020;396(10252): 649.

9. Chudasama YV, Gillies CL, Zaccardi F, et al. Impact of COVID-19 on routine care for chronic diseases: a global survey of views from healthcare professionals. Diabetes Metab Syndr 2020;14(5):965–7.

10. McMahon DE, Peters GA, Ivers LC, et al. Global resource shortages during COVID-19: bad news for low-income countries. Plos Negl Trop Dis 2020; 14(7):e0008412.

11. Mitjà O, Marks M, Bertran L, et al. Integrated control and management of neglected tropical skin diseases. Plos Negl Trop Dis 2017;11(1):e0005136.

12. WHO/Department of control of neglected tropical diseases: ending the neglect to attain the Sustainable Development Goals: a road map for neglected tropical diseases 2021–2030. WHO reference number WHO/UCN/NTD/2020.01.

13. Engelman D, Fuller LC, Solomon AW, et al. Opportunities for integrated control of neglected tropical diseases that affect the skin. Trends Parasitol 2016; 32(11):843–54.

14. Abdela SG, van Griensven J, Seife F, et al. Neglecting the effect of COVID-19 on neglected tropical diseases: the Ethiopian perspective. Trans R Soc Trop Med Hyg 2020. https://doi.org/10.1093/trstmh/traa072.

15. Simon GG. Impacts of neglected tropical disease on incidence and progression of HIV/AIDS,

tuberculosis, and malaria: scientific links. Int J Infect Dis 2016;42:54–7.

16. Jewell BL, Mudimu E, Stover J, et al. Potential effects of disruption to HIV programmes in sub-Saharan Africa caused by COVID-19: results from multiple mathematical models. Lancet HIV 2020;7(9): e629–40.

17. Lagat H, Sharma M, Kariithi E, et al. Impact of the COVID-19 pandemic on HIV testing and assisted partner notification services, western Kenya. AIDS Behav 2020;1–4.

18. Introcaso CE, Kovarik CL. Dermatology in Botswana: the American Academy of Dermatology's Resident International Grant. Dermatol Clin 2011;29(1):63–7.

19. Available at: http://pasha4health.org. Accessed: January 23, 2021.

20. Citrin D, Mehanni S, Acharya B, et al. Power, potential, and pitfalls in global health academic partnerships: review and reflections on an approach in Nepal. Glob Health Action 2017;10(1):1367161.

21. Pinto AD, Cole DC, ter Kuile A, et al. A case study of global health at the university: implications for research and action. Glob Health Action 2014;7. https://doi.org/10.3402/gha.v7.24526.

22. Available at: https://pacificdermatology.org.au/dermatology-diploma-fiji-national-university/. Accessed: January 23, 2021.

23. Perkins S, Cohen JM, Nelson CA, et al. Teledermatology in the era of COVID-19: experience of an academic department of dermatology. J Am Acad Dermatol 2020;83(1):e43–4.

24. Hollander JE, Carr BG. Virtually perfect? Telemedicine for COVID-19. N Engl J Med 2020;382(18): 1679–81.

25. Bajowala SS, Milosch J, Bansal C. Telemedicine pays: billing and coding update. Curr Allergy Asthma Rep 2020;20(10):60.

26. Bakhtiar M, Elbuluk N, Lipoff JB. The digital divide: how COVID-19's telemedicine expansion could exacerbate disparities. J Am Acad Dermatol 2020; 83(5):e345–6.

27. Campagna M, Naka F, Lu J. Teledermatology: an updated overview of clinical applications and reimbursement policies. Int J Womens Dermatol 2017; 3(3):176–9.

28. Rabin TL, Mayanja-Kizza H, Barry M. Global health education in the time of COVID-19: an opportunity to restructure relationships and address supremacy. Acad Med 2020. https://doi.org/10.1097/ACM. 0000000000003911.

Effect of the COVID-19 Pandemic on Delayed Skin Cancer Services

Sarem Rashid, BS[a,b], Hensin Tsao, MD, PhD[a,*]

KEYWORDS

- Surgical delay • Evidence-based guidelines • Time to surgery • Skin cancer • COVID-19
- COVID-19 delays • Survival

KEY POINTS

- Guidelines during the pandemic suggest that surgical treatment of melanoma in situ may be deferred for up to 2 to 3 months, with priority given to T1-T4 lesions.
- Operating rooms should be used sparingly during lockdown periods to limit potential virus transmission and to maximize ventilator capacity.
- Sentinel lymph node biopsy may be delayed for certain skin cancers according to the NCCN guidelines.
- Dermatologists should evaluate skin cancer lesions on a case-by-case basis when following these guidelines.
- Longer term studies are needed to determine if the COVID-19 lockdown had any impact on skin cancer outcomes.

INTRODUCTION

The COVID-19 pandemic has dramatically impacted implementation of health care services in the United States. Since the first reported US cases in January 2020, the virus has surpassed 25 million infections causing more than 525,000 deaths nationally. A state of emergency was declared by the World Health Organization on March 11, 2020, followed shortly in the United States with state-sanctioned lockdown orders starting from March 19, 2020.[1] During lockdown, hospitals reported a substantial decrease in surgical volume when compared with previous years to accommodate pandemic-related medical resources and personnel.[2] As a result, health care systems have been pressured to manage essential supplies and human capital while mitigating risk of viral transmission.[3]

For all patients with cancer, many faced delays in obtaining a diagnosis, whereas others experienced delays in starting or maintaining treatment.[2–4] Patient compliance toward scheduled but deferable visits also reportedly contributed to these totals.[5] For skin cancer, the total number of lesions diagnosed and treated during lockdown periods decreased, with clinical priority given to tumors with high-risk histopathologic features.[6–9] To date, we could not find any studies reporting outcomes for patients with skin cancer affected by COVID-19.

Evidence-based recommendations from several dermatologic research centers have been proposed to facilitate delivery of care to patients with skin cancer.[10–14] In this review, we summarize available 2020 pandemic guidelines from the National Comprehensive Cancer Network (NCCN), the American College of Mohs Surgery (ACMS), the European Society of Medical Oncology, Society of Surgical Oncology (SSO), the British Association of Dermatologists (BAD), and the British Society for Dermatologic Surgery

[a] Department of Dermatology, Wellman Center for Photomedicine, Massachusetts General Hospital, Boston, MA 02466, USA; [b] Boston University School of Medicine, Boston, MA, USA
* Corresponding author. Massachusetts General Hospital, Edwards 211, 50 Blossom Street, Boston, MA 02114.
E-mail address: htsao@mgh.harvard.edu

Dermatol Clin 39 (2021) 627–637
https://doi.org/10.1016/j.det.2021.05.015

(BSDS) and describe the general impact of COVID-19 on skin cancer diagnosis and treatment recognizing that information regarding the impact on long-term outcomes is still limited. Although these guidelines were written for COVID-19 surges and may not be active at the time of this publication, future surges with potentially new COVID-19 variants or new viruses may lead to a reactivation of these recommendations.

MELANOMA TREATMENT GUIDELINES DURING THE PANDEMIC

In 2020, melanoma comprised approximately 5.6% of all US cancer cases, and caused most deaths from skin cancer.[15,16] The risk of metastasis is approximated by histopathologic features, such as primary tumor thickness, ulceration, anatomic location, and regional lymph node involvements.[17] Mortality has been shown to vary significantly based on pathologic stage. From 2010 to 2016, Surveillance, Epidemiology, and End Results data showed a 5-year survival rate of 99% and 66% in localized and regional disease, respectively, and 27% for melanomas with distant metastases.[18]

Skin cancers diagnosed during lockdown also differed from prelockdown tumors in several notable ways. Ricci and colleagues[19] compared histopathologic features for melanomas diagnosed before and after Italy's 54-day lockdown period and observed increased thickness (mean thickness of 0.88 mm and 1.96 mm, respectively), ulceration (odds ratio [OR], 4.9; 95% confidence interval [CI], 1.4–17.3), and nodular subtype (OR, 5.5; 95% CI, 1.3–25.1) in postlockdown melanomas compared with prelockdown melanomas. Although these factors have been previously described as independent adverse prognostic factors, further investigation is required to thoroughly characterize and examine the effect of pandemic delays on long-term survival.[12,20]

Wide local excision (WLE) remains the mainstay treatment of early and localized lesions. Current guidelines recommend 1-cm margins for melanomas less than or equal to 2 mm, and 2-cm margins for thicker lesions greater than 2 mm.[21] In the absence of delays, complete surgical excision should be performed 4 to 6 weeks after the initial diagnosis. Mohs surgery is used for melanomas with poorly distinguished visible margins (ie, lentigo maligna melanoma and acral melanoma), including those in cosmetically sensitive areas.[22]

Appropriate intervals for melanoma time to definitive surgery have been widely studied, although there is a lack of consensus.[23] A 2020 literature review of surgical delay and mortality in primary cutaneous melanoma yielded five total studies that addressed surgical delays of 1 month or longer.[24] From this sample, only two studies reported an association between delayed WLE and poor survival outcomes, both of which derived samples from the National Cancer Database. Conic and colleagues[25] stratified National Cancer Database melanomas by pathologic stage and discovered a significant mortality risk among stage 1 melanomas exclusively (30–50 days: hazard ratio, 1.05; 95% CI, 1.01–1.1; 60–89 days: hazard ratio, 1.16; 95% CI, 1.07–1.25). Basnet and colleagues[26] independently found a significant increase in overall survival for time to definitive surgery intervals less than 60 days, compared with after 60 days.

According to the NCCN, surgical treatment of T0 (melanoma in-situ) and T1 melanomas could have been delayed during pandemic surges for up to 3 months, with priority given to T3 and T4 melanomas.[14] If a substantial proportion of residual lesion remained after biopsy for T1 melanomas, then a complete biopsy with narrow surgical margins or elliptical excision with 1-cm surgical margins was recommended. In the setting of limited operating room capacity, sentinel lymph node biopsy (SLNB) for lesions greater than 0.8 mm were recommended for deferral for up to 3 months. For melanomas staged N1 and higher, the NCCN recommended deferral of lymphadenectomy if regional lymph nodes were palpable. Likewise, the BAD and BSDS suggested deferral of WLE for stage T0 and T1a melanomas based on histopathologic features of the biopsy.[11] The ACMS suggested deferral of melanoma in situ for up to 2 to 3 months, and reiterated NCCN guidelines for management of T0 and T1a melanomas.[12] The European Society of Medical Oncology endorsed a tiered system (high, high/medium, low) for guidelines based on value-based prioritization.[27] High priority surgeries included any curative resection for stage III lesions, procedures associated with neoadjuvant trials. High/medium priority surgeries included WLE and SLNB for new invasive melanomas staged T1b or higher, WLE alone for T1a or lower tumors, and resection of oligometastatic disease. There were no surgeries designated in the low priority category. Lastly, the SSO endorsed a case-by-case evaluation of melanomas before surgery.[28] WLE for T0 melanomas could have been deferred for up to 3 months. Surgical treatment of T3 and T4 melanomas held priority over T1 and T2 melanomas, although gross complete resection recommended for any melanoma with a large degree of residual lesion present because of incomplete biopsy. SLNB should have been performed for lesions with greater than 1 mm thickness and could otherwise be deferred for up to 3 months. The SSO guidelines included precise language to recommend documentation of tumor anatomic location in the event of surgical delay and encouraged that surgeries occur in the outpatient setting. Pandemic guidelines for all skin cancers are summarized in **Table 1**.

KERATINOCYTE CANCER TREATMENT GUIDELINES DURING THE PANDEMIC

Keratinocyte cancers (KC), primarily comprised of basal cell carcinomas (BCC) and squamous cell carcinomas (SCC), represent the most common malignancy in fair-skinned populations.[29] Predisposing factors for KCs include chronic exposure to UV radiation, male gender, and an immunocompromised state. Risk of metastasis correlates to histologic factors, such as subtype (eg, superficial, nodular, or infiltrative) and depth of the primary tumor.[15,16] Generally, BCCs are slow-growing tumors that have a small estimated risk of metastasis (0.003%–0.55%),[30] whereas SCCs are fast-growing tumors with considerable likelihood to metastasize (0.5%–16%).[31]

Primary management for KC includes WLE, electrodessication and curettage, and Mohs micrographic surgery. Mohs surgery has been shown to be the most effective treatment modality for high-risk or recurrent KC in some reports.[17] A meta-analysis of treatments used in KC reported an aggregated 5-year cure rate of 99% and 97% for previously untreated BCC and SCC, respectively.[32] A more recent prospective study from the Netherlands found no statistical difference in recurrence rates between surgical excision and Mohs surgery for treatment of BCC.[33] For SCC in particular, surgical delays longer than 18 months were associated with significantly increased likelihood of thicker and invasive tumors (OR, 4.18; 95% CI, 2.45–7.13), although this association is not yet well-established for delays relevant to pandemic lockdown periods.[20]

The NCCN recommended deferral of KC, including BCC, SCC, dermatofibrosarcoma protuberans, and other rare tumors, unless the physician estimated a high risk of metastasis or debilitating progression within 3 months. Following local excision, adjuvant therapy should be postponed for N0 and N1 tumors without extension invasion of large caliber nerves. The ACMS recommended deferral of BCC management for up to 3 months for small and well-differentiated lesions unless the patient was symptomatic.[12] Deferral of slowly enlarging and well-differentiated SCC/SCC in situ was also

recommended, although no discrete time period is suggested. SCC that was symptomatic or contained significant risk factors, such as rapid growth, poor differentiation, ulceration, and perineural invasion, should have been prioritized. The BAD and BSDS recommended deferring surgical excisions of BCC for 3 to 6 months unless the patient was highly symptomatic or endorsed high potential for significant growth.[11] Surgical treatment of SCC/SCC in situ that were small and well-differentiated may have also been reasonably deferred unless the lesion demonstrated rapid growth, poor differentiation, ulceration, and/or perineural invasion. High-priority lesions should have been carefully evaluated on a case-by-case basis to assess the risks and benefits of treatment with the concurrent risk of COVID-19 exposure.

MERKEL CELL CARCINOMA TREATMENT GUIDELINES DURING THE PANDEMIC

Merkel cell carcinoma (MCC) is a highly aggressive neuroendocrine-derived skin cancer that resides within the basal layer of the epidermis (eg, deep skin and hair follicles).[34] This lesion commonly affects individuals who are elderly (median age of diagnosis, 75–80 years) and immunocompromised.[35,36] These underlying conditions have been associated with increased risk of requiring intensive care because of COVID-19,[37] thus extra precautions should be taken during treatment to limit potential exposure to the virus in this patient population.

Treatment of MCC requires careful consideration of tumor stage and patient-specific factors. WLE with clear margins is performed to prevent local recurrence and regional metastasis of early stage tumors, although has not been shown effective in stand-alone treatment.[38,39] Mohs micrographic surgery has been recommended to effectively remove smaller lesions in cosmetically sensitive areas, or to monitor local recurrence during adjuvant therapy.[40] To note, Brisset and colleagues[41] reported lower survival of patients treated with Mohs excision when compared with those treated with radical excision supplemented by cervical block dissection, although the chart review was limited to 22 patients. Surgical treatment is usually accompanied by adjuvant radiation therapy, particularly in patients suspectable to local-nodal recurrence. Because of the high-risk nature of the lesion, there are limited studies available to date that describe outcomes related to surgical delay in MCC.

According to the NCCN, treatment should not have been deferred because of the COVID-19

Table 1
Summary of surgical treatment guidelines for skin cancer

		NCCN[10,14]	BAD/BSDS[11]	ACMS[12]	ESMO[27]	SSO[28]
MCC		Do not defer treatment with the exception of lesions <1 cm in elderly populations. Given low OR capacity, delay SLNB from excision if wound is allowed to granulate.	Prioritize rapidly enlarging tumors, poorly differentiated tumors, perineural tumors, ulcerated and symptomatic lesions.			
KC	BCC	Defer up to 3 mo unless the physician estimates a high risk of metastasis or debilitating progression.	Defer up to 3–6 mo unless the patient is highly symptomatic or endorses high potential for significant growth.	Defer up to 3 mo for small and well-differentiated lesions unless the patient is symptomatic.		
	SCC	Defer up to 3 mo unless the physician estimates a high risk of metastasis or debilitating progression.	Defer SCC/SCC in situ unless the lesion demonstrates rapid growth, poor differentiation, ulceration, and/or perineural invasion.	Prioritize SCC that are symptomatic or contain significant risk factors, such as rapid growth, poor differentiation, ulceration, and perineural invasion.		

Melanoma	Defer T0/T1 melanomas up to 3 mo, with priority given to T3/T4 melanomas. Prioritize complete biopsy with narrow surgical margins or elliptical excision with 1 cm surgical margins if large amount of residual lesion remains. Given low OR capacity, defer SLNB >0.8 mm for up to 3 mo. Defer lymphadenectomy for N1+ tumors if regional lymph nodes are palpable.	Defer T0/T1a melanomas based on histopathologic features.	Defer T0 up to 2–3 mo. Defer T0/T1a melanomas based on histopathologic features.	High priority: any curative stage III melanoma resection, procedures associated with neoadjuvant trials, procedures addressing postsurgical complications. High/medium priority: WLE and SLNB for new invasive melanomas staged T1b or higher, WLE alone for T1a or lower tumors, and resection of oligometastatic disease.	Defer T0 up to 3 mo, with priority given to T1/T2 melanomas. Prioritize gross complete resection for residual lesion in the setting of incomplete biopsy. SLNB performed only for >1 mm melanomas, otherwise defer for up to 3 mo.

Guidelines uniformly endorse urgent surgical excision, particularly for when high-risk features, such as increased thickness, poor differentiation, ulceration, and/or perineural invasion, are present. When evaluating a biopsy for high-risk features, specimen size and depth should be appropriate to provide the recommended clinical information.

Abbreviations: ACMS, American College of Mohs Surgery; BAD/BSDS, British Association of Dermatologists/British Society for Dermatological Surgery; BCC, basal cell carcinoma; ESMO, European Society of Medical Oncology; KC, Keratinocyte cancer; MCC, Merkel cell carcinoma; NCCN, National Comprehensive Cancer Network; OR, operating room; SCC, squamous cell carcinoma; SLNB, sentinel lymph node biopsy; SSO, Society of Surgical Oncology; WLE, wide local excision.

Table 2
Synopsis of studies for the impact of COVID-19 on skin cancer outcomes

Paper	Study Characteristics	Key Findings
Barruscotti et al, 2020[6]	Retrospective review of all surgical excisions performed in the dermatologic surgery room at Fondazione IRCCS Policlinico San Matteo from February 22–May 3, 2020 (n = 163).	Melanoma diagnoses in the 2020 lockdown period was reduced 60% from previous years (prevalence, 3.7%; 95% CI, 1–8). 30% relative decrease in all dermatologic surgical activity.
Earnshaw et al, 2020[7]	Retrospective review of a cancer tracking database in the UK from February to April 2020.	34.3% reduction in urgent skin cancer referrals during the study period. Largest decrease observed in April 2020 (56.4% lower cases than April 2019). Lower total skin cancers diagnosed in March 2020 compared with previous years.
Nolan et al, 2020[8]	Prospective cohort of patients undergoing skin cancer surgery from 32 plastic surgery units in the United Kingdom from March 16–June 14, 2020 (n = 1549). Retrospective patient data on melanoma surgery (March 23–June 14, 2020) from 20 plastic surgery units (n = 501).	Treatment of KC decreased by 27%–47% throughout April and May 20. SCCs prioritized over BCCs, and at the pandemic's peak SCCs comprised 71% of excisions. 77% of Mohs micrographic surgeons stopped procedures.
Filoni et al, 2021[9]	Retrospective review of all dermatologic and surgical activity performed in an Italy-based melanoma skin unit from February 23–May 21, 2020.	When compared with the previous calendar year, surgical excisions during lockdown increased 31.7% and SLNBs decreased 29%. Dermatologic follow-up decreased 30.2%, whereas surgical follow-up decreased 37%.
Ferrara et al, 2021[4]	Standards-based audit retrospective review comparing the number first diagnoses of tumors finalized during weeks 11–20 of 2020 at an Italian pathology unit (n = 2751).	All cancer diagnoses fell in 2020 by 44.9% compared with 2018 and 2019. Melanoma and KC represented 56.7% of all missing diagnoses.
Nicholson et al, 2020[48]	Survey study for all BSDS members practicing Mohs over the course of 3 wk starting April 27, 2020 (n = 47).	49% of respondents stopped Mohs surgery. When Mohs was performed, 35% reported decrease use of grafts/flaps, 81% reported increased use of dissolvable sutures, and 29% reported increase prescribing of prophylactic antibiotics.

(continued on next page)

Table 2
(continued)

Paper	Study Characteristics	Key Findings
Schauer et al, 2020[47]	Retrospective study of a UK hospital laboratory database January 27–March 22, 2020; and March 23–May 18, 2020 (inclusive) (n = 17).	Most cases represented early or thin melanomas (7% and 44% for prelockdown and during lockdown). Malignant melanoma detection rates were higher during lockdown (5.73%).
Ricci et al, 2020[19]	Cross-sectional study of all consecutive primary malignant melanomas from the Pathology Registry of IDI-IRCCS (Rome, Italy) during the COVID-19 pandemic (n = 237).	Mean number of melanomas diagnosed per day: 0.6 during lockdown vs 2.3 prelockdown vs 1.3 postlockdown. Mean Breslow thickness was 0.88 (95% CI, 0.50–1.26) prelockdown and 1.96 (95% CI, 1.16–2.76) postlockdown. Proportion of ulceration was 5.9% (95% CI, 2.4%–11.7%) prelockdown and 23.5% (95% CI, 10.8%–41.2%) postlockdown.
Valenti 2021[46]	Retrospective study of excised advanced melanoma and keratinocyte cancers in an Italian dermatosurgery division from May 18–November 18, 2020 (n = 265).	The number of advanced skin cancers was significantly higher during lockdown (54 vs 22; OR, 2.64; 95% CI, 1.56–4.47; P = .0003). The number of advanced SCCs (OR, 4.60; 95% CI, 1.31–16.18; P = .0175) and BCCs (OR, 2.15; 95% CI, 1.14–4.07; P = .0187) was significantly higher during lockdown.
Marson 2021[43]	Retrospective study of 143 US dermatology practices (350 providers) covering 4.7 million patients across 13 geographically distributed states.	Average monthly number of skin cancers decreased during lockdown compared with before (cutaneous melanoma mean difference, −126.5; cSCC, −2086.6; BCC, −3305.8) and immediately after (cutaneous melanoma, −144.7; cSCC, −2057.7; BCC, −3370.0). Largest decreases were observed during April 2020 (cutaneous melanomas, −69.6%; SCCs, −77.7%; BCCs, −85.9%).
Andrew 2021[44]	Retrospective review of data from the Northern Cancer Network from March 23–June 23, 2020 compared with the same period in 2019.	Skin cancer diagnoses decreased 68.61% (P<.01). Waiting times were decreased during COVID-19 compared with before (median 8 d and 12 d, respectively; P<.0001).

We found 11 studies that reported short-term skin cancer outcomes because of the pandemic, only one of which was based in the United States. At the time of this review, no studies were found reporting long-term patient outcomes because of surgical treatment delay.

Abbreviation: BCC, basal cell carcinoma; BSDS, British Society for Dermatological Surgery; KC, Keratinocyte cancer; SCC, squamous cell carcinoma.

pandemic because of high risk of disease progression,[10] with the exception of lesions less than 1 cm in elderly populations (favorable T1 tumors with no immunosuppression or angioinvasion).[42] Delayed surgery of MCC may increase the likelihood that the patient requires adjuvant radiotherapy. In the setting of limited operating room capacity, SLNB could be deferred from WLE or Mohs excision if the wound was allowed to granulate. NCCN guidelines also emphasized cutoffs in pathologic stage to guide treatment. For example, MCC diagnosed at stage III (or higher) should require careful evaluation of patient comorbidities by the physician to determine treatment (eg, definitive resection with complete lymphadenectomy or off-label immunotherapy). The BAD and BSDS recommended prioritizing treatment of all "rapidly-enlarging tumors, poorly-differentiated tumors, perineural tumors, ulcerated and symptomatic lesions" in addition to careful multidisciplinary evaluation of complex cases.[11]

DISRUPTIONS IN SKIN CANCER CARE DURING THE COVID-19 PANDEMIC

Several clinical observations suggest that COVID-19 lockdown periods have caused disruptions in skin cancer care. There has been a substantial decrease in the number of skin cancers diagnosed[6–9,43,44] and treated[8,9,45] during lockdown (**Table 2**). In the United Kingdom, a prospective cohort study of 2050 patients found a 27% to 47% weekly decrease in the number of keratinocyte cancers treated during their COVID-19 lockdown period (March 16, 2020 to June 14, 2020).[8] SCC were prioritized over BCC, comprising approximately 71% of all excisions during this study period. Andrew and colleagues[44] found a 68.61% decrease in overall skin cancers diagnosed in the United Kingdom when compared with the previous calendar year ($P<.01$). In Italy, Valenti and colleagues found no decrease in total skin cancers diagnosed from May to November 2020 but reported a significant increase of advanced skin cancers diagnosed (54 vs 22; OR, 2.64; 95% CI, 1.56–4.47; $P = .0003$).[46] In this study, advanced skin cancers were defined as melanomas staged T1b or higher (according to TNM staging) or KC with high-risk clinical and histopathologic features as determined by the clinician. Another study reported improved detection of earlier stage during lockdown in London, suggesting the importance of maintained skin referral pathways during pandemics.[47]

In the United States, a multicenter study reported significantly decreased average monthly number of skin cancers diagnosed during pandemic months (March to May 2020), with only a modest increase during the recovery period (BCC, +1.4%; SCC, +3.1%; melanoma, +9.2%) from June to August 2020. A US retrospective chart study found a 43.1%, 44.1%, and 51.2% decrease in cutaneous melanomas, SCC, and BCC diagnosed respectively from March to May 2020. The authors also proposed that the backlog of undiagnosed cancers during the recovery period (June to August 2020) may lead to average diagnostic delays of 1.8 months, 2.1 months, and 1.9 months for melanomas, SCC, and BCC diagnosed, respectively.[43]

In a UK-based survey, approximately half of Mohs surgeons reported discontinuing care during lockdown because of reallocated resources, lack of personal protective equipment, or concerns regarding viral transmission.[48] Postsurgical management was modified by limiting referrals for external reconstruction procedures and the increasing use of dissolvable sutures. In Italy, Filoni and colleagues[9] surprisingly found a 31.7% increase in surgical excisions accompanied by a 29% increase and 64% decrease in SLNB and lymph node dissections, respectively. The increase in surgical excisions was attributed to the reallocation of personnel from elective surgeries into oncologic referral pathways.

Data on skin cancer outcomes during the pandemic are limited because of short follow-up. It has previously been reported that modest delays in cancer care may significantly affect long-term survival. In a model-based study of cancer outcomes affected by the pandemic, a recent study reported an average loss of 0.97 and 2.19 life-years gained per person with surgery delays of 3 and 6 months, respectively, for all cancers.[45]

SUMMARY

The COVID-19 pandemic has had a profound impact on the routine management of skin cancer services. Surgical delays in cancer have historically decreased long-term survival. Consequently, a significant reduction in skin cancer surgery may manifest as increased morbidity and mortality because of undetected tumors, although no outcomes during COVID-19 have been reported yet. Patients with high-risk underlying conditions, such as old age, immunosuppression, and/or previous malignancy history, should be carefully triaged by a multidisciplinary team to mitigate potential COVID-19 exposure.

CLINICS CARE POINTS

- When interpreting these guidelines, tumor-specific factors should be carefully examined in the context of patient history and pandemic status.
- Three cancer centers have made recommendations for the surgical management of MCC. All guidelines endorse urgent surgical excision, particularly for high-risk features, such as increased thickness, poor differentiation, ulceration, and/or perineural invasion present.
- Surgical excision of BCC may be deferred 3 to 6 months for slow-growing and well-differentiated lesions according to the NCCN, BAD/BSDS, and ACMS guidelines.
- Treatment of SCC may be deferred unless significant risk factors are present according to the NCCN, BAD/BSDS, and ACMS.
- Guidelines for melanoma patients suggest deferral of melanoma in situ for up to 2 to 3 months, with priority given to T1-T4 lesions.
- A normal throughput of surgical and diagnostic processes for skin cancer should be maintained to avoid negative consequences associated with postlockdown backlog.
- When triaging cases during lockdown periods, the survival benefit for skin cancer surgery should outweigh the possible risk of COVID-related mortality.

DISCLOSURE

The authors have nothing to disclose.

REFERENCES

1. Qamar MA. COVID-19: a look into the modern age pandemic. Z Gesundheitswissenschaften 2020; 1–4. https://doi.org/10.1007/s10389-020-01294-z.
2. Meredith JW, High KP, Freischlag JA. Preserving elective surgeries in the COVID-19 pandemic and the future. JAMA 2020;324(17):1725.
3. Patt D, Gordan L, Diaz M, et al. Impact of COVID-19 on cancer care: how the pandemic is delaying cancer diagnosis and treatment for American seniors. Clin Cancer Inform 2020;(4):1059–71.
4. Ferrara G, De Vincentiis L, Ambrosini-Spaltro A, et al. Cancer diagnostic delay in Northern and Central Italy during the 2020 lockdown due to the coronavirus disease 2019 pandemic. Am J Clin Pathol 2020. https://doi.org/10.1093/ajcp/aqaa177.
5. Harper CA, Satchell LP, Fido D, et al. Functional fear predicts public health compliance in the COVID-19 pandemic. Int J Ment Health Addict 2020;1–14. https://doi.org/10.1007/s11469-020-00281-5.
6. Barruscotti S, Giorgini C, Brazzelli V, et al. A significant reduction in the diagnosis of melanoma during the COVID-19 lockdown in a third-level center in the Northern Italy. Dermatol Ther 2020;33(6):e14074.
7. Earnshaw CH, Hunter HJA, McMullen E, et al. Reduction in skin cancer diagnosis, and overall cancer referrals, during the COVID-19 pandemic. Br J Dermatol 2020;183(4):792–4.
8. Nolan GS, Dunne JA, Kiely AL, et al. The effect of the COVID-19 pandemic on skin cancer surgery in the United Kingdom: a national, multi-centre, prospective cohort study and survey of plastic surgeons. BJS Br J Surg 2020;107(12):e598–600. https://doi.org/10.1002/bjs.12047.
9. Filoni A, Fiore PD, Cappellesso R, et al. Management of melanoma patients during COVID-19 pandemic in an Italian skin unit. Dermatol Ther 2021;e14908. https://doi.org/10.1111/dth.14908.
10. National Comprehensive Cancer Network (NCCN). Clinical practice guidelines in oncology: NMSC. National Comprehensive Cancer Network. Available at: https://www.nccn.org/covid-19/pdf/NCCN-NMSC.pdf. Accessed February 25, 2021.
11. British Association of Dermatologists & British Society for Dermatological Surgery COVID-19: skin cancer surgery guidance. Br Assoc Dermatol Br Soc Dermatol Surg. 2020;1:4.
12. COVID-19 (Coronavirus) Preparedness. American College of Mohs Surgery. Available at: https://www.mohscollege.org/UserFiles/AM20/Member%20Alert/COVIDAlert3March20.pdf. Accessed February 26, 2021.
13. Garbe C, Amaral T, Peris K, et al. European consensus-based interdisciplinary guideline for melanoma. Part 2: Treatment – Update 2019. Eur J Cancer 2020;126:159–77.
14. National Comprehensive Cancer Network (NCCN). Clinical practice guidelines in oncology: melanoma. National Comprehensive Cancer Network. Available at: https://www.nccn.org/covid-19/pdf/Melanoma.pdf. Accessed February 25, 2021.
15. Quaedvlieg PJF, Creytens DHKV, Epping GG, et al. Histopathological characteristics of metastasizing squamous cell carcinoma of the skin and lips. Histopathology 2006;49(3):256–64.
16. Randle HW. Basal cell carcinoma. Identification and treatment of the high-risk patient. Dermatol Surg 1996;22(3):255–61.
17. Samarasinghe V, Madan V. Nonmelanoma skin cancer. J Cutan Aesthet Surg 2012;5(1):3–10.

18. Melanoma of the Skin - Cancer Stat Facts. SEER. Available at: https://seer.cancer.gov/statfacts/html/melan.html. Accessed March 8, 2021.

19. Ricci F, Fania L, Paradisi A, et al. Delayed melanoma diagnosis in the COVID-19 era: increased Breslow thickness in primary melanomas seen after the COVID-19 lockdown. J Eur Acad Dermatol Venereol 2020;34(12):e778–9.

20. Renzi C, Mastroeni S, Mannooranparampil T, et al. Delay in diagnosis and treatment of squamous cell carcinoma of the skin. Acta Derm Venereol 2010; 90(6):595–601.

21. Sladden MJ, Nieweg OE, Howle J, et al. Updated evidence-based clinical practice guidelines for the diagnosis and management of melanoma: definitive excision margins for primary cutaneous melanoma. Med J Aust 2018;208(3):137–42.

22. Beaulieu D, Fathi R, Srivastava D, et al. Current perspectives on Mohs micrographic surgery for melanoma. Clin Cosmet Investig Dermatol 2018;11: 309–20.

23. Matthews NH, Li W-Q, Qureshi AA, et al. Epidemiology of melanoma. In: Ward WH, Farma JM, editors. Cutaneous melanoma: etiology and therapy. Codon Publications; 2017. Available at: http://www.ncbi.nlm.nih.gov/books/NBK481862/. Accessed November 30, 2020.

24. Guhan S, Boland G, Tanabe K, et al. Surgical delay and mortality for primary cutaneous melanoma. J Am Acad Dermatol 2020. https://doi.org/10.1016/j.jaad.2020.07.078.

25. Conic RZ, Cabrera CI, Khorana AA, et al. Determination of the impact of melanoma surgical timing on survival using the National Cancer Database. J Am Acad Dermatol 2018;78(1):40–6.e7.

26. Basnet A, Wang D, Sinha S, et al. Effect of a delay in definitive surgery in melanoma on overall survival: a NCDB analysis. J Clin Oncol 2018;36(15_suppl): e21586.

27. ESMO. ESMO management and treatment adapted recommendations in the COVID-19 era: melanoma. Available at: https://www.esmo.org/guidelines/cancer-patient-management-during-the-covid-19-pandemic/melanoma-in-the-covid-19-era. Accessed February 26, 2021.

28. Resource for Management Options of Melanoma During COVID-19. Society of Surgical Oncology. Available at: https://www.surgonc.org/wp-content/uploads/2020/03/Melanoma-Resource-during-COVID-19-3.30.20.pdf. Accessed March 1, 2021.

29. Xiang F, Lucas R, Hales S, et al. Incidence of nonmelanoma skin cancer in relation to ambient UV radiation in white populations, 1978-2012: empirical relationships. JAMA Dermatol 2014;150(10):1063–71.

30. Robinson JK. Basal cell carcinoma with pulmonary and lymph node metastasis causing death. Arch Dermatol 2003;139(5):643.

31. Cherpelis BS, Marcusen C, Lang PG. Prognostic factors for metastasis in squamous cell carcinoma of the skin. Dermatol Surg 2002;28(3): 268–73.

32. Rowe DE, Carroll RJ, Day CL. Long-term recurrence rates in previously untreated (primary) basal cell carcinoma: implications for patient follow-up. J Dermatol Surg Oncol 1989;15(3):315–28.

33. Smeets NWJ, Krekels GAM, Ostertag JU, et al. Surgical excision vs Mohs' micrographic surgery for basal-cell carcinoma of the face: randomised controlled trial. Lancet Lond Engl 2004;364(9447): 1766–72.

34. Becker JC, Stang A, DeCaprio JA, et al. Merkel cell carcinoma. Nat Rev Dis Primer 2017;3(1):1–17.

35. Youlden DR, Soyer HP, Youl PH, et al. Incidence and survival for Merkel cell carcinoma in Queensland, Australia, 1993-2010. JAMA Dermatol 2014;150(8): 864–72.

36. Zaar O, Gillstedt M, Lindelöf B, et al. Merkel cell carcinoma incidence is increasing in Sweden. J Eur Acad Dermatol Venereol 2016;30(10):1708–13.

37. Perrotta F, Corbi G, Mazzeo G, et al. COVID-19 and the elderly: insights into pathogenesis and clinical decision-making. Aging Clin Exp Res 2020;1–10. https://doi.org/10.1007/s40520-020-01631-y.

38. Fields RC, Busam KJ, Chou JF, et al. Recurrence after complete resection and selective use of adjuvant therapy for stage I through III Merkel cell carcinoma. Cancer 2012;118(13):3311–20.

39. Frohm ML, Griffith KA, Harms KL, et al. Recurrence and survival in patients with Merkel cell carcinoma undergoing surgery without adjuvant radiation therapy to the primary site. JAMA Dermatol 2016; 152(9):1001–7.

40. Kline L, Coldiron B. Mohs micrographic surgery for the treatment of Merkel cell carcinoma. Dermatol Surg 2016;42(8):945–51.

41. Brissett AE, Olsen KD, Kasperbauer JL, et al. Merkel cell carcinoma of the head and neck: a retrospective case series. Head Neck 2002;24(11):982–8. https://doi.org/10.1002/hed.10153.

42. Baumann BC, MacArthur KM, Brewer JD, et al. Management of primary skin cancer during a pandemic: multidisciplinary recommendations. Cancer 2020. https://doi.org/10.1002/cncr.32969.

43. Marson JW, Maner BS, Harding TP, et al. The magnitude of COVID-19's effect on the timely management of melanoma and nonmelanoma skin cancers. J Am Acad Dermatol 2021. https://doi.org/10.1016/j.jaad.2020.12.065.

44. Andrew TW, Alrawi M, Lovat P. Reduction in skin cancer diagnoses in the UK during the COVID-19 pandemic. Clin Exp Dermatol 2021;46(1): 145–6.

45. Sud A, Jones ME, Broggio J, et al. Collateral damage: the impact on outcomes from cancer surgery

of the COVID-19 pandemic. Ann Oncol 2020;31(8):
1065–74.

46. Valenti M, Pavia G, Gargiulo L, et al. Impact of delay
in follow-up due to COVID-19 pandemic on skin cancer progression: a real-life experience from an Italian hub hospital. Int J Dermatol 2021. https://doi.
org/10.1111/ijd.15501.

47. Schauer AA, Kulakov EL, Martyn-Simmons CL, et al.
Melanoma defies "lockdown": ongoing detection
during Covid-19 in central London. Clin Exp Dermatol 2020;45(7):900.

48. Nicholson P, Ali FR, Mallipeddi R. Impact of COVID-
19 on Mohs micrographic surgery: UK-wide survey
and recommendations for practice. Clin Exp Dermatol 2020. https://doi.org/10.1111/ced.14356.

How Coronavirus Disease 2019 Changed Dermatology Practice in 1 Year Around the World
Perspectives from 11 Countries

Qisi Sun, MD[a], Devon E. McMahon, MD[b], Pearl O. Ugwu-Dike, BS[b],
Qiuning Sun, MD[c], Keyun Tang, BS[c], Hanlin Zhang, BS[c],
Poonkiat Suchonwanit, MD[d], Choon Chiat Oh, MD[e],
Alvin H. Chong, MBBS, MMed[f,g], Anneliese Willems, MBBS, FRACGP[f],
Cristina Galván, MD[h], Roni P. Dodiuk-Gad, MD[i,j,k], Fabrizio Fantini, MD[l],
Sebastiano Recalcati, MD[l], Joao Avancini, MD[m], Denise Miyamoto, MD, PhD[m],
Jose A. Sanches, MD, PhD[m], Noufal Raboobee, MD[n], Francisco Bravo, MD[o,p],
Esther E. Freeman, MD, PhD[b],*

KEYWORDS
- COVID-19 • SARS-CoV-2 • China • Italy • Spain • Peru • Brazil • South Africa

KEY POINTS
- COVID-19 has affected the global dermatology workforce, as many dermatologists were redeployed to the frontlines, managed a broad array of COVID-19-associated dermatologic conditions, and adopted telemedicine practices.
- Globally, there are differences in the morphology and prevalence of COVID-19-associated skin lesions.
- Just as the pandemic unevenly impacted various communities across the world, the COVID-19 telemedicine expansion also widened the digital divide, exacerbating disparities among the dermatology patient population.

Dr. Freeman is the principal investigator for the AAD/ILDS COVID-19 Dermatology Registry. The authors have nothing to disclose.

[a] Department of Dermatology, Yale University School of Medicine, 333 Cedar Street, New Haven, CT 06510, USA; [b] Department of Dermatology, Massachusetts General Hospital, Harvard Medical School, 55 Fruit Street, Boston, MA 02114, USA; [c] Department of Dermatology, Peking Union Medical College Hospital, Peking Union Medical College, Chinese Academy of Medical Sciences, 9 Dongdan 3rd Alley, Dong Dan, Dongcheng Qu, Beijing Shi, China; [d] Division of Dermatology, Faculty of Medicine, Ramathibodi Hospital, Mahidol University, 270 Thanon Rama VI, Khwaeng Thung Phaya Thai, Khet Ratchathewi, Krung Thep Maha Nakhon 10400, Thailand; [e] Department of Dermatology, Singapore General Hospital, Singapore, Outram Rd, Singapore 169608, Singapore; [f] Skin Health Institute, level 1/80 Drummond St, Carlton, VIC 3053, Australia; [g] Department of Medicine (Dermatology), St Vincent's Hospital Melbourne, University of Melbourne, Parkville, VIC 3010, Australia; [h] Department of Dermatology, Hospital Universitario de Móstoles, Calle Río Júcar, S/N, 28935 Móstoles, Madrid, Spain; [i] Bruce Rappaport Faculty of Medicine, Technion - Institute of Technology, Haifa, 3200003, Israel; [j] Department of Dermatology, Emek Medical Center, Yitshak Rabin Boulevard 21, Afula, 1834111, Israel; [k] Division of Dermatology, Department of Medicine, Sunnybrook Health Sciences Centre, University of Toronto, 2075 Bayview Ave, Toronto, ON M4N 3M5, Canada; [l] Department of Dermatology, Dermatology Unit, ASST Lecco, Alessandro Manzoni Hospital, Via dell'Eremo, 9/11, 23900 Lecco LC, Italy; [m] Department of Dermatology, Hospital das Clínicas of the University of Sao Paulo, Rua, Av. Dr. Enéas Carvalho de Aguiar, 255-Cerqueira César, São Paulo-SP, 05403-000, Brazil; [n] Department of Dermatology, Westville Hospital, 7 Harry Gwala Rd, Westville, Durban, 3630, South Africa; [o] Department of Dermatology, Universidad Peruana Cayetano Heredia, Hospital Cayetano Heredia, Av. Honorio Delgado 430, San Martín de Porres 15102, Peru; [p] Department of Pathology, Universidad Peruana Cayetano Heredia, Hospital Cayetano Heredia, 1 CV Zac, Av. Honorio Delgado 262, San Martín de Porres 15102, Peru

* Corresponding author.
E-mail address: Efreeman@mgh.harvard.edu

Dermatol Clin 39 (2021) 639–651
https://doi.org/10.1016/j.det.2021.05.014
0733-8635/21/© 2021 Elsevier Inc. All rights reserved.

INTRODUCTION

When cases of a mysterious pneumonia debuted in Wuhan, Hubei province, China, in early December 2019, few people could have anticipated the outbreak's trajectory.[1] Within 2 weeks, scientists identified the responsible pathogen as a novel virus that is 96% identical to the bat coronavirus BatCoV RaTG13.[2] On January 13, 2020, the first case outside of mainland China was reported in Thailand, and 1 month later, the disease had swept across the world, impacting 36 countries in 6 continents.[3] As hospitalizations and deaths skyrocketed, the respiratory disease, later renamed coronavirus disease 2019 (COVID-19), exposed the ugly underbelly of societal inequities and threatened to collapse world economies and the sturdiest of health care systems. By March 11, 2020, the World Health Organization (WHO) declared COVID-19 a pandemic.[4]

Dermatologists have played an important role in the treatment of patients since the beginning of the pandemic. From redeployment onto the frontlines to managing cutaneous manifestations of COVID-19 and patients on biologics and immunosuppressants, dermatologists around the world rapidly adapted to overcome the unique challenges in their region. An international perspective of the unique trends, trials, and lessons learned can not only inform response to future challenges in the pandemic but also enhance quality of care.

In this article, we present an overview of the impact of COVID-19 on each region from an epidemiologic standpoint, followed by unique insights from local dermatologists on how the specialty has evolved over the past year (**Figs. 1** and **2**).

China

Although China was initially the pandemic epicenter, the nation has since managed to avoid many of the surges seen elsewhere. After the severe acute respiratory syndrome (SARS) outbreak, China implemented the "Regulations on Preparedness for the Response to Emergent Public Health Hazards," a mechanism allowing for rapid mobilization of resources in the event of a medical disaster.[5] The COVID-19 outbreak occurred just before Chinese New Year, when billions of residents travel home. The government announced a travel quarantine on January 23, 2020, in the Hubei province, affecting approximately 45 million people.[5] All public transportation was suspended and all outdoor businesses closed. Through a centralized effort on behalf of the government,

food, medicine, and supplies were deployed and distributed to all residents by community committees. As hospitals became overwhelmed in Wuhan, 2 emergency field hospitals with approximately 2400 beds and 10 mobile hospitals were constructed in 10 days.[5] In addition, other provinces dispatched multiple teams of over 42,600 medical staff to help frontline workers in Wuhan.[5]

Other measures such as the "grid closed management" allowed only 1 resident from each household to venture outside of the community every 2 days, and Health Code (a QR color code displaying the individual's health status) allowed for rapid contact tracing and isolation.[5] After 76 days, China lifted the lockdown and allowed Wuhan residents to return to work. As of February 1, 2021, there were 101,039 confirmed cases in China and 4826 deaths (case fatality rate 4.8%).[6]

In the heavily affected regions, dermatologists were redeployed to care for patients with COVID-19; others helped analyze COVID-19 swab tests and served as consultants at fever clinics.[7] Dermatologists also stepped into an educational role, guiding health care workers on how to manage and prevent skin injuries from personal protective equipment (PPE) and educating the public on knowing which types of skin disorders must be seen urgently.[7,8]

Skin manifestations of COVID-19 were not common during this time. In fact, only one multicentered study focused on cutaneous manifestations of Chinese patients infected with COVID-19. Of the 586 Chinese patients and 92 Italian patients in the study, 53 patients (7.8%) had new skin manifestations detected at admission or during hospitalization. Among the 53 patients, the most common skin finding related to COVID-19 was erythematous rash (70%), such as macular, papular, maculopapular, and erythema multiforme-like eruptions, followed by diffuse urticaria (26%) and scattered vesicular, varicelliform eruptions (4%).[9] In contrast to findings in Western nations but consistent with those seen in other Asian countries, there was a lack of chilblainslike lesions among SARS coronavirus 2 (SARS-CoV-2)-positive patients; this may be because pernio is quite common in the region during winter, so frontline physicians may have overlooked those lesions to focus on respiratory issues. Another explanation may be genetic differences among various populations. Lipoprotein A, a major player in thrombo-occlusive vasculopathy, and factor V Leiden mutations are lower among people of Asian descent compared with those of European descent.[10] These differences may partly explain

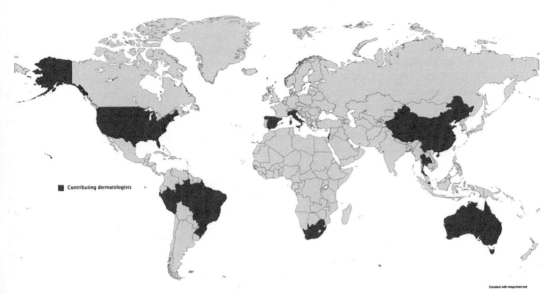

Fig. 1. Map of the international perspectives represented. In this article, 11 countries (China, Thailand, United States, Singapore, Australia, Spain, Israel, Italy, Brazil, South Africa, and Peru) contributed their insights on the impact of COVID-19 on the field of dermatology.

the lack of chilblainslike lesions among patients with COVID-19 in Asia.

Teledermatology was widely used throughout this period, and hospitals advertised telemedicine services on social media. At the Peking Union Medical College Hospital, 618 teleconsultations were received in the first week alone.[11] Most issues revolved around treatment adjustment of severe diseases (bullous pemphigoid, systematic lupus erythematosus, etc) and management of common, chronic, and refractory diseases (eczema, acne, dermatitis, etc). The incidence of pet-related dermatophytosis and irritant contact dermatitis also increased.[12]

Despite the overall success of teledermatology, its expansion exacerbated existing disparities. For instance, some patients with skin conditions

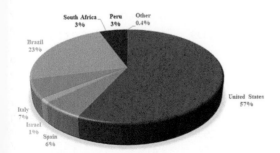

Fig. 2. Distribution of COVID-19 cases among the 11 countries as of March 31, 2021. The Other category includes Thailand, China, Singapore, and Australia. (*Data from* www.worldometers.info/.)

experienced delays in medication adjustment, which resulted in side effects, because they lived in rural areas with unreliable Internet connection or were more elderly with limited Internet literacy.

Thailand

Thailand was the first country outside of China to report a new case of COVID-19 on January 13, 2020.[3] The number of cases increased exponentially until mid-April 2020, but a second wave emerged in mid-December 2020. As of March 18, 2021, there were 27,494 confirmed cases, 89 (0.32%) deaths, 26,377 (95.93%) recovered patients, and 61,791 vaccinated people as reported by the Department of Disease Control, Ministry of Public Health, Govt. of Thailand.[13]

Following the initial outbreak, the Thai government imposed the National Emergency Decree on March 26, 2020.[14] Travel restrictions, physical distancing, and working from home were mandated. Most hospitals discharged their inpatients and reassigned intensive care units and wards for COVID-19 cases. Outpatient departments also minimized their appointments to reduce hospital crowding and conserve PPE. Moreover, the Department of Disease Control widely broadcasted updated protocols on managing COVID-19 among health care professionals and the general population.

Many dermatologists in Thailand worked alongside frontline physicians, especially at designated areas, to screen potential COVID-19 cases. The

Faculty of Medicine Ramathibodi Hospital at Mahidol University is an advanced referral center in Bangkok and was converted into a pandemic response center (Ramathibodi Chakri Naruebodindra Hospital) for accepting COVID-19 cases referred from various regions. Dermatology consults decreased significantly, and all nonessential procedures were postponed. Apart from serving on the frontlines, dermatologists also educated their colleagues and patients regarding skin problems associated with preventive measures such as irritant contact dermatitis from hand hygiene and pressure-related symptoms due to PPE usage.

Dermatologists were often consulted for cutaneous problems in hospitalized patients with COVID-19 through in-person visits and inpatient teledermatology. At the Ramathibodi Chakri Naruebodindra Hospital, 5 of 218 (2.3%) COVID-19 cases manifested skin lesions, including maculopapular eruption (n = 3, 1.4%), urticaria (n = 2, 0.9%), and petechiae (n = 1, 0.5%). The findings are consistent with a previous study in Thai individuals but showed lower incidence than another study that used telephone interviews.[15,16] Unlike reports from other Western countries, there have been no reported chilblainslike lesions among SARS-CoV-2-positive Thai patients.[17,18] Thailand's tropical climate and/or genetic differences between racial groups may explain this discordance. Notably, clinicians were cautious about misdiagnosing dengue fever as COVID-19 because both can initially present with fever and petechiae and dengue is endemic in Thailand.[18]

The lack of adequate telecommunication infrastructure and unclear legal status of telemedicine rendered teledermatology challenging in Thailand.

Therefore, dermatologists mainly conducted telephone consultations for patients with a prior confirmed diagnosis to assess clinical progression. At present, the Ministry of Public Health is actively working to address technical problems and medicolegal liabilities. The significant challenges posed by the pandemic have served as a wake-up call for Thailand to improve its health care systems for the well-being of its current population and future generations.

United States

With its leaders initially dubious about the gravity of the COVID-19 outbreak, the United States missed opportunities to act swiftly, allowing the coronavirus to gain a foothold since the country's first case on January 19, 2020, in Washington state.[19] Slow decision making, fueled in part by partisan politics, resulted in an overall decentralized response. One study showed that if the United States had enacted control measures just 1 week earlier, the nation could have prevented more than 35,000 COVID-19 deaths.[20] By April 7, 2020, New York surpassed Italy to become the global epicenter with 138,836 cases.[21] Eventually, poor coordination of containment measures, inability to conduct rapid testing on a grand scale, and tension to restart the economy catapulted the United States to the top as the nation with more cases and deaths than any other country in the world. As of March 31, 2021, more than 31 million people were infected and 564,399 died (**Table 1**).[22]

COVID-19 exploited existing inequities in the United States. Already disproportionately targeted

Table 1
The COVID-19 landscape in 11 countries as of March 31, 2021

Region/Country	Date of First Case	Cases	Deaths	Case Fatality	Recovered
China	December 12, 2019[a]	90,201	4636	5.14%	85,385
Thailand	January 13, 2020	28,863	94	0.33%	27,426
United States	January 20, 2020	31,109,108	564,399	1.81%	23,588,100
Singapore	January 23, 2020	60,381	30	0.05%	60,149
Australia	January 26, 2020	29,304	909	3.10%	26,288
Spain	January 31, 2020	3,284,353	75,459	2.30%	3,042,352
Israel	February 21, 2020	833,040	6203	0.74%	819,564
Italy	February 21, 2020	3,584,899	109,346	3.05%	2,913,045
Brazil	February 25, 2020	12,664,058	317,936	2.51%	11,074,483
South Africa	March 5, 2020	1,543,079	52,602	3.41%	1,469,565
Peru	March 6, 2020	1,540,077	51,801	3.36%	1,459,886

[a] Estimated date.
Data from www.worldometers.info.

by the virus, the elderly faced stricter lockdowns, loss of social support, and a digital divide.[23] Women were more likely to be underemployed and shoulder caregiver burden while facing increasing rates of domestic violence.[24,25] Blacks, Latinos, and Native Americans were approximately 3 to 4 times more likely to be hospitalized with COVID-19 and approximately 2 times more likely to die of COVID-19 than white, non-Hispanic individuals, whereas Asians and Asian Americans faced a surge of racist and xenophobic abuse.[26–30]

On the frontlines, a surge of critically ill patients and shortage of hospital staff required rapid reassignment of physicians to new roles. In the United States, dermatologists worked alongside internists in COVID-19 wards and described some of the initial cutaneous manifestations of COVID-19, including morphologies such as morbiliform, perniolike, urticarial, macular erythema, vesicular, papulosquamous, and retiform purpura.[31] Perniolike lesions were associated with a milder COVID-19 course, whereas retiform purpura were only seen in severe cases.[31] To further understand and characterize the relationship between the virus and skin, researchers in the United States created the American Academy of Dermatology COVID-19 and International League of Dermatologic Societies COVID-19 Registry to collate cases of COVID-19-associated cutaneous manifestations from around the world, with more than 2000 case entries from 52 countries by the end of March 2021.[32]

The pandemic also transformed dermatology practice in the United States. During the pandemic, teledermatology became the primary means of delivering care. In contrast, before the pandemic, only 15% of dermatologists worked in a practice that used telemedicine in 2016.[33] In response to the pandemic, the Centers for Medicare and Medicaid Services (CMS) and other private payers have also expanded telehealth coverage.[34] Coupled with findings that teledermatology is an effective and reliable means of care delivery, it is likely that telemedicine will remain a major feature of patient care in dermatology.[35,36]

Guidelines for how to provide treatment of patients living with other skin conditions during the pandemic evolved during the past year.[37] Initially, many dermatologists engaged in difficult conversations with their patients regarding the use of biologics in the setting of COVID-19 with limited data. It was not until December 2020 that the National Psoriasis Foundation released guidance for the management of psoriasis during the pandemic.[38] Patients with cutaneous T cell lymphoma requiring photophoresis and those with psoriasis needing phototherapy experienced treatment disruptions. Patients at high risk for skin cancer also experienced delays in routine care.[39]

Singapore

Singapore reported its first case on January 23, 2020.[40] Having learned from the SARS outbreak in 2003, Singapore instituted border control measures in the first week of January 2020. This swift response prevented the deluge of hospitalized patients with COVID-19 seen in other nations. After the SARS epidemic, Singapore created a disease outbreak plan called the color-coded Disease Outbreak Response System Condition (DORSCON), which raised national awareness of the necessity of coordinated efforts during an outbreak.[41] Therefore, residents were already more prepared and receptive to restrictions. In addition to border control, Singapore also scaled up rapid testing, contact tracing, and isolation to contain the pandemic. In April 2020, Singapore initiated the Circuit Breaker—a series of significantly stricter measures to curb widespread community transmission. In March 2021, Singapore has a case fatality rate of 0.05% and fewer than 20 new cases per day.

Many dermatologists volunteered to care for the acutely ill in COVID-19 wards, whereas others reduced in-person clinic sessions and turned to telemedicine. Teledermatology was a relatively new concept for Singapore in early 2020, and most patients, unaccustomed to this new platform, preferred face-to-face visits. To incentivize its usage, patients were offered fee reductions if they opted for teledermatology. According to dermatologists in Singapore, COVID-19-associated skin findings were uncommon. There were early case reports of maculopapular exanthem, skin conditions from prolonged PPE usage, and hand dermatitis, but chilblainslike lesions were rare.[42]

Australia

Australia confirmed its first case in late January 2020.[43] Two months later, the country ordered a national lockdown and restricted all international, interstate and, in some cases, intrastate travel. With a population of 25 million divided into 6 states and 2 territories, Australia reported approximately 29,000 COVID-19 cases with 909 deaths (3% case fatality rate) at the time of writing, in early March 2021.[44] Victoria, the most severely affected state, had 4-fold the number of cases compared with other states and 75% of the fatalities.[45] Victoria's capital city, Melbourne, suffered a second wave in late June 2020, resulting in 18,000 infections and more than 800 deaths.[46] In response, Victoria issued a second lockdown on July 9, 2020, that lasted for 112 days.[47] The lockdown, one of the world's strictest, involved curfews, closure of all schools and nonessential businesses, mask wearing, and travel restrictions. The aggressive measures allowed Melbourne to descend from a daily caseload of approximately 725 to zero cases in late October 2020.[46,48]

The experiences of dermatologists varied from state to state. Most in private practice used a mixture of telehealth and in-person visits, with the latter reserved for urgent cases. Before COVID-19, there were approximately 150,000 teledermatology consultations in Australia per year.[49] In 2020, its usage increased by nearly 24-fold.[50] However, teledermatology remains challenging because there are often technical issues, and it can be difficult to use with elderly and non-English-speaking patients. Telehealth was most useful in the follow-up of inflammatory skin diseases such as acne and psoriasis. Patients with skin cancer often had to attend face-to-face appointments for tissue biopsies after the initial teledermatology assessment. One of the many advantages of teledermatology was that it afforded patients in remote locations increased access to expert skin care. Ultimately, the shift to telehealth corresponded to a 32% drop in the number of samples sent for pathologic testing.[51] In Victoria, there was a 10% reduction in the number of cancer diagnoses throughout this period, leading to an estimated 2530 undiagnosed cancers.[52] Melanoma, in particular, had a 13% drop in diagnosis with an estimated 511 undiagnosed melanomas.[52] Dermatologists anticipate an increase in skin cancer diagnoses in 2021. Aside from an increase in hand dermatitis and mask-induced acne and rosacea, there are few reports of cutaneous manifestations in Australian patients with COVID-19. In addition, unlike many other countries, dermatologists were not deployed to the frontlines.

Spain

Spain's first official case of COVID-19 was reported on January 31, 2020. Exactly 2 months later, there were more than 85,199 cases and 7424 deaths, surpassing that of mainland China.[53] During the height of the pandemic in late March 2020, Spain had a case fatality rate of 6.16%. Over the course of the year, the nation experienced 3 major waves of infection. The first wave marked the beginning of the pandemic, the second major wave occurred around early November,

and the third wave spiked around late January 2021.[54] At the time of writing (March 24, 2021), there have been a total of 3,183,704 confirmed cases and 72,258 deaths in Spain.[54]

Despite the creation of a Centre for Coordination of Health Alerts and Emergency in 2004, the pandemic exposed the fragility of Spain's governance, medical workforce, and health care delivery. In addition to understaffed and underresourced health services, Spain had the lowest nurse to patient ratio in the European Union.[55] Perhaps unsurprisingly, given the importance of regional autonomy in Spain, there was a lack of strong, centralized effort aimed at mitigating the pandemic.[55] Regional disparities were also pronounced when analyzed by socioeconomic characteristics; there was significant negative correlation between mean income and COVID-19 incidence rate.[56]

Dermatologists in Spain were mobilized to manage patients on the COVID-19 wards and included in treatment committees because their expertise on managing the cytokine storm and perspectives on immune function proved invaluable.[57] Dermatologists were also consulted on skin lesions associated with the novel virus. From an analysis of 375 patients in Spain with COVID-19 and unexplained skin findings, 5 major patterns emerged: pseudochilblains on acral areas, vesicular eruptions, urticaria, other maculopapules, and livedo or necrosis—each with associated demographics and prognoses.[58] Pseudochilblains and vesicular eruptions were associated with younger patients and better prognosis, whereas urticaria and maculopapular lesions were seen in older patients with more severe disease.[58] Livedoid or necrotic lesions were more variable but were typically seen in older patients and associated with a 10% mortality rate.[58] These patterns suggest the activation of multiple pathways in COVID-19 infection.

Unlike many of its counterparts, Spain had a robust teledermatology program before the pandemic, with 25% of hospitals using teledermatology in 2014.[59] Therefore, despite the associated challenges such as delayed diagnosis of skin cancers, dermatologists in Spain were overall more accustomed to this technology and welcomed it as a new means to facilitate patient care.[60]

Israel

Following the first case of COVID-19 in Israel on February 21, 2020, the Israeli Ministry of Health implemented aggressive containment measures amid political unrest.[61] After these restrictions were relaxed in May 2020, Israel saw a viral resurgence that forced the nation into a second lockdown in September 2020.[62] The nation entered its third lockdown in January 2021. At the time of writing in April 2021, there were 836,334 COVID-19 cases and 6309 deaths among the country's 9 million inhabitants.[63]

Israel managed the pandemic in the midst of a constitutional crisis. Members of parliament struggled to work cohesively, and an interim prime minister sometimes made critical decisions regarding the pandemic without consulting his cabinet.[64] At the same time, Israel's health care system was already under strain from lack of resources even before the pandemic.[65] To address the limited intensive care unit capacity and PPE shortages, Israel enforced travel restrictions, shuttered schools and nonessential businesses, and mandated local and national curfews. Sick contacts were traced through mobile phone surveillance. However, compliance with these measures came at a high price for many. A multiethnic country, Israel has a significant number of individuals living in poverty, particularly among the Arab and ultra-Orthodox Jewish populations.[66] These 2 communities experienced double the incidence of COVID-19 compared with groups of higher socioeconomic status.[66]

One unique aspect of Israel's COVID-19 management is the unprecedented efficiency of its vaccine rollout. The Israeli government approved the BNT162b2 COVID-19 vaccine (manufactured by Pfizer, Pfizer-BioNTech) and initiated the national immunization campaign on December 20, 2020. Individuals aged 60 years and older were prioritized, including nursing home residents, people at high risk due to medical conditions, and frontline health care workers.[67] Israel's 4 large, competing, nonprofit health plans also scheduled hundreds of thousands of vaccination appointments for their members in a short period. By February 2021, 84% of those aged 70 years and older had received both doses of the vaccine, and the ratio of patients with COVID-19 aged 70 years and older requiring mechanical ventilation to those younger than 50 years declined 67% from October–December 2020 to February 2021.[68]

COVID-19 also changed dermatology practice in Israel. At several medical centers, residents were redeployed to COVID-19 emergency departments. Outpatient clinics moved online, and although in-person visits were permitted for those needing phototherapy and/or urgent dermatologic care, many hesitated to attend their appointments. One study showed that among dermatologic patients in Emek Medical Center, more than 50% of patients stopped phototherapy treatment from March 1, 2020, to April 30, 2020, for fear of contracting COVID-19.[69] During this time, teledermatology was widely used for nonurgent consultations, expanding access to care and facilitating new collaborations. A group of independent dermatologists from Israel and Canada also established the "International Dermatologists Fighting Coronavirus Together," a collective effort enabling rapid transfer of knowledge and insights among clinicians regarding COVID-19's impact on the skin.

Italy

Although the country's first case of COVID-19 was officially registered in February 2020, Italy's patient zero may have been a young dermatology patient who presented with urticarial plaquelike dermatosis on the arms and a mild sore throat in November 2019.[70] The recent retrospective study confirmed the presence of SARS-CoV-2 in a biopsy done at that time, suggesting that the virus may have circulated surreptitiously for months before the first case was reported.[70]

Since then, the number of cases in Italy has soared exponentially. The hardest hit areas were initially in northern Italy, with Lombardy at the epicenter reporting the highest number of cases. As the medical and humanitarian emergency unfolded, it became clear that a shift from patient-centered to community-focused care was required to battle the pandemic. Stringent lockdowns were issued, and the Italian National Health Service expanded intensive care units and converted entire medical units into COVID-19 wards. At the time of writing (March 13, 2021), Italy has reported 3,164,484 cases, 100,459 deaths (3.2% case fatality rate), and 2,343,087 recoveries.[71]

Initially, dermatologists in Italy were redeployed to the frontlines, where they directly cared for patients with COVID-19 on the wards and in triage stations.[72] The biggest challenge was lack of PPE.[73] Before long, dermatologists were sought for their expertise on novel findings among coronavirus patients. The first reports of cutaneous manifestations of COVID-19 emerged from Italy. According to a study using data from 345 infected patients in Lombardy, the skin findings can be classified into 3 main groups: exanthems, vascular lesions, and other cutaneous manifestations.[74] Exanthems, characteristic of an early viremic phase, were the most common (67.3%)[74]; they included maculopapular rash, urticarial rash, vesicular rash, and erythema multiforme eruptions. Vascular lesions were the second most commonly reported and included vasculitic lesions in more severely affected patients and chilblainslike lesions.[74] The latter were mostly seen in young patients and portended a good prognosis. The third group, other cutaneous manifestations, included alopecia (particularly telogen effluvium) and indirect cutaneous manifestations such as herpes simplex, zoster, and drug reactions. Aggravation of preexisting skin conditions due to PPE and hand hygiene was also common.

Scarcely used before the pandemic, teledermatology became the new means of diagnosing, treating, and following up with patients. However, the quality of photographs was frequently inadequate and the lack of proper physical examination and dermoscopy made it difficult to diagnose pigmented and nonpigmented lesions.[75] Furthermore, second-order analysis such as biopsies and swabs could not be performed. Most impacted were dermatologic oncology patients. The diagnosis of skin cancers was delayed and surgical excisions were postponed, resulting in an increased incidence of advanced skin cancer with poorer prognoses.[76]

As the pandemic evolved, dermatologists adapted. Initially, dermatology consultations decreased drastically by 80% to 90% in Italy, and many private clinics closed.[73] By 2021, many dermatologists in Italy have been redeployed again, this time to administer COVID-19 vaccinations.

Brazil

Brazil announced its first COVID-19 case on February 25 in Sao Paulo.[77] Since then, more than 12 million confirmed cases have been registered with more than 301,000 deaths.[78] At the height of the pandemic during the first wave, Brazil had a case fatality rate of 5.68%, likely due in part to a greater elderly population (13.5%).[79] Between September and December 2020, cases dipped slightly, but in January 2021, a new outbreak of SARS-CoV-2 variants erupted in the city of Manaus.[80] At the time of writing, in March 2021, Brazil is facing one of the worst waves in the pandemic yet, with more than 2000 deaths per day.[80]

COVID-19 spotlighted deep-rooted social, ethnic, and economic disparities. For instance, "favelas," or low-income urban conglomerates, comprise a significant portion of the population in some regions, and these communities often lived in close quarters with little access to financial support or medical care.[81] The Brazilian health system consists of a public system that provides universal care to all residents and a private system funded by individual and corporate contributions. Most Brazilian inhabitants rely exclusively on the public infrastructure, which was already deficient before the pandemic.

During the first peak, many dermatology residents were redeployed to the frontlines. Beds for patients with skin disease were drastically reduced in favor of COVID-19 cases. At the University of São Paulo Medical School Hospital, the largest referral center in Brazil, a group of experienced dermatologists was fully dedicated to evaluating hospitalized patients with COVID-19 from April to July 2020. Linear blisters and ulcerations presenting in unusual pressure sites were a common finding in patients treated with prone ventilation. In Brazil, there was no evidence of specific cutaneous manifestations in critical patients that could definitively be attributed to SARS-CoV-2 infection.[82] Since then, a minority of mild cases demonstrating exanthema, urticaria, pruritus sine materia, vasculitis, and telogen effluvium have been observed and could arguably be related to COVID-19.[3]

Outpatient clinic visits dropped from March to August 2020 and then increased again until the current wave of infection as of March 2021. Interruption of dermatology referrals and a lack of medication for chronic and infectious diseases such as leprosy prevented quality care. Flares in patients with eczema, pemphigus vulgaris, psoriasis, and other diseases were common, leading to an increase in demand for hospitalization. The delay of surgical excisions and routine appointments also impacted proper diagnosis and treatment of cutaneous lymphoma, melanoma, and other skin cancers.

Teledermatology became an important tool, especially in the care of chronic patients in private clinics. Nevertheless, the lack of technological infrastructure in the hospital and patients' houses made it challenging for teledermatology to achieve popularity.

South Africa

South Africa, the epicenter of Africa's outbreak, confirmed its first case on March 5, 2020.[83] Although only accounting for 5% of Africa's population, South Africa comprised 54% of total cases and 44% of deaths in the WHO African region by the end of 2020.[84] Although South Africa had a high infection rate, there was an unusually lower death rate compared with some European nations, likely due to early aggressive lockdown measures and a much younger average age. In December 2020, a more contagious new variant 501Y.V2 emerged. By March 12, 2021, the country with its population of 59 million had 1.53 million confirmed cases and 51,261 deaths.[85]

As a country that champions human rights, South Africa is a popular destination for asylum seekers and refugees. This already vulnerable population was disproportionately impacted in the pandemic. In addition to already weakened social support and isolation, many foreign-born migrants in South Africa are business owners but most of their businesses are not considered for the Business Relief Fund because to qualify, the businesses must be majority South African owned.[86] Migrants who were employed in the formal sector were also not eligible to receive Unemployment Insurance Funds due to the electronic system's inability to recognize foreign passport numbers.[86] Patient populations such as those with human immunodeficiency virus and tuberculosis were also impacted because hospitals reduced nonurgent admissions and impeded access to chronic medications.[87]

Income-related health inequalities were also exacerbated. Approximately 84% of South Africans depend on an underresourced and overcrowded public health sector, whereas the rest are attended to by a private sector.[88] Huge disparities exist between the 2 tiers. During the height of the pandemic in 2020, the average COVID-19 test turnaround time in the private sector was 24 to 48 hours compared with 12 days in the public sector.[89] This difference had a major impact on patients who were admitted to the hospital, including patients with skin disorders, such as patients with pemphigus who had to remain in an isolation ward until the results were negative before they could begin pulse therapy.

Dermatologists took advantage of teledermatology and attended educational seminars on telemedicine. In March 2020, the government published a set of Telemedicine Guidelines to help practitioners navigate the unfamiliar realm of virtual consults.[90,91] In the beginning, live video was popular. Over time, the store-and-forward method of patients taking photographs to send to their dermatologists became preferred for its flexibility. Access to Internet and electronics remained a challenge in poorer communities, likely further accentuating disparities. The most common skin manifestations of COVID-19 seen in South Africa included urticaria, erythema multiforme-like lesions, and vasculitis, as well as papular, morbiliform, and vesicular eruptions. Chilblains ("COVID toes") were also common, although most reports came from Johannesburg in the winter and many were never tested for COVID-19. Hand dermatitis, perioral dermatitis, and postinflammatory hyperpigmentation in skin of color due to irritation from the N95 mask were also common.

Peru

In the southern hemisphere, Peru confirmed its first case, a young man returning from Europe,

just days before the WHO declared COVID-19 a pandemic.[92] With growing international alarm, Peru closed its borders on March 16, 2020. By April 15, 2020, there were 11,475 cases and 254 deaths in the nation, with 8412 cases in Lima alone.[92] Since then, Peru has experienced 2 major waves of infection, and at the time of writing (March 3, 2021), 1,349,847 cases and 47,306 deaths (3.5% case fatality rate) have been reported.

Although Peru was lauded for rapidly implementing comprehensive control measures, the country's transmission rate remained high, and as of June 2020, Peru's mortality rates were among the highest internationally.[93] Together with the shortcomings of the Peru health care system, the pandemic exposed deeply ingrained gender, socioeconomic, and ethnic inequalities. For instance, limited oxygen supplies forced some relatives of patients with COVID-19 to buy oxygen at exorbitant prices on the open market, whereas those with fewer means had to do without.[93] The indigenous communities, which had already been ravaged by a dengue outbreak right before the pandemic, were more heavily impacted given challenges with maintaining sanitary conditions and lack of access to medical care.[93]

With the overwhelming number of COVID-19 cases and shortage of physicians, younger dermatologists were sent to the frontlines, where many encountered several COVID-19 skin manifestations, such as urticaria and morbiliform eruptions. In outpatient settings, the most common consultations were telogen effluvium, perioral dermatitis, and irritant contact dermatitis of the hands in addition to a significant number of chilblainslike cases. Teledermatology was widely used to manage common pathologic conditions such as acne, eczema, and mild to moderate psoriasis but was less suitable for evaluation of pigmented lesions. Those with pemphigus and other bullous diseases requiring close monitoring were often lost to follow-up, forcing some dermatologists to temporarily reopen their clinics for patients with severe skin conditions. Other aspects of dermatologic patient care remained the same. Dermatology consult services for endemic infectious diseases such as leishmaniasis remained robust in Peru. At the time of writing, in March 2021, most hospital-based dermatologists continue to rely on telemedicine.

SUMMARY

COVID-19 knows no borders. During an international medical crisis, the global perspectives and insights from those in our field are invaluable. For instance, the regional differences observed in regard dermatologic manifestations of COVID-19, such as pernio-like lesions, could provide insight into various pathogenic mechanisms of COVID-19. Furthermore, it seems that a hybrid of teledermatology and in-person visits may be most ideal to reduce contact and potential transmission while also ensuring timely diagnosis and treatment of urgent skin disorders. Although responses to the pandemic varied depending on government leadership, culture, and resources, the lessons learned and experiences of dermatologists during this time can serve as a guidepost to help our field address new challenges as cases continue to escalate in parts of the world.

CLINICS CARE POINTS

- Dermatologists around the globe have played a significant role in the COVID-19 pandemic, from adopting teledermatology and restructuring clinics to serving on the front lines and identifying new skin manifestations of SARS-CoV-2 infection.
- COVID-19 has also impacted the care of dermatologic patients around the world, resulting in delays in skin cancer management and decreased usage of phototherapy for inflammatory diseases.

ACKNOWLEDGEMENTS

The AAD/ILDS Dermatology Registry is supported by a grant from the ILDS to Massachusetts General Hospital (Freeman, PI), and by in-kind support from the AAD.

REFERENCES

1. Huang C, Wang Y, Li X, et al. Clinical features of patients infected with 2019 novel coronavirus in Wuhan, China. Lancet 2020;395:497–506.
2. Zhou P, Yang XL, Wang XG, et al. A pneumonia outbreak associated with a new coronavirus of probable bat origin. Nature 2020;579:270–3.
3. Burke RM, Midgley CM, Dratch A, et al. Active monitoring of persons exposed to patients with confirmed COVID-19 - United States, January-February 2020. MMWR Morb Mortal Wkly Rep 2020;69:245–6.
4. Cucinotta D, Vanelli M. WHO declares COVID-19 a pandemic. Acta Biomed 2020;91:157–60.
5. Liu W, Yue X-G, Tchounwou PB. Response to the COVID-19 epidemic: the chinese experience and implications for other countries. Int J Environ Res Public Health 2020;17:2304.
6. Wang C, Wang Z, Wang G, et al. COVID-19 in early 2021: current status and looking forward. Signal Transduct Target Ther 2021;6:114.
7. Zhang H, Tang K, Fang R, et al. What dermatologists could do to cope with the novel coronavirus (SARS-CoV-2): a dermatologist's perspective from China. J Eur Acad Dermatol Venereol 2020;34:e211–2.
8. Tao J, Song Z, Yang L, et al. Emergency management of 2019 novel coronavirus: implications for the dermatology department. Br J Dermatol 2020; 182:e195.
9. De Giorgi V, Recalcati S, Jia Z, et al. Cutaneous manifestations related to coronavirus disease 2019 (COVID-19): a prospective study from China and Italy. J Am Acad Dermatol 2020;83:674–5.
10. Tan SW, Tam YC, Oh CC. Skin manifestations of COVID-19: a worldwide review. JAAD Int 2021;2: 119–33.
11. Tang K, Zhang H, Jin H. Resuming work gradually in the context of COVID-19: experience from a tertiary dermatology department in China. Dermatol Ther 2020;33:e13554.
12. Gao C, Liu B, Xie Y, et al. Change of dermatological practice after the COVID-19 outbreak resolves. J Dermatolog Treat 2020;1–3.
13. Government RT. Coronavrus disease 2019 (COVID-19) report. Thailand: Department of Disease Control, Ministry of Health, Government of Thailand; 2019; 2021.
14. Mahikul W, Chotsiri P, Ploddi K, et al. Evaluating the impact of intervention strategies on the first wave and predicting the second wave of COVID-19 in Thailand: a mathematical modeling study. Biology (Basel) 2021;10:80.
15. Punyaratabandhu P, Chirachanakul P. Cutaneous eruption in COVID-19-infected patients in Thailand: an observational descriptive study. J Dermatol 2021;48:14–20.
16. Rerknimitr P, Theerawattanawit C, Lertpichitkul P, et al. Skin manifestations in COVID-19: the tropics experience. J Dermatol 2020;47:e444–6.
17. Suchonwanit P, Leerunyakul K, Kositkuljorn C. Diagnostic and prognostic values of cutaneous manifestations in COVID-19. Dermatol Ther 2020;33: e13650.
18. Suchonwanit P, Leerunyakul K, Kositkuljorn C. Cutaneous manifestations in COVID-19: lessons learned from current evidence. J Am Acad Dermatol 2020; 83:e57–60.
19. Holshue ML, DeBolt C, Lindquist S, et al. First Case of 2019 novel coronavirus in the United States. N Engl J Med 2020;382:929–36.
20. Pei S, Kandula S, Shaman J. Differential effects of intervention timing on COVID-19 spread in the

United States. medRxiv 2020. 2020.2005.2015. 20103655.

21. Konda SR, Dankert JF, Merkow D, et al. COVID-19 response in the global epicenter: converting a New York City level 1 orthopedic trauma service into a hybrid orthopedic and medicine COVID-19 management team. J Orthop Trauma 2020;34:411–7.

22. WorldOMeter. United States coronavirus cases. US: WorldOMeter; 2021.

23. Martins Van Jaarsveld G. The effects of COVID-19 among the elderly population: a case for closing the digital divide. Front Psychiatry 2020;11:577427.

24. Usher K, Bhullar N, Durkin J, et al. Family violence and COVID-19: increased vulnerability and reduced options for support. Int J Ment Health Nurs 2020;29: 549–52.

25. Connor J, Madhavan S, Mokashi M, et al. Health risks and outcomes that disproportionately affect women during the Covid-19 pandemic: a review. Soc Sci Med 2020;266:113364.

26. Thakur N, Lovinsky-Desir S, Bime C, et al. The structural and social determinants of the racial/ethnic disparities in the U.S. COVID-19 pandemic. What's our role? Am J Respir Crit Care Med 2020;202: 943–9.

27. Gover AR, Harper SB, Langton L. Anti-Asian hate crime during the COVID-19 pandemic: exploring the reproduction of inequality. Am J Crim Justice 2020;1–21.

28. Price-Haywood EG, Burton J, Fort D, et al. Hospitalization and mortality among black patients and white patients with Covid-19. N Engl J Med 2020;382: 2534–43.

29. Holmes L, Enwere M, Williams J, et al. Black–white risk differentials in COVID-19 (SARS-COV2) transmission, mortality and case fatality in the United States: translational epidemiologic perspective and challenges. Int J Environ Res Public Health 2020; 17:4322.

30. Centers for Disease C. Risk for COVID-19 infection, hospitalization, and death by race/ethnicity. Online. US: Centers for Disease Control; 2021.

31. Freeman EE, McMahon DE, Lipoff JB, et al. The spectrum of COVID-19-associated dermatologic manifestations: An international registry of 716 patients from 31 countries. J Am Acad Dermatol 2020;83:1118–29.

32. Freeman EE, McMahon DE, Fitzgerald ME, et al. The American Academy of Dermatology COVID-19 registry: crowdsourcing dermatology in the age of COVID-19. J Am Acad Dermatol 2020;83:509–10.

33. Richardson VL, Garcia-Albea VR, Bort NL, et al. Reflections of COVID-19 on dermatology practice. J Dermatol Nurses Assoc 2021;13:49–53.

34. Chuchvara N, Patel R, Srivastava R, et al. The growth of teledermatology: expanding to reach the underserved. J Am Acad Dermatol 2020;82: 1025–33.

35. Piccolo D, Smolle J, Wolf IH, et al. Face-to-face diagnosis vs telediagnosis of pigmented skin tumors: a teledermoscopic study. Arch Dermatol 1999;135:1467–71.

36. Arzberger E, Curiel-Lewandrowski C, Blum A, et al. Teledermoscopy in high-risk melanoma patients: a comparative study of face-to-face and teledermatology visits. Acta Derm Venereol 2016;96:779–83.

37. Freeman EE, McMahon DE. Creating dermatology guidelines for COVID-19: the pitfalls of applying evidence-based medicine to an emerging infectious disease. J Am Acad Dermatol 2020;82:e231–2.

38. Gelfand JM, Armstrong AW, Bell S, et al. National psoriasis foundation COVID-19 task force guidance for management of psoriatic disease during the pandemic: version 1. J Am Acad Dermatol 2020; 83:1704–16.

39. Marson JW, Maner BS, Harding TP, et al. The magnitude of COVID-19's effect on the timely management of melanoma and nonmelanoma skin cancers. J Am Acad Dermatol 2021;84:1100–3.

40. Lee WC, Ong CY. Overview of rapid mitigating strategies in Singapore during the COVID-19 pandemic. Public Health 2020;185:15–7.

41. Chen JI, Yap JC, Hsu LY, et al. COVID-19 and Singapore: from early response to circuit breaker. Ann Acad Med Singap 2020;49:561–72.

42. Ho WYB, Wang D, Tan LYC, et al. Two cases of cutaneous eruptions due to CoVID-19 infection in Singapore: new insights into the spectrum of clinical presentation and histopathology. J Eur Acad Dermatol Venereol 2020;34:e576–9.

43. Andrikopoulos S, Johnson G. The Australian response to the COVID-19 pandemic and diabetes - Lessons learned. Diabetes Res Clin Pract 2020; 165:108246.

44. Australian Government Department of Health. Coronavirus (COVID-19) current situation and case numbers. Australia: Australian Government Department of Health; 2021.

45. Australian Government Department of Health. Coronavirus (COVID-19) at a glance – 10 March 2021. Australia: Australian Government Department of Health; 2021.

46. Tsirtsakis A. Ending the second wave: how did Victoria get to zero active cases? NewsGP 2020.

47. Manipis K, Street D, Cronin P, et al. Exploring the trade-off between economic and health outcomes during a pandemic: a discrete choice experiment of lockdown policies in Australia. Patient 2021;1–13.

48. Patrick A. Australia has almost eliminated the coronavirus — by putting faith in science. Washington, DC: The Washington Post; 2020.

49. Snoswell C, Mehrotra A, Thomas A, et al. Making the most of telehealth in COVID-19 responses, and

beyond. 2020 [March 11, 2021]. Available at: https://croakey.org/making-the-most-of-telehealth-in-covid-19-responses-and-beyond/. Accessed March, 11, 2021.

50. Snoswell CL, Caffery LJ, Hobson G, et al. Centre for Online Health, The University of Queensland. Telehealth and coronavirus: Medicare Benefits Schedule (MBS) activity in Australia. 2020 [March 11 2021]. Available at: https://coh.centre.uq.edu.au/telehealth-and-coronavirus-medicare-benefits-schedule-mbs-activity-australia. Accessed March, 11, 2021.

51. Scott A. The impact of COVID-19 on GPs and non-GP specialists in private practice. Melbourne: Melbourne Institute: Applied Economic & Social Research; 2020.

52. Te Marvelde L, Wolfe R, McArthur G, et al. Decline in cancer pathology notifications during the 2020 COVID-19-related restrictions in Victoria. Med J Aust 2021;6:281–3.

53. Oliver N, Barber X, Roomp K, et al. Assessing the Impact of the COVID-19 Pandemic in Spain: Large-Scale, Online, Self-Reported Population Survey. J Med Internet Res 2020;22:e21319.

54. Ministerio de Sanidad cybsdE. Curva epidemica COVID-19 España. Internet. Spain: Ministero de Sanidad; 2021.

55. The Lancet Public Health. COVID-19 in Spain: a predictable storm? Lancet Public Health 2020;5:e568.

56. Baena-Díez JM, Barroso M, Cordeiro-Coelho SI, et al. Impact of COVID-19 outbreak by income: hitting hardest the most deprived. J Public Health (Oxf) 2020;42:698–703.

57. Romani S, Illi B, De Mori R, et al. The ciliary proteins Meckelin and Jouberin are required for retinoic acid-dependent neural differentiation of mouse embryonic stem cells. Differentiation 2014;87:134–46.

58. Galván Casas C, Català A, Carretero Hernández G, et al. Classification of the cutaneous manifestations of COVID-19: a rapid prospective nationwide consensus study in Spain with 375 cases. Br J Dermatol 2020;183:71–7.

59. Pasquali P, Romero-Aguilera G, Moreno-Ramírez D. Teledermatology before, during, and after the COVID-19 pandemic. Actas Dermo-Sifiliográficas (English Edition). Spain: Actas Dermo-Sifiliográficas; 2021.

60. Gómez Arias PJ, Abad Arenas E, Arias Blanco MC, et al. Aspectos medicolegales de la práctica de la teledermatología en España. Actas Dermosifiliogr (Engl Ed) 2021;112:127–33.

61. Last M. The first wave of COVID-19 in Israel—initial analysis of publicly available data. PLoS One 2020;15:e0240393.

62. Rossman H, Meir T, Somer J, et al. Hospital load and increased COVID-19 related mortality in Israel. Nat Commun 2021;12:1904.

63. WorldOMeter. Israel coronavirus cases. US: WorldOMeter; 2021.

64. Gesser-Edelsburg A, Cohen R, Hijazi R, et al. Analysis of public perception of the israeli government's early emergency instructions regarding COVID-19: online survey study. J Med Internet Res 2020;22:e19370.

65. Leshem E, Afek A, Kreiss Y. Buying time with COVID-19 outbreak response, Israel. Emerg Infect Dis 2020;26:2251–3.

66. Saban M, Myers V, Shachar T, et al. Effect of socioeconomic and ethnic characteristics on COVID-19 infection: the case of the ultra-orthodox and the Arab Communities in Israel. J Racial Ethn Health Disparities 2021;1–8.

67. Rosen B, Waitzberg R, Israeli A. Israel's rapid rollout of vaccinations for COVID-19. Isr J Health Policy Res 2021;10:6.

68. Rinott E, Youngster I, Lewis YE. Reduction in COVID-19 patients requiring mechanical ventilation following implementation of a national COVID-19 vaccination program - Israel, December 2020-February 2021. MMWR Morb Mortal Wkly Rep 2021;70:326–8.

69. Fisher S, Ziv M. COVID-19 effect on phototherapy treatment utilization in dermatology. J Dermatolog Treat 2020;1–3.

70. Gianotti R, Barberis M, Fellegara G, et al. COVID-19-related dermatosis in November 2019: could this case be Italy's patient zero? Br J Dermatol. 2019; 184(5):970-1.

71. WorldOMeter. Italy coronavirus cases. US: WorldOMeter; 2021.

72. Recalcati S. Cutaneous manifestations in COVID-19: a first perspective. J Eur Acad Dermatol Venereol 2020;34:e212–3.

73. Gisondi P, Piaserico S, Conti A, et al. Dermatologists and SARS-CoV-2: the impact of the pandemic on daily practice. J Eur Acad Dermatol Venereol 2020; 34:1196–201.

74. Recalcati S, Gianotti R, Fantini F. COVID-19: the experience from Italy. Clin Dermatol 2020;39(1): 12–22.

75. Bergamo S, Calacione R, Fagotti S, et al. Teledermatology with general practitioners and pediatricians during COVID-19 outbreak in Italy: Preliminary data from a second-level dermatology department in North-Eastern Italy. Dermatol Ther 2020;33:e14040.

76. Valenti M, Pavia G, Gargiulo L, et al. Impact of delay in follow-up due to COVID-19 pandemic on skin cancer progression: a real-life experience from an Italian hub hospital. Int J Dermatol 2021;7:860–3.

77. Neiva MB, Carvalho I, Costa Filho EDS, et al. Brazil: the emerging epicenter of COVID-19 pandemic. Rev Soc Bras Med Trop 2020;53:e20200550.

78. WorldOMeter. Brazil Coronavirus Cases. Online. US: WorldOMeter; 2021.

79. Marson FAL, Ortega MM. COVID-19 in Brazil. Pulmonology 2020;26:241–4.

80. Sabino EC, Buss LF, Carvalho MPS, et al. Resurgence of COVID-19 in Manaus, Brazil, despite high seroprevalence. Lancet 2021;397:452–5.

81. Pereira RJ, Nascimento GNLd, Gratão LHA, et al. The risk of COVID-19 transmission in favelas and slums in Brazil. Public Health 2020;183:42–3.

82. Avancini J, Miyamoto D, Arnone M, et al. Absence of specific cutaneous manifestations of severe acute respiratory syndrome coronavirus 2 in a reference center in Brazil. J Am Acad Dermatol 2021;84:e67.

83. Giandhari J, Pillay S, Wilkinson E, et al. Early transmission of SARS-CoV-2 in South Africa: An epidemiological and phylogenetic report. Int J Infect Dis 2021;103:234–41.

84. Gu X, Mukherjee B, Das S, et al. COVID-19 prediction in South Africa: understanding the unascertained cases – the hidden part of the epidemiological iceberg. medRxiv 2020. 2020.2012.2010.20247361.

85. WorldOMeter. South Africa coronavirus cases. Online. US: WorldOMeter; 2021.

86. Mukumbang FC, Ambe AN, Adebiyi BO. Unspoken inequality: how COVID-19 has exacerbated existing vulnerabilities of asylum-seekers, refugees, and undocumented migrants in South Africa. Int J Equity Health 2020;19:141.

87. Abdool Karim Q, Abdool Karim SS. COVID-19 affects HIV and tuberculosis care. Science 2020;369:366–8.

88. Maphumulo WT, Bhengu BR. Challenges of quality improvement in the healthcare of South Africa post-apartheid: a critical review. Curationis 2019;42:e1–9.

89. Baxter C, Abdool Karim Q, Abdool Karim SS. Identifying SARS-CoV-2 infections in South Africa: balancing public health imperatives with saving lives. Biochem Biophys Res Commun 2021;538:221–5.

90. Christoff Pienaar LS. Digital health and health care IT. South Africa: digital health laws and regulations 2021. ICLG.com. Washington DC: Global Legal Group; 2021.

91. Board of Heathcare Funders. COVID-19-Guidelines: telehealth and telemedicine as a result of South African state of disaster. South Africa: Web: Board of Healthcare Funders; 2020.

92. Munayco CV, Tariq A, Rothenberg R, et al. Early transmission dynamics of COVID-19 in a southern hemisphere setting: Lima-Peru: February 29(th)-March 30(th), 2020. Infect Dis Model 2020;5:338–45.

93. Gianella C, Iguiñiz-Romero R, Romero MJ, et al. Good health indicators are not enough: lessons from COVID-19 in Peru. Health Hum Rights 2020;22:317–9.

COVID-19 Vaccines and the Skin

The Landscape of Cutaneous Vaccine Reactions Worldwide

Qisi Sun, MD[a,1], Ramie Fathy, AB[b,1], Devon E. McMahon, MD[c], Esther E. Freeman, MD, PhD[c,*]

KEYWORDS

- COVID-19 • Vaccines • Cutaneous • Reactions • Urticaria • Side effects • Adverse • Moderna

KEY POINTS

- The most common cutaneous reactions cited in the clinical trial data of COVID-19 vaccines are local injection site reactions.
- The most common cutaneous reactions cited in nontrial literature are delayed large local reactions.
- Dermatologic side effects of COVID-19 vaccines range from morbilliform rash and pernio to pityriasis rosea and erythema multiforme.
- As vaccine reactogenicity reports continue to surface, dermatologists and other health care providers should understand the landscape of the latest cutaneous reactions to guide and address patients' concerns.

INTRODUCTION

As of April 22, 2021, the novel coronavirus disease 2019 (COVID-19) has sickened more than 142 million people and taken more than 3 million lives worldwide.[1] Although restrictions such as physical distancing are crucial to containment, these measures are only temporary solutions. One silver lining amid this crisis is that the tragedy has become a catalyst. Scientists around the globe have raced to develop a long-term solution to impede viral transmission. On March 13, 2020, just 63 days after the genetic sequence of severe acute respiratory syndrome novel coronavirus 2 (SARS-CoV-2) was published, researchers began testing the first doses of a human COVID-19 vaccine.[2] By December 2, 2020, the United Kingdom became the first country to approve of and distribute the Pfizer-BioNTech BNT162b2 vaccine.[3] The United States followed suit days later, with the Food and Drug Administration (FDA) issuing Emergency Use Authorizations for both the Pfizer-BioNTech and Moderna vaccines.

Since then, several COVID-19 vaccines have been authorized and approved for distribution around the globe, with many more in the pipeline. Of significance to dermatologists are the increasing reports of cutaneous reactions associated with these vaccines. The American Academy of Dermatology and the International League of Dermatologic Societies COVID-19 Registry began collecting such cases in late December 2020. The cases submitted ranged from delayed large local reactions to pityriasis-rosea–like eruptions and reactivation of herpes simplex and varicella zoster.[4] Mass vaccination is key to achieving herd

[a] Department of Dermatology, Yale University School of Medicine, 333 Cedar Street, New Haven, CT 06510, USA; [b] Department of Dermatology, Perelman School of Medicine, University of Pennsylvania, 3400 Civic Center Blvd, Philadelphia, PA 19104, USA; [c] Department of Dermatology, Massachusetts General Hospital, Harvard Medical School, 55 Fruit Street, Boston, MA 02114, USA
[1] Co-first authors.
* Corresponding author.
E-mail address: efreeman@mgh.harvard.edu

Dermatol Clin 39 (2021) 653–673
https://doi.org/10.1016/j.det.2021.05.016

immunity and ending the pandemic. Therefore, it is critical that providers are aware of and understand the cutaneous side effects among the approved vaccines to better educate patients and provide proper counseling.

In this article, we evaluate the landscape of dermatologic side effects from COVID-19 vaccines worldwide. We first summarize the latest skin reactions reported in clinical trial data following the administration of 11 different approved COVID-19 vaccines, before describing additional skin findings in reports outside of clinical trials.

CUTANEOUS MANIFESTATIONS OF COVID-19 VACCINATION IN CLINICAL TRIALS

As of April 15, 2021, 13 vaccines have achieved regulatory authorization and approval: Pfizer-BioNTech's BNT162b2, Moderna's mRNA-1273, Oxford-AstraZeneca's AZD1222, Gamaleya's Sputnik V, Johnson & Johnson's Janssen's Ad26.COV2.S, Sinovac's CoronaVac, Sinopharm's BBIBP-CorV, The Vector Institute's EpiVacCorona, CanSino's Convidecia, Bharat's Covaxin, Sinopharm's WIBP-CorV, Chumakov's CoviVac and Anhui Zhifei Longcom's ZF2001 (**Table 1**).[5] Of these vaccines, 11 have published trial data (**Table 2**).

The most common adverse cutaneous reactions noted were local injection site reactions such as erythema, swelling, tenderness, pain, induration, and pruritus within 7 days after injection. Mild to moderate injection site pain was the most prevalent event among all 11 COVID-19 vaccine trials, with up to 88% of participants experiencing pain that typically resolved within 24 to 48 hours after onset. Erythema, swelling, induration, and itch were less common, and reported in up to 20%, 15%, 25%, and 35% of participants, respectively (see **Table 2**). An emerging trend is the higher incidence of these local injection site reactions in the younger population compared with participants age 60 years and older.[6–8]

Delayed large local reactions, with a typical onset of 8 days or more after vaccination and consisting of erythema, induration, and tenderness, were specifically reported in Moderna's phase III trial.[6] After the first dose, 244 participants (0.8%) in the vaccinated cohort developed mild, delayed injection reactions that resolved over the course of 4 to 5 days.[6] After the second dose, 68 participants (0.2%) developed delayed large local reactions.[6] There was no mention, however, of whether those who had reactions after the first dose experienced a recurrence after the second dose.

Although infrequent, a series of other dermatologic manifestations with varying severity have been reported. Less than 0.2% of Moderna's vaccinated cohort developed rashes, including allergic, atopic and contact dermatitis; eczema; exfoliative rash; hypersensitivity reactions; injection site urticaria; papular urticaria; and vesicular rash, among others (see **Table 2**).[6] Although specific characteristics such as timing and duration were not reported, none of these skin findings were labeled as severe.[6] Similarly, acneiform and allergic dermatitis, alopecia, petechial rash and eczema were seen in less than 0.1% of Sputnik V's vaccinated participants.[9] One participant developed an unspecified rash in the BBIBP-CorV vaccine trial and another developed a mild unspecified rash in the Covaxin trial.[8,10] Vaccine-related buccal ulceration and oral herpes were also noted in the Convidecia vaccine cohort.[11]

Three cases of serious cutaneous reactions were observed among these 11 vaccines. One participant in the CoronaVac trial developed a severe, acute hypersensitivity reaction with urticaria 48 hours after the first dose.[12] The rash resolved within 3 days after the administration of chlorphenamine and dexamethasone, and a similar reaction was not observed after the second dose.[12] Among the 11 recipients of the ZF2001 vaccine who developed unspecified rashes, 1 case was labeled as severe (grade 3 or higher).[13] The AZD1222 trial reported 1 case of severe cellulitis in addition to one case each of vaccine-induced psoriasis, rosacea, vitiligo, and Raynaud phenomenon.[14]

CUTANEOUS MANIFESTATIONS OF COVID-19 VACCINATION IN REAL-WORLD SETTINGS

Dermatologic reactions to COVID-19 vaccines may be largely uncommon among clinical trial participants, but as we enter global mass vaccination, these adverse events will increase and new cutaneous reactions will emerge. In fact, numerous observational reports and case series of COVID-19 vaccine-related dermatoses have been published recently. An increased awareness of these manifestations can help dermatologists to identify potential risks, engage in anticipatory guidance, and initiate appropriate management. Here, we present an overview of the latest nontrial literature on reactive dermatoses to COVID-19 vaccines.

Delayed Large Local Reactions

A delayed large local reaction, defined as the onset of an erythematous and edematous patch at the injection site at least 4 days or more after vaccine administration, was the most commonly noted adverse cutaneous event in nontrial literature.[4] Across all 6 observational studies, 350 participants experienced at least one episode of delayed large local reaction (**Table 3**). Of these

Table 1
Characteristics of 13 authorized/approved COVID-19 vaccines as of April 21, 2021

Vaccine Name(s)	Manufacturer(s)	Type	Country of Origin	Trial Phase with Published Data	Trial Time Frame	Age Group Tested
BNT162b2, Comirnaty	Pfizer-BioNTech, Fosun Pharma	mRNA	US, Germany	III	7/27/2020—11/14/2020	16+
mRNA-1273	Moderna, National Institute of Allergy and Infectious Diseases	mRNA	US	III	7/27/2020—10/23/2020	18+
AZD1222, ChAdOx1 nCoV-19	Oxford-AstraZeneca	Adenovirus	UK	I/II	4/23/2020—11/4/2020	18+
Sputnik V, Gam-COVID-Vac	Gamaleya Research Institute; Health Ministry of the Russian Federation	Recombinant adenovirus (rAd26, rAd5)	Russia	III	9/7/2020—11/24/2020	18+
Ad26.COV2.5, JNJ-78436735	Johnson & Johnson's Janssen Biotech	Nonreplicating viral vector	The Netherlands, US	I/IIa	7/22/2020—11/7/2020	18–55, 65+
CoronaVac	Sinovac Biotech	Inactivated (formalin with alum adjuvant)	China	I/II	Phase I: 4/16/2020—4/25/2020 Phase II: 5/3/2020—5/5/2020	18–59
BBIBP-CorV	China National Pharmaceutical Group (Sinopharm); Beijing Institute of Biological Products	Inactivated	China	I/IIa	5/18/2020—7/30/2020	18–59
EpiVacCorona	Federal Budgetary Research Institution State Research Center of Virology and Biotechnology	Peptide	Russia	I/II[a]	7/27/2020—Present	18–60
Convidicea, Ad5-nCoV	CanSino Biologics	Recombinant (adenovirus type 5 vector)	China	III	4/11/2020—4/16/2020	18+

(continued on next page)

Table 1
(continued)

Vaccine Name(s)	Manufacturer(s)	Type	Country of Origin	Trial Phase with Published Data	Trial Time Frame	Age Group Tested
Covaxin, BBV152	Bharat Biotech; Indian Council of Medical Research	Inactivated	India	I/II	9/5/2020—9/12/2020	12–65
WIBP-CorV	China National Pharmaceutical Group (Sinopharm); Wuhan Institute of Biological Products	Inactivated	China	I/II	4/12/2020—5/2/2020	18–59
CoviVac	Chumakov Federal Scientific Center for Research and Development of Immune and Biological Products	Inactivated	Russia	I/II[a]	N/A	N/A
ZF2001	Anhui Zhifei Longcom Biopharmaceutical; Institute of Microbiology of the Chinese Academy of Sciences	Recombinant	China, Uzbekistan	I/II	Phase I: 6/22/2020—7/3/2020 Phase II: 7/12/2020—7/17/2020	18–59

[a] No data published yet as of April 22, 2021.

Table 2
Cutaneous side effects reported in the trial data of 11 authorized COVID-19 vaccines

Vaccine name(s)	Erythema	Swelling	Tenderness	Pain	Induration	Pruritus	Other Skin Findings	Serious Cutaneous Reactions
BNT162b2, Comirnaty	Dose 1: 16–55 y: 5% >55 y 5% Dose 2: 16–55 y 6% >55 y 7%	Dose 1: 16–55 y 6% >55 y 7% Dose 2: 16–55 y 6% >55 y 7%	N/A	Dose 1: 16–55 y 83% >55 y 71% Dose 2: 16–55 y 78% >55 y 66%	N/A	N/A	N/A	None
mRNA-1273	Dose 1: 2.8% Dose 2: 8.6%	Dose 1: 6.1% Dose 2: 12.2%	Dose 1: 10.2% Dose 2: 14.2%	Dose 1: 83.7% Dose 2: 88.2%	N/A	N/A	Allergic, hand, atopic and contact dermatitis; eczema; exfoliative rash; hypersensitivity; injection site urticaria; erythematous rash; macular rash; maculopapular rash; pruritic rash; vesicular rash; urticaria; papular urticaria (<0.2%)	None
AZD1222, ChAdOx1 nCoV-19	Group 1a, 1b, 2a, 2b: Without paracetamol prophylaxis: 3% With paracetamol prophylaxis: 2%	Group 1a, 1b, 2a, 2b: Without paracetamol prophylaxis: 4% With paracetamol prophylaxis: 2%	Group 1a, 1b, 2a, 2b: Without paracetamol prophylaxis: 83% With paracetamol prophylaxis: 77%	Group 1a, 1b, 2a, 2b: Without paracetamol prophylaxis: 67% With paracetamol prophylaxis: 50%	Group 1a, 1b, 2a, 2b: Without paracetamol prophylaxis: 3% With paracetamol prophylaxis: 0%	Group 1a, 1b, 2a, 2b: Without paracetamol prophylaxis: 7% With paracetamol prophylaxis: 12%	One case each of psoriasis, rosacea, vitiligo and Raynaud phenomenon (<0.1%)	One case of severe cellulitis

(continued on next page)

Table 2
(continued)

Vaccine name(s)	Erythema	Swelling	Tenderness	Pain	Induration	Pruritus	Other Skin Findings	Serious Cutaneous Reactions
	Group 3 None	Group 3 None	Group 3 Dose 1: 50% Dose 2: 50%	Group 3 Dose 1: 50% Dose 2: 20%	Group 3 None	Group 3 Dose 1: 10% Dose 2: 10%		
Sputnik V, Gam-COVID-Vac	N/A	N/A	N/A	N/A	N/A	N/A	Acneiform dermatitis, allergic rash, alopecia, indeterminate rash, petechial rash, and eczema ($<0.1\%$)	None
Ad26.COV2.S, JNJ-78436735	7.3%	5.3%	N/A	48.6%	N/A	N/A	N/A	None
CoronaVac	0/14 schedule: Dose 1: 3μg group: 0.8% 6μg group: None Dose 2: 3μg group: None 6μg group: 1.7% 0/28 schedule: Dose 1: 3μg group: None 6μg group: 0.8% Dose 2: None	0/14 schedule: Dose 1: 3μg group: 0.8% 6μg group: None Dose 2: 3μg group: 0.8% 6μg group: 2.5% 0/28 schedule: Dose 1: None Dose 2: 3μg group: None 6μg group: 0.9%	N/A	0/14 schedule: Dose 1: 3μg group: 9.2% 6μg group: 16.7% Dose 2: 3μg group: 13.3% 6μg group: 11.8% 0/28 schedule: Dose 1: 3μg group: 7.5% 6μg group: 10% Dose 2: 3μg group: 2.6% 6μg group: 5.9%	0/14 schedule: Dose 1: None Dose 2: 3μg group: 0.8% 6μg group: 0.8% 0/28 schedule: None	0/14 schedule: Dose 1: None Dose 2: 3μg group: 0.8% 6μg group: 0.8% 0/28 schedule: None	N/A	One case of acute hypersensitivity with urticaria 48 h after dose 1 (6 μg group)

	1%	2%	N/A	16%	N/A	2%	Unspecified rash in 1 participant (<1%)
BBIBP-CorV	1%	2%	N/A	16%	N/A	2%	None
Convidicea, Ad5-nCoV	Low dose: 2% High dose: 1%	Low dose: 4% High dose: 4%	N/A	Low dose: 57% High dose: 56%	Low dose: 2% High dose: 2%	Low dose: 6% High dose: 2%	One case of buccal ulceration within 14 d One case of oral herpes
Covaxin, BBV152	Dose 1: 3µg group: 1% 6µg group: 1% Dose 2: None	N/A	N/A	Dose 1: 3µg group: 3% 6µg group: 3% Dose 2: 3µg group: 4% 6µg group: 2%	N/A	Dose 1: 3µg group: 1% 6µg group: 1% Dose 2: 3µg group: None 6µg group: 1%	One case of mild unspecified rash after dose 2 (3 µg group)
WIBP-CorV	Phase I (0, 28, 56-d group): Low dose: None Medium dose: None High dose: 4.2% Phase II 0 and 14-d group: Medium dose: None 0 and 21-d group: Medium dose: None	Phase I (0, 28, 56-d group): Low dose: 4.2% Medium dose: None High dose: 4.2% Phase II 0 and 14-d group: Medium dose: None 0 and 21-d group: Medium dose: 1.2%	N/A	Phase I (0, 28, 56-d group): Low dose: 20.8% Medium dose: 4.2% High dose: 25% Phase II 0 and 14-d group: Medium dose: 2.4% 0 and 21-d group: Medium dose: 14.3%	N/A	Phase I (0, 28, 56-d group): Low dose: None Medium dose: None High dose: None Phase II 0 and 14-d group: Medium dose: None 0 and 21-d group: Medium dose: 1.2%	N/A

(continued on next page)

Table 2
(continued)

Vaccine name(s)	Erythema	Swelling	Tenderness	Pain	Induration	Pruritus	Other Skin Findings	Serious Cutaneous Reactions
ZF2001	Phase I 25 µg group: 20% 50 µg group: 20% Phase II Two-dose group: 25 µg group: 8% 50 µg group: 8% Three-dose group: 25 µg group: 16% 50 µg group: 14%	Phase I 25 µg group: 5% 50 µg group: 15% Phase II Two-dose group: 25 µg group: 4% 50 µg group: 6% Three-dose group: 25 µg group: 14% 50 µg group: 13%	N/A	Phase I 25 µg group: 20% 50 µg group: 55% Phase II Two-dose group: 25 µg group: 3% 50 µg group: 5% Three-dose group: 25 µg group: 12% 50 µg group: 12%	Phase I 25 µg group: 10% 50 µg group: 25% Phase II Two-dose group: 25 µg group: 3% 50 µg group: 5% Three-dose group: 25 µg group: 9% 50 µg group: 7%	Phase I 25 µg group: 20% 50 µg group: 35% Phase II Two-dose group: 25 µg group: 6% 50 µg group: 9% Three-dose group: 25 µg group: 19% 50 µg group: 17%	One case of unspecified rash in the phase I trial (50 µg group) Three cases of unspecified rash in the phase II trial, 2-dose schedule, 25 µg group Four cases of unspecified rash in the phase II trial, 2-dose schedule, 50 µg group 2 cases of unspecified rash in phase II trial, three-dose schedule, 25 µg group One case of unspecified rash in phase II trial, three-dose schedule, 50 µg group	One case of unspecified grade ≥3 rash (50 µg group)

Abbreviation: N/A, not applicable.

Table 3
Reactive dermatoses to authorized COVID-19 vaccines reported in the nontrial literature[a]

Article Reference	Study Design	Study Size	Study Period	Vaccine Name(s)	Cutaneous Reactions	Dose Number	Time to Onset after Vaccination	Time to Resolution	Intervention
Delayed large local reactions									
Fernandez-Nieto et al,[24] 2021	Retrospective study at a tertiary referral hospital in Spain	4775	1/11/2021–2/12/2021	BNT162b2/Comirnaty	103 participants with delayed large local reactions	Dose 1: 49/103 (47.6%) Dose 2: 54/103 (52.4%)	N/A	<8 h: 23/103 (22.3%) 8–24 h: 27/103 (26.2%) 48–72 h: 38/103 (36.9%) >72 h: 14/103 (13.6%)	N/A
Blumenthal et al,[23] 2021	Case series	12	N/A	mRNA-1273	12 participants with delayed large local reactions after dose 1 3 participants with similarly severe reactions, 3 participants with less severe reactions after dose 2	Dose 1: 12/12 (100%) Dose 2: 6/12 (50%)	Dose 1: 4–11 d (median 8 d) Dose 2: 1–3 d (median 2 d)	Dose 1: 2–11 d after onset (median, 6 d) Dose 2: N/A	Ice, antihistamines, glucocorticoids (topical, oral or both), antibiotics
McMahon et al,[4] 2021	Retrospective review of AAD/ILDS registry of vaccine-related cutaneous reactions	414	12/24/2020–2/14/2021	BNT162b2/Comirnaty mRNA-1273	BNT162b2/Comirnaty: 12 reports of delayed large local reactions mRNA-1273 206 reports of delayed large local reactions	BNT162b2/Comirnaty: Dose 1: 5/34 (15%) Dose 2: 7/40 (18%) mRNA-1273 Dose 1: 175/267 (66%) Dose 2: 31/102 (30%)	BNT162b2/Comirnaty: N/A mRNA-1273: median 7 d after dose 1, median 3 d after dose 2	BNT162b2/Comirnaty: N/A mRNA-1273: median 4 d after dose 1; median 3 d after dose 2	Topical corticosteroids, oral antihistamines, pain relievers, antibiotics

(continued on next page)

Table 3
(continued)

Article Reference	Study Design	Study Size	Study Period	Vaccine Name(s)	Cutaneous Reactions	Dose Number	Time to Onset after Vaccination	Time to Resolution	Intervention
Wei et al,[25] 2021	Case series	4	N/A	mRNA-1273	Delayed large local reactions	Dose 1	Case 1: 8 d, Case 2: 8 d, Case 3: 7 d, Case 4: 10 d	Case 1: N/A, Case 2: 3 d, Case 3: 4 d, Case 4: 2 d	Case 1 and 2: topical corticosteroids, oral antihistamine; Case 3 and 4: None
Ramos et al,[27] 2021	Case series	12	N/A	BNT162b2/Comirnaty mRNA-1273	BNT162b2/Comirnaty: 1 report of delayed large local reaction; mRNA-1273 11 reports of delayed large local reactions	BNT162b2/Comirnaty: 1 case of delayed large local reaction after dose 2 only; mRNA-1273 11 case of delayed large local reaction after dose 1 only	5–11 d (average 7 d)	3–8 d (average 5 d)	Topical corticosteroids, ice, oral antihistamines, pain relievers
Morbilliform rashes									
Baeck et al., 2021	Case report	1	N/A	BNT162b2/Comirnaty	Delayed large local reaction	Dose 1 only	6 d	5 d	N/A
Jedlowski et al,[30] 2021	Case report	1	N/A	BNT162b2/Comirnaty	Morbilliform rash on lower back	Dose 1 and dose 2	Dose 1 and 2: 48 h	Dose 1 and 2: 24 h	None
CDC COVID-19 Response Team and FDA[37]	Case series	10	12/21/2020–1/10/2021	mRNA-1273	4 cases of morbilliform rash	Dose 1	5–45 min	N/A	Intramuscular epinephrine
CDC COVID-19 Response Team and FDA[37]	Case series	21	12/14/2020–12/23/2020	BNT162b2/Comirnaty	7 cases of morbilliform rash	Dose 1	2–25 min	N/A	Intramuscular epinephrine

									Corticosteroids
Ackerman et al,[29] 2021	Case report	1	N/A	BNT162b2/Comirnaty	Maculopapular exanthema (30% body surface area)	Dose 1 (dose 2 avoided)	3 h	>1 mo	None
Corbeddu et al., 2021	Case series	11	N/A	BNT162b2/Comirnaty	3 cases of morbilliform rashes	Dose 2: 3/3 (100%)	Dose 2: 5 hours–3 days	2–3 d	None
McMahon et al,[4] 2021	Retrospective review of AAD/ILDS registry of vaccine-related cutaneous reactions	414	12/24/2020–2/14/2021	BNT162b2/Comirnaty mRNA-1273	BNT162b2/Comirnaty 9 reports of morbilliform rash mRNA-1273 18 reports of morbilliform rash	BNT162b2/Comirnaty: Dose 1: 6/9 (67%) Dose 2: 3/9 (33%) mRNA-1273 Dose 1: 11/18 (61%) Dose 2: 7/18 (39%)	Dose 1: Median of 3 d Dose 2: Median of 2 d	Dose 1: Median of 4.5 d Dose 2: Median of 2.5 d	Topical corticosteroids, oral antihistamines, pain relievers, antibiotics
Urticaria									
CDC COVID-19 Response Team and FDA[37]	Case series	10	12/21/2020–1/10/2021	mRNA-1273	1 case of urticaria	Dose 1	11 min	N/A	Intramuscular epinephrine
CDC COVID-19 Response Team and FDA[37]	Case series	21	12/14/2020–12/23/2020	BNT162b2/Comirnaty	10 cases of urticaria	Dose 1	5–54 min	N/A	Intramuscular epinephrine
John M. Kelso, 2021	Case series	4	N/A	mRNA-1273	1 case of urticaria	Dose 1 (dose 2 refused)	1 min	N/A	Diphenhyramine, IV epinephrine, diazepam
Corbeddu et al., 2021	Case series	11	N/A	BNT162b2/Comirnaty	2 cases of urticaria	Dose 1: 2/2 (100%)	Dose 1: 1 hour–2 days	2–3 d	None
Park et al,[38] 2021	Case report	1	N/A	BNT162b2/Comirnaty	Urticaria with immediate anaphylaxis	Dose 1 only	3 min	2 d	Intramuscular epinephrine and diphenhydramine

(continued on next page)

Table 3
(continued)

Article Reference	Study Design	Study Size	Study Period	Vaccine Name(s)	Cutaneous Reactions	Dose Number	Time to Onset after Vaccination	Time to Resolution	Intervention
McMahon et al,[4] 2021	Retrospective review of AAD/ILDS registry of vaccine-related cutaneous reactions	414	12/24/2020–2/14/2021	BNT162b2/ Comirnaty mRNA-1273	BNT162b2/ Comirnaty: 17 reports of urticaria mRNA-1273 23 reports of urticaria	BNT162b2/ Comirnaty: Dose 1: 9/17 (53%) Dose 2: 8/17 (47%) mRNA-1273 Dose 1: 16/23 (70%) Dose 2: 7/23 (30%)	BNT162b2/ Comirnaty: Dose 1: 9 cases after 24 h Dose 2: 1 case within 24 h, 7 cases after 24 h mRNA-1273 Dose 1: 13 cases after 24 h 3 cases of unknown timing Dose 2: 2 cases within 24 h, 5 cases after 24 h	Dose 1: Median 5 d Dose 2: Median 3 d	Topical corticosteroids, oral antihistamines, pain relievers, antibiotics
EM									
Gambichler et al., 2021	Case report	1	N/A	BNT162b2/ Comirnaty	Rowell's syndrome	Dose 1	1 d	N/A	Oral corticosteroids
McMahon et al,[4] 2021	Retrospective review of AAD/ILDS registry of vaccine-related cutaneous reactions	414	12/24/2020–2/14/2021	mRNA-1273	3 reports of EM	mRNA-1273 Dose 1: 3/3 (100%)	N/A	N/A	N/A

DIRs to hyaluronic acid dermal fillers

Study	Study type	N	Dates	Findings	Dose (%)	Onset	Resolution	Medications
Munavalli et al,[40] 2021	Case series	2	N/A	BNT162b2/Comirnaty 1 report of DIR to hyaluronic acid dermal fillers mRNA-1273 1 report of DIRs to hyaluronic acid dermal fillers	BNT162b2/Comirnaty: Dose 2: 1/2 (50%) mRNA-1273 Dose 1: 1/2 (50%)	BNT162b2/Comirnaty: Dose 2: 24 h mRNA-1273 Dose 1: 48 h	BNT162b2/Comirnaty: Dose 2: 24 h mRNA-1273 Dose 1: Initiation of lisinopril at 48 h, resolved after 24 h	BNT162b2/Comirnaty: Corticosteroids mRNA-1273: Antihistamines, acetaminophen, lisinopril
Munavalli et al,[41] 2021	Case series	4	N/A	BNT162b2/Comirnaty 2 reports of DIRs to hyaluronic acid dermal fillers mRNA-1273 2 reports of DIRs to hyaluronic acid dermal fillers	BNT162b2/Comirnaty: Dose 1: 1/2 (50%) Dose 2: 1/2 (50%) mRNA-1273 Dose 1: 16/23 (70%) Dose 2: 1/2 (50%)	BNT162b2/Comirnaty: Dose 1: 10 d Dose 2: 2 d mRNA-1273 Dose 1: 18 h (recurred with dose 2) Dose 2: 24 h	BNT162b2/Comirnaty: Dose 1: 7 d Dose 2: Initiation of lisinopril at 72 h, resolved after 24 h mRNA-1273 Dose 1: Initiation of lisinopril at 48 h, resolved after 24 h Dose 2: Initiation of lisinopril at 48 h, resolved after 72 h	Low-dose lisinopril
McMahon et al,[4] 2021	Retrospective review of AAD/ILDS registry of vaccine-related cutaneous reactions	414	12/24/2020–2/14/2021	BNT162b2/Comirnaty 1 report of DIR to hyaluronic acid dermal fillers mRNA-1273 8 reports of DIR to hyaluronic acid dermal fillers	BNT162b2/Comirnaty: Dose 2: 1/1 (100%) mRNA-1273 Dose 1: 3/8 (38%) Dose 2: 5/8 (63%)	N/A	N/A	N/A

(continued on next page)

Table 3
(continued)

Article Reference	Study Design	Study Size	Study Period	Vaccine Name(s)	Cutaneous Reactions	Dose Number	Time to Onset after Vaccination	Time to Resolution	Intervention
Local injection site reactions									
McMahon et al,[4] 2021	Retrospective review of AAD/ILDS registry of vaccine-related cutaneous reactions	414	12/24/2020–2/14/2021	BNT162b2/ Comirnaty mRNA-1273	BNT162b2/ Comirnaty: 16 reports of local injection site reactions mRNA-1273 186 reports of local injection site reactions	BNT162b2/ Comirnaty: Dose 1: 8/16 (50%) Dose 2: 8/16 (50%) mRNA-1273 Dose 1: 117/186 (63%) Dose 2: 69/186 (37%)	Dose 1: Median day 1 Dose 2: Median day 1	Dose 1: Median days 4 Dose 2: Median days 3	N/A
Erythromelalgia									
McMahon et al,[4] 2021	Retrospective review of AAD/ILDS registry of vaccine-related cutaneous reactions	414	12/24/2020–2/14/2021	BNT162b2/ Comirnaty mRNA-1273	BNT162b2/ Comirnaty: 3 reports of erythromelalgias mRNA-1273 11 reports of erythromelalgias	BNT162b2/ Comirnaty: Dose 1: 1/3 (33%) Dose 2: 2/3 (67%) mRNA-1273 Dose 1: 5/11 (45%) Dose 2: 6/11 (55%)	Dose 1: Median day 7 Dose 2: Median day 1	Dose 1: Median days 5.5 Dose 2: Median days 3	N/A
Lichen planus									
Hiltun et al., 2021	Case report	1	N/A	BNT162b2/ Comirnaty	Lichen planus flare	Dose 2	48 h	N/A	Topical corticosteroids
Varicella zoster									
Bostan et al., 2021	Case report	1	N/A	N/A	Varicella zoster flare	N/A	5 d	1 wk	Oral valacyclovir

McMahon et al,[4] 2021	Retrospective review of AAD/ILDS registry of vaccine-related cutaneous reactions	414	12/24/2020–2/14/2021	BNT162b2/Comirnaty mRNA-1273	5 reports of varicella zoster mRNA-1273 5 reports of varicella zoster	BNT162b2/Comirnaty: Dose 1: 1/5 (20%) Dose 2: 4/5 (80%) mRNA-1273 Dose 1: 5/5 (100%)	N/A	N/A	N/A
Herpes simplex									
McMahon et al,[4] 2021	Retrospective review of AAD/ILDS registry of vaccine-related cutaneous reactions	414	12/24/2020–2/14/2021	N/A	4 reports of herpes simplex flares	N/A	N/A	N/A	N/A
Pityriasis rosea									
McMahon et al,[4] 2021	Retrospective review of AAD/ILDS registry of vaccine-related cutaneous reactions	414	12/24/2020–2/14/2021	BNT162b2/Comirnaty mRNA-1273	3 reports of pityriasis rosea mRNA-1273 1 report of pityriasis rosea	BNT162b2/Comirnaty: Dose 1: 2/3 (67%) Dose 2: 1/3 (33%) mRNA-1273 Dose 1: 1/1 (100%)	N/A	N/A	N/A
Busto-Leis et al,[47] 2021	Case series	2	N/A	BNT162b2/Comirnaty	2 reports of pityriasis rosea	Dose 2	24 h, 7 d	N/A	N/A
Pernio/chilblains									
Kha et al,[45] 2021	Case report	1	N/A	mRNA-1273	1 report of pernio/chilblains	Dose 1 and 2	Dose 1: 2 d Dose 2: 3 d	Dose 1: 14 d Dose 2: 7 d	Topical corticosteroids

(continued on next page)

Table 3
(continued)

Article Reference	Study Design	Study Size	Study Period	Vaccine Name(s)	Cutaneous Reactions	Dose Number	Time to Onset after Vaccination	Time to Resolution	Intervention
McMahon et al,[4] 2021	Retrospective review of AAD/ILDS registry of vaccine-related cutaneous reactions	414	12/24/2020–2/14/2021	BNT162b2 Comirnaty mRNA-1273	BNT162b2/Comirnaty: 5 reports of pernio/chilblains mRNA-1273 3 reports of pernio/chilblains	BNT162b2/Comirnaty: Dose 1: 3/5 (60%) Dose 2: 2/5 (40%) mRNA-1273 Dose 1: 3/3 (100%)	N/A	N/A	N/A
Lopez et al,[44] 2021	Case report	1	1/2021	BNT162b2	Pernio/chilblains	Dose 2	3 d	>28 d	Clobetasol as needed, avoidance of cold exposure
Petechiae									
McMahon et al,[4] 2021	Retrospective review of AAD/ILDS registry of vaccine-related reactions	414	12/24/2020–2/14/2021	BNT162b2 Comirnaty mRNA-1273	BNT162b2/Comirnaty: 1 report of petechiae mRNA-1273 3 reports of petechiae	BNT162b2/Comirnaty: Dose 1: 1/1 (100%) mRNA-1273 Dose 1: 1/3 (33%) Dose 2: 2/3 (67%)	N/A	N/A	N/A
Purpura									
Malayala et al,[48] 2021	Case report	1	3/2021	mRNA-1273	Brown to red purpuric, nonblanchable rash	Dose 1	1 d	N/A	Monitoring of platelet, liver, renal function panels; antihypertensives

Abbreviations: AAD, American Academy of Dermatology; *CDC,* Centers for Disease Control and Prevention; *DIRs,* delayed inflammatory reaction; *EM,* erythema multiforme; *FDA,* Food and Drug Administration; *ILDS,* International League of Dermatologic Societies; *N/A,* not applicable.

[a] Articles within each morphology group are organized in order of publication date.

350 individuals, 117 (33.4%) received the BNT162b2 vaccine and 233 (66.6%) received the mRNA-1273 vaccine (see **Table 3**).

Of note, female patients younger than 65 years of age consistently composed the majority of these delayed large local reactions, prompting the question of sex's role in vaccine response. Notably, women also comprise an overwhelming majority (>70%) of the national and international health care workforce.[15–17] Therefore, the observation may reflect a reporting bias, given that vaccination campaigns initially targeted health care professionals and that women may be more likely to visit their doctor. However, the cause is likely multifactorial, because biology is also at play. Women have stronger immune responses to foreign antigens than men, and decades of research have shown that although women exhibit a greater immune response to vaccines, they also experience more adverse events.[18–22]

Although studies varied in their reporting of characteristics, most of the delayed large local reactions were mild and transient, with few recurrences after the second dose. All delayed large local reactions reported in the nontrial literature resolved within 11 days. In the study by McMahon and associates,[4] only 11 participants developed reactions after both doses; all were mRNA-1273 vaccine recipients, and reactions after the second dose were frequently smaller in size with an earlier onset at a median of 2 days. Six of the 12 patients who received the mRNA-1273 vaccine in Blumenthal and colleagues[23] had recurrent reactions that were of lesser severity than those after the first dose and also occurred at a median of 2 days. Likewise, of the 11 patients who received the mRNA-1273 vaccine in Ramos and Kelso, 4 developed similar local reactions after the second dose with an onset of 2 to 3 days after injection. Although most delayed large local reaction reports in nontrial literature occurred with the mRNA-1273 vaccine, these findings have also been observed with the BNT162b2 vaccine. Of the 103 patients reported on by Fernandez-Nieto and colleagues[24] and who developed delayed large local reactions after the first dose of BNT162b2, one-half experienced similar recurrent reactions after the second dose (onset not reported).

The morphology of these delayed large local reactions ranged from erythematous targetoid patches to large plaques.[4,24] In 2 studies of mRNA-1273 vaccine recipients, lesion diameters ranged from 5.0 to 19.5 cm, with 7 of the 16 lesions labeled as grade 3 plaques ($\geq$10 cm in diameter).[23,25] Histology of these skin lesions revealed superficial and deep perivascular lymphocytic infiltrates with rare eosinophils and scattered mast cells, confirming a delayed type, T-cell–mediated hypersensitivity reaction.[23,24,26] To date, no such findings have been reported with other non-mRNA COVID-19 vaccines and the exact etiology is still unknown. However, a delayed hypersensitivity reaction to polyethylene glycol, an allergen, may be one explanation because both BNT162b2 and mRNA-1273 vaccines contain this excipient.[25]

Treatment has not been necessary; most reactions are mild and resolve spontaneously. Although some patients were treated with ice, antihistamines, pain relievers, and glucocorticoids (topical, oral, or both), others received no intervention.[4,23,24,26,27] However, some patients received unnecessary antibiotics owing to concern for cellulitis or other infections, highlighting the need for more providers to recognize that these delayed large local reactions are benign and not a contraindication to the second dose.

Morbilliform Rashes

Morbilliform and maculopapular exanthems have been described in 43 participants across 3 observational studies (see **Table 3**). Of these 43 individuals, 21 (49%) received the BNT162b2 vaccine and 22 (51%) received the mRNA-1273 vaccine (see **Table 3**). Of these cases, 11 (4 associated with mRNA-1273; 7 associated with BNT162b2) had been submitted to the Vaccine Adverse Event Reporting System (VAERS) and labeled by the Centers for Disease Control and Prevention (CDC) as part of an anaphylaxis reaction.[28]

Among the cases not characterized as anaphylaxis, most rashes occurred within 2 to 3 days after injection and resolved within 1 week. One recipient of the BNT162b2 vaccine developed a pruritic, maculopapular exanthem that persisted for more than 1 month. This patient, who had no significant past medical history or drug allergy, erupted in an erythematous rash over 30% of his body, including the face, trunk, upper extremities, and thighs, but sparing the oral and genital mucosa.[29] Histologic examination revealed lymphocytic perivascular infiltrates, consistent with maculopapular toxidermia.[29] Despite a lack of other systemic manifestations, the patient developed concomitant liver injury with slightly elevated aspartate transaminase and gamma-glutamyl transferase enzymes.[29] Given the persistence of this exanthem, the patient was advised to avoid the second dose, and gradually the rash and elevated liver enzymes improved with corticosteroids.[29] Another BNT162b2 vaccine recipient developed a pruritic morbilliform rash across his lower back 48 hours after injection; the rash self-resolved within

24 hours.[30] Upon receiving the second dose, he developed a recurrent and more robust morbilliform eruption involving not only the lower back, but also the flanks, proximal extremities, and upper back.[30] This rash also resolved within 24 hours without intervention.

Notably, morbilliform rashes have been reported in several cases of COVID-19 infection in both pediatric and adult populations.[31–34] Histologic examinations of such cases have revealed spongiosis and mild dermal perivascular lymphocytic infiltrates, suggesting an immune-mediated etiology rather than a direct viral effect.[35] Therefore, although the exact mechanism of COVID-19 vaccine-induced morbilliform rashes remains unknown, it is plausible that these cutaneous manifestations are also the result of an immune activation.

Urticaria

Urticaria is defined as wheals (hives) that typically resolve within 24 hours.[36] It can either present as part of immediate hypersensitivity reactions, defined by the CDC as an onset within 4 hours after injection, or occur as similar reactions 4 hours after injection.[37] This delineation is important to recognize because the former are potential contraindications to the second dose.

There are 55 cases of urticaria among the 6 observational reports in nontrial literature (see **Table 3**). Of these 55 individuals, 30 (55%) received the BNT162b2 vaccine and 25 (45%) received the mRNA-1273 vaccine (see **Table 3**). Of these cases, 11 (1 associated with mRNA-1273 and 10 associated with BNT162b2) had been submitted to the Vaccine Adverse Event Reporting System (VAERS) and labeled by the CDC as part of an anaphylaxis reaction.[28] In contrast, in an analysis of 414 COVID-19 dermatology registry cases, none of the 40 urticaria reactions (17 associated with BNT162b2, 23 associated with mRNA-1273) were classified as an immediate hypersensitivity rash.[4]

One female patient in the report from Park and colleagues[38] developed pruritic urticaria on her extremities and face within 3 minutes after administration of the BNT162b2 vaccine. However, history and test results demonstrated a baseline proclivity to allergic reactions and revealed a previously undiagnosed, underlying cholinergic urticaria.[38] Given that she felt overheated while waiting in line for the dose, the anaphylaxis likely arose from heat-induced rather than vaccine-induced cholinergic urticaria. As such, she received the second dose in a cool, temperature-controlled room without incident.[38] This case illustrates that categorically denying patients a second dose based solely on an anaphylactic reaction may erroneously prevent patients from reaping the benefits of immunization, because not all cases of anaphylaxis are directly vaccine related.

Delayed Inflammatory Reactions to Dermal Hyaluronic Acid Fillers

Hyaluronic acid fillers are increasingly resistant to biodegradation, resulting in longevity and more delayed inflammatory reactions (DIRs) to these implants. Among the known triggers of DIRs to fillers include viral illness, low-quality products, dental procedures, influenza vaccines, and, most recently, COVID-19 vaccines.[4,39,40] To date, 15 cases have been reported across 3 observational studies. Of these reports, 11 (73%) are associated with the mRNA-1273 vaccine and 4 (27%) are associated with the BNT162b2 vaccine (see **Table 3**).

In many cases, DIRs occurred to fillers that had been injected more than 1 to 2 years before the COVID-19 vaccination.[40] These reactions developed rapidly, often within 24 to 48 hours, and presented as swelling and inflammation focused around areas previously treated with fillers.[39,40] Most cases were recalcitrant to antihistamines, hyaluronidase, and acetaminophen.[39,40]

However, a novel mechanism for these reactions has been proposed, generating a potential pathogenesis-based treatment. Previous research revealed high expression of angiotensin-converting enzyme (ACE) 2 receptors in adipose tissue, where most fillers are injected.[40] These receptors are targeted by the SARS-CoV-2 spike protein, and the resulting interaction in the skin releases a proinflammatory cascade, which may explain the DIRs to hyaluronic acid fillers seen in COVID-infection.[41] By blocking the production of angiotensin II and thus reducing the substrate for ACE2, ACE inhibitors (ACE-I) in effect promote an anti-inflammatory response.[39,40] Indeed, upon initiation with oral lisinopril, all DIRs resolved completely within 24 to 72 hours.[39,40] Despite the success of ACE-Is in treating DIRs, further research on the proposed mechanism of action is warranted.

Important factors to consider when treating these reactions with ACE-Is include laboratory tests to assess for metabolic disturbances, especially if a patient is on medications that could interact with ACE-Is.[39,40] Given that treatment of DIRs to hyaluronic acid fillers do not require a long course of ACE-Is, a brief discontinuation of concurrent drugs may suffice.

Pernio and Chilblains

Pernio-like lesions have been observed in COVID-19 infected individuals since the beginning of the pandemic.[42,43] Only recently have they also been associated with COVID-19 vaccines. Of the 10 cases described across 3 observation studies, 6 (60%) were associated with the BNT162b2 vaccine, and the rest were associated with the mRNA-1273 vaccine.

Pernio-like lesions tend to present as painless, erythematous, and violaceous papules and macules on the hands and feet, with some cases exacerbated by cold exposure.[44,45] Histopathologic examinations of these vaccine-associated lesions reveal dense, perivascular lymphocytic infiltrates in the superficial to deep dermis, confirming the pernio diagnosis.[44,45] With topical corticosteroids, these lesions can resolve in 1 week to 1 month.[44,45]

The appearance of pernio lesions not just during COVID-19 infection, but also after vaccination suggests that the vaccines and SARS-CoV-2 activate a similar immune pathway. Although the mechanism remains unclear, these findings suggest that the pernio lesions seen in COVID-19 infection and after vaccination may be less directly related to viral effects.

Other Reactions

Reports of other cutaneous reactions include early-onset local injection site reactions, erythromelalgia, erythema multiforme, lichen planus, varicella zoster and herpes simplex reactivation, pityriasis rosea-like reactions, petechial rash, and purpuric rash (see **Table 3**). Local injection site reactions occurring within 3 days of vaccination were the second most common skin manifestations observed in the analysis of 414 COVID-19 dermatology registry cases.[4] Of the 202 cases of local injection site reactions, 186 (92%) were attributed to the mRNA-1273 vaccine.[4] These findings were also widely reported in clinical trial data, but less frequently discussed in the nontrial literature, likely because this pattern of reactogenicity is commonly observed in other vaccines.[46]

Some reactions, such as erythromelalgia, erythema multiforme, and pityriasis rosea, mimic known cutaneous manifestations of COVID-19 infection. Of the 14 reports of erythromelalgia, 11 (79%) were associated with the mRNA-1273 vaccine.[4] Of the 4 cases of erythema multiforme, 3 (75%) were associated with the mRNA-1273 vaccine, and among the 6 reports of pityriasis rosea, 5 (83%) were associated with the BNT162b2 vaccine.[4,40,47] Similarly, varicella zoster and herpes simplex reactivations have also been reported with COVID-19 infection cases and after COVID-19 vaccinations (see **Table 3**). Rarer reactions include a flare of previously well-controlled lichen planus, as well as petechial and purpuric rash, the latter of which has been associated with thrombocytopenia after the mRNA-1273 vaccine.[48]

SUMMARY

As of April 2021, more than 1 billion COVID-19 vaccine doses have been administered worldwide.[49] Although these vaccines are instrumental against the pandemic, important knowledge gaps remain, such as our understanding of the mechanistic relationship between these vaccines and their associated cutaneous side effects.

Currently, no reactive dermatoses have been recorded outside of trial data for vaccines other than BNT162b2 and mRNA-1273. However, the COVID-19 vaccine frontier is evolving rapidly. We have summarized the latest clinical trial data for authorized COVID-19 vaccines as of April 15, 2021, and described the associated cutaneous manifestations reported in nontrial literature. Recognition of these common and emerging reactions has key implications for vaccine strategy because concerns about reactogenicity can significantly influence an individual's willingness to return for a second dose. Because the benefits of immunization far outweigh the risks, it is crucial for health care providers, particularly dermatologists, to recognize our role in encouraging vaccine completion, educating our patients, and allaying their fears.

CLINICS CARE POINTS

- The most common cutaneous manifestations of COVID-19 vaccination in clinical trials were local injection site reactions, of which there is a higher incidence in individuals younger than 60 years.

- The most common cutaneous manifestation of COVID-19 vaccination in real-world settings is delayed large local reactions, of which two-thirds were associated with the mRNA-1273 vaccine and one-third was associated with the BNT162b2 vaccine.

- Other reactive dermatoses to COVID-19 vaccines in real-world settings include morbiliform rashes, urticaria, erythema multiforme, delayed inflammatory reactions to dermal fillers, erythromelalgia, lichen planus, varicella zoster, herpes simplex, pityriasis rosea, petechiae, purpura. Most are self-limiting and resolve with topical steroids or oral medications.

ACKNOWLEDGEMENTS

The International League of Dermatologic Societies (ILDS) provides grant support to Massachusetts General Hospital for the AAD/ILDS COVID-19 Dermatology Registry. AAD provides in-kind support.

DISCLOSURE

Dr. Freeman is the Principal Investigator of the AAD/ILDS COVID-19 Dermatology Registry. The authors have nothing to disclose.

REFERENCES

1. WHO Coronavirus (COVID-19) Dashboard.
2. Tregoning JS, Brown ES, Cheeseman HM, et al. Vaccines for COVID-19. Clin Exp Immunol 2020;202: 162–92.
3. Ledford H, Cyranoski D, Van Noorden R. The UK has approved a COVID vaccine - here's what scientists now want to know. Nature 2020;588:205–6.
4. McMahon DE, Amerson E, Rosenbach M, et al. Cutaneous reactions reported after Moderna and Pfizer COVID-19 vaccination: a registry-based study of 414 cases. J Am Acad Dermatol 2021;85(1): 46–55.
5. Craven J. COVID-19 vaccine tracker. April 15, 2021, . Online: regulatory Affairs Professionals Society.
6. Baden LR, El Sahly HM, Essink B, et al. Efficacy and safety of the mRNA-1273 SARS-CoV-2 vaccine. New Engl J Med 2020;384:403–16.
7. Polack FP, Thomas SJ, Kitchin N, et al. Safety and efficacy of the BNT162b2 mRNA Covid-19 vaccine. N Engl J Med 2020;383:2603–15.
8. Xia S, Zhang Y, Wang Y, et al. Safety and immunogenicity of an inactivated SARS-CoV-2 vaccine, BBIBP-CorV: a randomised, double-blind, placebo-controlled, phase 1/2 trial. Lancet Infect Dis 2021; 21:39–51.
9. Logunov DY, Dolzhikova IV, Shcheblyakov DV, et al. Safety and efficacy of an rAd26 and rAd5 vector-based heterologous prime-boost COVID-19 vaccine: an interim analysis of a randomised controlled phase 3 trial in Russia. Lancet 2021;397:671–81.
10. Ella R, Reddy S, Jogdand H, et al. Safety and immunogenicity of an inactivated SARS-CoV-2 vaccine, BBV152: interim results from a double-blind, randomised, multicentre, phase 2 trial, and 3-month follow-up of a double-blind, randomised phase 1 trial. Lancet Infect Dis 2021;21(7):950–61.
11. Zhu FC, Guan XH, Li YH, et al. Immunogenicity and safety of a recombinant adenovirus type-5-vectored COVID-19 vaccine in healthy adults aged 18 years or older: a randomised, double-blind, placebo-controlled, phase 2 trial. Lancet 2020;396: 479–88.
12. Zhang Y, Zeng G, Pan H, et al. Safety, tolerability, and immunogenicity of an inactivated SARS-CoV-2 vaccine in healthy adults aged 18–59 years: a randomised, double-blind, placebo-controlled, phase 1/ 2 clinical trial. The Lancet Infect Dis 2021;21: 181–92.
13. Yang S, Li Y, Dai L, et al. Safety and immunogenicity of a recombinant tandem-repeat dimeric RBD-based protein subunit vaccine (ZF2001) against COVID-19 in adults: two randomised, double-blind, placebo-controlled, phase 1 and 2 trials. The Lancet Infect Dis 2021.
14. Voysey M, Clemens SAC, Madhi SA, et al. Safety and efficacy of the ChAdOx1 nCoV-19 vaccine (AZD1222) against SARS-CoV-2: an interim analysis of four randomised controlled trials in Brazil, South Africa, and the UK. Lancet 2021;397:99–111.
15. Alobaid AM, Gosling CM, Khasawneh E, et al. Challenges faced by female healthcare professionals in the workforce: a scoping review. J Multidiscip Healthc 2020;13:681–91.
16. World Health O. Gender equity in the health workforce: analysis of 104 countries 2019.
17. Your health care is in women's hands. United States Census Bureau.
18. Klein SL, Flanagan KL. Sex differences in immune responses. Nat Rev Immunol 2016;16:626–38.
19. Fink AL, Klein SL. Sex and gender impact immune responses to vaccines among the elderly. Physiology (Bethesda) 2015;30:408–16.
20. Fink AL, Klein SL. The evolution of greater humoral immunity in females than males: implications for vaccine efficacy. Curr Opin Physiol 2018;6:16–20.
21. Fischinger S, Boudreau CM, Butler AL, et al. Sex differences in vaccine-induced humoral immunity. Semin Immunopathol 2019;41:239–49.
22. Flanagan KL, Fink AL, Plebanski M, et al. Sex and gender differences in the outcomes of vaccination over the life course. Annu Rev Cell Dev Biol 2017; 33:577–99.
23. Blumenthal KG, Freeman EE, Saff RR, et al. Delayed large local reactions to mRNA-1273 vaccine against SARS-CoV-2. New Engl J Med 2021;384:1273–7.
24. Fernandez-Nieto D, Hammerle J, Fernandez-Escribano M, et al. Skin manifestations of the BNT162b2 mRNA COVID-19 vaccine in healthcare workers. 'COVID-arm': a clinical and histological characterization. J Eur Academy of Dermatology and Venereology. 2021;35(7):425-7.
25. Wei N, Fishman M, Wattenberg D, et al. "COVID arm": a reaction to the Moderna vaccine. JAAD case Rep 2021;10:92–5.
26. Blumenthal KG, Freeman EE, Saff RR, et al. Delayed large local reactions to mRNA vaccines. New Engl J Med 2021;284:1273–7.
27. Ramos CL, Kelso JM. "COVID Arm": very delayed large injection site reactions to mRNA COVID-19

vaccines. J Allergy Clin Immunol Pract 2021;9(6): 2480–1.

28. CDC COVID-19 Response Team, FDA. Allergic reactions including anaphylaxis after receipt of the first dose of Pfizer-BioNTech COVID-19 vaccine — United States, December 14–23, 2020. MMWR Morb Mortal Wkly Rep 2021;70(2):46–51.

29. Ackerman M, Henry D, Finon A, et al. Persistent maculopapular rash after the first dose of Pfizer-BioNTech COVID-19 vaccine. J Eur Acad Dermatol Venereol. 2021;35(7):423-5.

30. Jedlowski PM, Jedlowski MF. Morbilliform rash after administration of Pfizer-BioNTech COVID-19 mRNA vaccine. Dermatol Online J 2021;27.

31. Almutairi M, Azizalrahman A. Febrile morbilliform rash as a clinical presentation of COVID-19 in a pediatric patient 2020.

32. Avellana Moreno R, Estela Villa LM, Avellana Moreno V, et al. Cutaneous manifestation of COVID-19 in images: a case report. J Eur Acad Dermatol Venereol : JEADV 2020;34:e307–9.

33. Kulkarni RB, Lederman Y, Afiari A, et al. Morbilliform rash: an uncommon herald of SARS-CoV-2. Cureus 2020;12:e9321.

34. Najarian DJ. Morbilliform exanthem associated with COVID-19. JAAD Case Rep 2020;6:493–4.

35. Fattori A, Cribier B, Chenard M-P, et al. Cutaneous manifestations in patients with coronavirus disease 2019: clinical and histological findings. Hum Pathol 2021;107:39–45.

36. McNeil MM, DeStefano F. Vaccine-associated hypersensitivity. The J Allergy Clin Immunol 2018;141: 463–72.

37. Centers for Disease C. Interim clinical considerations for use of mRNA COVID-19 vaccines currently authorized in the United States 2021.

38. Park HJ, Montgomery JR, Boggs NA. Anaphylaxis after the Covid-19 vaccine in a patient with cholinergic urticaria. Mil Med 2021.

39. Munavalli GG, Guthridge R, Knutsen-Larson S, et al. COVID-19/SARS-CoV-2 virus spike protein-related delayed inflammatory reaction to hyaluronic acid

dermal fillers: a challenging clinical conundrum in diagnosis and treatment. Arch Dermatol Res 2021; 1–15.

40. Munavalli GG, Knutsen-Larson S, Lupo MP, et al. Oral angiotensin-converting enzyme inhibitors for treatment of delayed inflammatory reaction to dermal hyaluronic acid fillers following COVID-19 vaccination-a model for inhibition of angiotensin II-induced cutaneous inflammation. JAAD Case Rep 2021;10:63–8.

41. Rowland-Warmann M. Hypersensitivity reaction to hyaluronic acid dermal filler following novel coronavirus infection – a case report. J Cosmet Dermatol 2021;20:1557–62.

42. Freeman EE, McMahon DE, Lipoff JB, et al. Pernio-like skin lesions associated with COVID-19: a case series of 318 patients from 8 countries. J Am Acad Dermatol 2020;83:486–92.

43. Freeman EE, McMahon DE, Fox LP. Emerging evidence of the direct association between COVID-19 and chilblains. JAMA Dermatol 2021;157:238–9.

44. Lopez S, Vakharia P, Vandergriff T, et al. Pernio after COVID-19 Vaccination. Br J Dermatol 2021.

45. Kha C, Itkin A. New-onset chilblains in close temporal association to mRNA-1273 (Moderna) vaccination. JAAD case Rep 2021. https://doi.org/10.1016/j.jdcr.2021.1003.1046.

46. Hervé C, Laupèze B, Del Giudice G, et al. The how's and what's of vaccine reactogenicity. NPJ Vaccin 2019;4:39.

47. Busto-Leis J, Servera-Negre G, Mayor-Ibarguren A, et al. "Pityriasis rosea, COVID-19 and vaccination: new keys to understand an old acquaintance". Journal of the European Academy of Dermatology and Venereology. n/a.

48. Malayala SV, Mohan G, Vasireddy D, et al. Purpuric rash and thrombocytopenia after the mRNA-1273 (Moderna) COVID-19 vaccine. Cureus 2021;13: e14099.

49. Hannah Ritchie EO-O, Beltekian D, Mathieu E, et al. Coronavirus (COVID-19) vaccinations. Online: our World in data 2021.

Statement of Ownership, Management, and Circulation (All Periodicals Publications Except Requester Publications)

UNITED STATES POSTAL SERVICE®

1. Publication Title: DERMATOLOGIC CLINICS

2. Publication Number: 000 – 705

3. Filing Date: 9/18/2021

4. Issue Frequency: JAN, APR, JUL, OCT

5. Number of Issues Published Annually: 4

6. Annual Subscription Price: $416.00

7. Complete Mailing Address of Known Office of Publication (Not printer) (Street, city, county, state, and ZIP+4®)
ELSEVIER INC.
230 Park Avenue, Suite 800
New York, NY 10169

Contact Person: Malathi Samayan
Telephone (Include area code): 91-44-4299-4507

8. Complete Mailing Address of Headquarters or General Business Office of Publisher (Not printer)
ELSEVIER INC.
230 Park Avenue, Suite 800
New York, NY 10169

9. Full Names and Complete Mailing Addresses of Publisher, Editor, and Managing Editor (Do not leave blank)

Publisher (Name and complete mailing address)
DOLORES MELONI, ELSEVIER INC.
1600 JOHN F KENNEDY BLVD. SUITE 1800
PHILADELPHIA, PA 19103-2899

Editor (Name and complete mailing address)
LAUREN BOYLE, ELSEVIER INC.
1600 JOHN F KENNEDY BLVD. SUITE 1800
PHILADELPHIA, PA 19103-2899

Managing Editor (Name and complete mailing address)
PATRICK MANLEY, ELSEVIER INC.
1600 JOHN F KENNEDY BLVD. SUITE 1800
PHILADELPHIA, PA 19103-2899

10. Owner (Do not leave blank. If the publication is owned by a corporation, give the name and address of the corporation immediately followed by the names and addresses of all stockholders owning or holding 1 percent or more of the total amount of stock. If not owned by a corporation, give the names and addresses of the individual owners. If owned by a partnership or other unincorporated firm, give its name and address as well as those of each individual owner. If the publication is published by a nonprofit organization, give its name and address.)

Full Name	Complete Mailing Address
WHOLLY OWNED SUBSIDIARY OF REED/ELSEVIER, US HOLDINGS	1600 JOHN F KENNEDY BLVD. SUITE 1800 PHILADELPHIA, PA 19103-2899

11. Known Bondholders, Mortgagees, and Other Security Holders Owning or Holding 1 Percent or More of Total Amount of Bonds, Mortgages, or Other Securities. If none, check box. ☐ None

Full Name	Complete Mailing Address
N/A	

12. Tax Status (For completion by nonprofit organizations authorized to mail at nonprofit rates) (Check one)
The purpose, function, and nonprofit status of this organization and the exempt status for federal income tax purposes:
☒ Has Not Changed During Preceding 12 Months
☐ Has Changed During Preceding 12 Months (Publisher must submit explanation of change with this statement)

PS Form **3526**, July 2014 (Page 1 of 4 (see instructions page 4)) PSN: 7530-01-000-9931 PRIVACY NOTICE: See our privacy policy on www.usps.com.

---

13. Publication Title: DERMATOLOGIC CLINICS

14. Issue Date for Circulation Data Below: JULY 2021

15. Extent and Nature of Circulation

		Average No. Copies Each Issue During Preceding 12 Months	No. Copies of Single Issue Published Nearest to Filing Date
a. Total Number of Copies (Net press run)		140	133
b. Paid Circulation (By Mail and Outside the Mail)	(1) Mailed Outside-County Paid Subscriptions Stated on PS Form 3541 (Include paid distribution above nominal rate, advertiser's proof copies, and exchange copies)	60	55
	(2) Mailed In-County Paid Subscriptions Stated on PS Form 3541 (Include paid distribution above nominal rate, advertiser's proof copies, and exchange copies)	0	0
	(3) Paid Distribution Outside the Mails Including Sales Through Dealers and Carriers, Street Vendors, Counter Sales, and Other Paid Distribution Outside USPS®	43	42
	(4) Paid Distribution by Other Classes of Mail Through the USPS (e.g., First-Class Mail®)	0	0
c. Total Paid Distribution (Sum of 15b (1), (2), (3), and (4))		103	97
d. Free or Nominal Rate Distribution (By Mail and Outside the Mail)	(1) Free or Nominal Rate Outside-County Copies included on PS Form 3541	19	17
	(2) Free or Nominal Rate In-County Copies Included on PS Form 3541	0	0
	(3) Free or Nominal Rate Copies Mailed at Other Classes Through the USPS (e.g., First-Class Mail)	0	0
	(4) Free or Nominal Rate Distribution Outside the Mail (Carriers or other means)	0	0
e. Total Free or Nominal Rate Distribution (Sum of 15d (1), (2), (3) and (4))		19	17
f. Total Distribution (Sum of 15c and 15e)		122	114
g. Copies not Distributed (See Instructions to Publishers #4 (page 43))		18	19
h. Total (Sum of 15f and g)		140	133
i. Percent Paid (15c divided by 15f times 100)		84.42%	85.08%

*If you are claiming electronic copies, go to line 16 on page 3. If you are not claiming electronic copies, skip to line 17 on page 3.

PS Form **3526**, July 2014 (Page 2 of 4)

16. Electronic Copy Circulation

	Average No. Copies Each Issue During Preceding 12 Months	No. Copies of Single Issue Published Nearest to Filing Date
a. Paid Electronic Copies		
b. Total Paid Print Copies (Line 15c) + Paid Electronic Copies (Line 16a)		
c. Total Print Distribution (Line 15f) + Paid Electronic Copies (Line 16a)		
d. Percent Paid (Both Print & Electronic Copies) (16b divided by 16c × 100)		

☒ I certify that 50% of all my distributed copies (electronic and print) are paid above a nominal price.

17. Publication of Statement of Ownership

☒ If the publication is a general publication, publication of this statement is required. Will be printed in the OCTOBER 2021 issue of this publication. ☐ Publication not required.

18. Signature and Title of Editor, Publisher, Business Manager, or Owner

Malathi Samayan

Malathi Samayan - Distribution Controller

Date: 9/18/2021

I certify that all information furnished on this form is true and complete. I understand that anyone who furnishes false or misleading information on this form or who omits material or information requested on the form may be subject to criminal sanctions (including fines and imprisonment) and/or civil sanctions (including civil penalties).

PS Form **3526**, July 2014 (Page 3 of 4) PRIVACY NOTICE: See our privacy policy on www.usps.com

Moving?

Make sure your subscription moves with you!

To notify us of your new address, find your **Clinics Account Number** (located on your mailing label above your name), and contact customer service at:

Email: journalscustomerservice-usa@elsevier.com

800-654-2452 (subscribers in the U.S. & Canada)
314-447-8871 (subscribers outside of the U.S. & Canada)

Fax number: 314-447-8029

Elsevier Health Sciences Division
Subscription Customer Service
3251 Riverport Lane
Maryland Heights, MO 63043

*To ensure uninterrupted delivery of your subscription, please notify us at least 4 weeks in advance of move.

CPI Antony Rowe
Eastbourne, UK
February 10, 2022